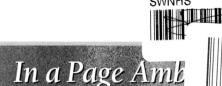

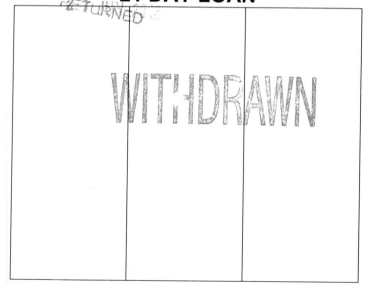

In a Page Ambulatory Medicine

RONALD J. WILLIAMS, MD, FAAP, FACP
Editor-in-Chief
Director, Combined Internal Medicine & Pediatrics Residency Program
Associate Director, Pediatrics Residency Program
Associate Professor of Pediatrics and Medicine
Pennsylvania State University Hershey Medical Center
Hershey, Pennsylvania

SCOTT KAHAN, MD, MPH
Editor-in-Chief
Series Editor
Research Fellow, The Johns Hopkins Hospital
Department of Preventive Medicine and Public Health
Johns Hopkins Bloomberg School of Public Health
Baltimore, Maryland
Director, Institute for Evidence-Based Nutrition
Baltimore, Maryland

Wolters Kluwer | Lippincott Williams & Wilkins
Health
Philadelphia · Baltimore · New York · London
Buenos Aires · Hong Kong · Sydney · Tokyo

Acquisitions Editor: Nancy Anastasi Duffy
Managing Editor: Elizabeth Stalnaker
Marketing Manager: Jennifer Kuklinski
Production Editor: Paula C. Williams
Designer: Risa J. Clow
Compositor: Nesbitt Graphics, Inc.

351 West Camden Street   530 Walnut Street
Baltimore, MD 21201   Philadelphia, PA 19106

9 8 7 6 5 4 3 2 1

Library of Congress Cataloging-in-Publication Data

In a page. Ambulatory medicine / Ronald J. Williams, editor-in-chief; Scott Kahan, editor-in-chief.
    p. ; cm.
    Includes index.
    ISBN-13: 978-0-7817-6495-7 (alk. paper)
    ISBN-10: 0-7817-6495-5 (alk. paper)
  1. Ambulatory medical care—Handbooks, manuals, etc. I. Williams, Ronald J.
(Ronald Jay), 1963-   II. Kahan, Scott, III. Title: Ambulatory medicine.
  [DNLM: 1. Ambulatory Care—Handbooks. WB 39 I348 2008]
  RC55.I4   2008
  362.12—dc22   2007022189

Contents

Section 1

Behavioral

Section 2

Gastrointestinal

Section **8**

Genitourinary

Section **9**

Endocrine

Section 10

Gynecology

Section 11

Rheumatology

Section 12

Dermatology

Section 13

Ophthalmology

Preface

The idea for this series came from the difficulty that I experienced during medical school and residency in weeding through the massive amount of medical information that confronted me. The problem wasn't that the material was too complex; rather, it was the challenge of separating the forest from the trees. Indeed, I still often feel overwhelmed by all there is to know.

I wanted a resource that would streamline the abundance of medical knowledge into a manageable nucleus, or as a resident once described it to me, "a book that tells me exactly what I need to know so my attending won't think I'm an idiot!"

That became the goal of this series: to present medical diseases in a high-yield, understandable fashion that makes it easier for readers to concentrate on the "big picture," without being distracted by the mountain of surrounding detail.

Reviews from medical students, residents, fellows, and other health professionals have been excellent. I hope readers will find the *In A Page* series to be a valuable tool on rounds, for board review, and for independent study. As always, I welcome your questions, comments, and suggestions.

SCOTT KAHAN, MD
drkahan@gmail.com

Acknowledgments

From Ron:

I would like to thank my friends and colleagues, especially the many residents and faculty at Pennsylvania State University who gave their time and expertise in contributing to this book. I am indebted to the many mentors and colleagues who have helped shape my medical career and the enthusiastic students and residents who inspire me to teach through their desire for learning.

I would also like to express gratitude to my mother and father Elaine and Milton Williams, Rick and Steve, and my siblings and family for their never-ending support and encouragement.

I will take this opportunity to deeply thank the three most important people in my life: my wonderful wife Caryn and two children, Arleen and Evan. Without their love, support, and understanding, this project could not have been completed. The pages of this book came out of their generous donation of personal time.

From Scott:

The greatest strength of this book is its diverse group of authors, all of whom have a special interest in ambulatory medicine. We sincerely thank all of them. In particular, I want to thank Phil Panzerella, who helped sow the initial seed of this book.

We are also grateful to the staff of Lippincott Williams & Wilkins, especially Nancy Duffy, Liz Stalnaker, Jennifer Kuklinski, and Betty Sun.

Finally, we thank our family, friends, and mentors for their support and guidance.

Contributors

David Adams, MD
Resident, Department of Surgery
Division of Urology
Pennsylvania State University Milton S.
Hershey Medical Center
Hershey, Pennsylvania

Shoaib Alam, MD
Assistant Professor of Medicine
Division of Pulmonary, Allergy and
Critical Care
Pennsylvania State University Milton S.
Hershey Medical Center
Hershey, Pennsylvania

Darryl P. Anderson, MD
Assistant Professor of Medicine
Division of General Internal Medicine
Pennsylvania State University Milton S.
Hershey Medical Center
Hershey, Pennsylvania

Punitha Arunkumar, MD
Assistant Professor of Medicine
Division of General Internal Medicine
Pennsylvania State University Milton S.
Hershey Medical Center
Hershey, Pennsylvania

Sonia Badreshia, MD
Chief Resident
Department of Dermatology
Pennsylvania State University Milton S.
Hershey Medical Center
Hershey, Pennsylvania

Sharon E. Banks, DO
Assistant Professor of Medicine
Division of Rheumatology
Pennsylvania State University Milton S.
Hershey Medical Center
Hershey, Pennsylvania

Tara Lynn Barto, MD
Resident
Combined Internal Medicine/Pediatrics
Residency Program
Pennsylvania State University Milton S.
Hershey Medical Center
Hershey, Pennsylvania

Rebecca Bascom, MD, MPH
Professor of Medicine
Division of Pulmonary, Allergy and
Critical Care Medicine
Department of Medicine
Pennsylvania State University Milton S.
Hershey Medical Center
Hershey, Pennsylvania

Femabelle Bautista, DO
Resident
Combined Internal Medicine/Pediatrics
Residency Program
Pennsylvania State University Milton S.
Hershey Medical Center
Hershey, Pennsylvania

Zachery Baxter, MD
Resident
Department of Urology
Pennsylvania State University Milton S.
Hershey Medical Center
Hershey, Pennsylvania

Karen S. Bell, MD
Assistant Professor
Section of General Internal Medicine
Pennsylvania State University Milton S.
Hershey Medical Center
Hershey, Pennsylvania

Caryn M. Brenner-Williams, MD
Specialist, Medical Record Documentation
Review
Health Information Services, HU24
Pennsylvania State University Milton S.
Hershey Medical Center
Hershey, Pennsylvania

Soheil Chegini, MD
Assistant Professor of Medicine &
Pediatrics
Section of Allergy and Immunology
Pennsylvania State University Milton S.
Hershey Medical Center
Hershey, Pennsylvania

Delia Chiaramonte, MD
Franklin Square Hospital Center
Baltimore, Maryland

Cynthia H. Chuang, MD MSc
Assistant Professor of Medicine and Health
Evaluation Sciences
Division of General Internal Medicine
Pennsylvania State University Milton S.
Hershey Medical Center
Hershey, Pennsylvania

Kristin L. Cox, MD
Resident
Department of Surgery
Pennsylvania State University Milton S.
Hershey Medical Center
Hershey, Pennsylvania

Timothy Craig, DO
Professor of Medicine and Pediatrics
Departments of Allergy/Medicine
Pennsylvania State University Milton S.
Hershey Medical Center
Hershey, Pennsylvania

Tonya J. Crook, MD, DTMH, MS
Assistant Professor
Division of Infectious Diseases
Department of Medicine
Pennsylvania State University Milton S.
Hershey Medical Center
Hershey, Pennsylvania

Lisa C. Cuff-Brenize, MSPAS, PA-C
Division of Gastroenterology
Department of Medicine
Pennsylvania State University Milton S.
Hershey Medical Center
Hershey, Pennsylvania

Michael Davies, MD
Fellow
Allergy and Immunology
Pennsylvania State University Milton S.
Hershey Medical Center
Hershey, Pennsylvania

Marcus Allan East, MD
Resident
Department of Ophthalmology
Pennsylvania State University Milton S.
Hershey Medical Center
Hershey, Pennsylvania

Latoya Edwards, MD
Greater Baltimore Medical
Center–Weinberg Center
Baltimore, Maryland

Niels Engberding, MD
Resident
Department of Medicine
Pennsylvania State University Milton S.
Hershey Medical Center
Hershey, Pennsylvania

Merritt L. Fajt, MD
Resident
Department of Medicine
Pennsylvania State University Milton S.
Hershey Medical Center
Hershey, Pennsylvania

Emmy M. Fernandez, MD
Resident
Department of Dermatology
Pennsylvania State University Milton S.
Hershey Medical Center
Hershey, Pennsylvania

Marius Figueredo, MD
Fellow
Division of Pulmonary, Allergy and
Critical Care
Pennsylvania State University Milton S.
Hershey Medical Center
Hershey, Pennsylvania

Laura Fisher, MD
Allergy Fellow
Section of Allergy, Asthma and
Immunology
Pennsylvania State University Milton S.
Hershey Medical Center
Hershey, Pennsylvania

Justin R. Fisher, MD
Fellow in Neurophysiology
Department of Neurology
Pennsylvania State University Milton S.
Hershey Medical Center
Hershey, Pennsylvania

Anneli Fogelberg, MD
Resident
Department of Dermatology
Pennsylvania State University Milton S.
Hershey Medical Center
Hershey, Pennsylvania

Gregory J. Fulchiero Jr., MD, MS Bio-Engineering
Resident
Department of Dermatology
Pennsylvania State University Milton S.
Hershey Medical Center
Hershey, Pennsylvania

Amir A. Gahremanpour, MD
Resident
Department of Medicine
Pennsylvania State University Milton S.
Hershey Medical Center
Hershey, Pennsylvania

Joseph M. Geskey, DO
Assistant Professor of Pediatrics and
Medicine
Divisions of General Pediatrics and
General Internal Medicine
Department of Pediatrics
Pennsylvania State University Milton S.
Hershey Medical Center
Hershey, Pennsylvania

Lauren Gordon, MD
Franklin Square Hospital Center
Baltimore, Maryland

Maryellen E. Gusic, MD
Associate Dean for Clinical Education
Pennsylvania State University College of
Medicine
Associate Professor of Pediatrics
Division of General Pediatrics
Pennsylvania State Children's Hospital
Hershey, Pennsylvania

Rehan Hague

Catherine M. Headley, MD
Resident
Department of Dermatology
Pennsylvania State University Milton S.
Hershey Medical Center
Hershey, Pennsylvania

Donald T. Hudak, MD
Assistant Professor of Surgery and
Ophthalmology
Departments of Surgery and
Ophthalmology
Division of Plastic Surgery
Ophthalmic Plastic and Reconstructive
Surgery
Pennsylvania State University Milton S.
Hershey Medical Center
Hershey, Pennsylvania

Virginia A. Imadojemu, MD
Associate Professor of Medicine
Division Pulmonary, Allergy and Critical
Care Medicine
Department of Medicine
Pennsylvania State University Milton S.
Hershey Medical Center
Hershey, Pennsylvania

Guillermo Infante, MD, MPH
Resident
Department of Family and Community
Medicine
Pennsylvania State University
Good Samaritan Family Practice Center
Cherry Hill, New Jersey

Faoud T. Ishmael, MD, PhD
Resident
Department of Medicine
Pennsylvania State University Milton S.
Hershey Medical Center
Hershey, Pennsylvania

Matthew Janiga, MD
Resident
Department of Surgery
Division of Urology
Pennsylvania State University Milton S.
Hershey Medical Center
Hershey, Pennsylvania

Lawrence H. Jones, MD
Assistant Professor of Medicine
Department of Medicine
Pennsylvania State University Milton S.
Hershey Medical Center
Hershey, Pennsylvania

Justina Ju, MD
Resident
Department of Medicine
Pennsylvania State University Milton S.
Hershey Medical Center
Hershey, Pennsylvania

Matthew Kaag, MD
Resident
Department of Surgery
Division of Urology
Pennsylvania State University Milton S.
Hershey Medical Center
Hershey, Pennsylvania

Scott Kahan, MD, MPH
Editor-in-Chief
Series Editor
Research Fellow, The Johns Hopkins
Hospital
Department of Preventive Medicine and
Public Health
Johns Hopkins Bloomberg School of Public
Health
Baltimore, Maryland
Director, Institute for Evidence-Based
Nutrition
Baltimore, Maryland

Pankaj Kapoor, MD
Fellow
Sleep Disorders Medicine
State University of New York at Buffalo
Buffalo, New York

Arash Karnama, DO
Cardiology Fellow
Oklahoma State University
Tulsa, Oklahoma

Rena Kass, MD
Assistant Professor
Department of Surgery
Section of Surgical Oncology
Pennsylvania State University Milton S.
Hershey Medical Center
Hershey, Pennsylvania

Leila Khan, MD
Resident
Department of Medicine
Pennsylvania State University Milton S.
Hershey Medical Center
Hershey, Pennsylvania

Milind J. Kothari, DO
Professor of Neurology
Vice Chair for Education and Training
Pennsylvania State College of Medicine
Hershey, Pennsylvania

Tri H. Le, MD
Assistant Professor of Medicine
Pennsylvania State College of Medicine
Division of Gastroenterology & Hepatology
Pennsylvania State University Milton S.
Hershey Medical Center
Hershey, Pennsylvania

Michael Lioudis, MD
Resident, Combined Internal
Medicine/Pediatrics Residency Program
Pennsylvania State University Milton S.
Hershey Medical Center
Hershey, Pennsylvania

Christine L. Mackley, MD
Assistant Professor of Dermatology
Department of Dermatology
Pennsylvania State University Milton S.
Hershey Medical Center
Hershey, Pennsylvania

Colin MacNeill, MD
Associate Professor
Department of Obstetrics and Gynecology,
H103
Division of Women's Health
Pennsylvania State University Milton S.
Hershey Medical Center
Hershey, Pennsylvania

Ather Mansoor, MD, MHA
Resident
Department of Medicine
Pennsylvania State University Milton S.
Hershey Medical Center
Hershey, Pennsylvania

Paul H. McCabe, MD
Associate Professor of Neurology
Director of Adult Epilepsy Program
Pennsylvania State University Milton S.
Hershey Medical Center
Hershey, Pennsylvania

Robert A. McCauley, MD
Resident
Combined Internal Medicine/Pediatrics
Residency Program
Pennsylvania State University Milton S.
Hershey Medical Center
Hershey, Pennsylvania

Johnathan D. McGinn, MD
Assistant Professor
Division Otolaryngology–Head & Neck
Surgery
Department Surgery
Pennsylvania State University Milton S.
Hershey Medical Center
Hershey, Pennsylvania

Elizabeth McIlmoyle, MD
Resident
Department of Internal Medicine
Pennsylvania State University Milton S.
Hershey Medical Center
Hershey, Pennsylvania

Ronald P. Miller, MD, FACP
Assistant Professor of Medicine
Division of Nephrology
Department of Medicine
Pennsylvania State University Milton S.
Hershey Medical Center
Hershey, Pennsylvania

Selma Mohammed, MD
Resident
Department of Medicine
Pennsylvania State University Milton S.
Hershey Medical Center
Hershey, Pennsylvania

Ai Mukai, MD
Resident Physician
Rehabilitation Institute of Chicago
Northwestern University
Chicago, Illinois

Aparna Mukherjee, MD
Fellow
Department of Gastroenterology and
Hepatology
Pennsylvania State University Milton S.
Hershey Medical Center
Hershey, Pennsylvania

Stanley J. Naides, MD
H. Thomas and Dorothy Willits Hallowell
Endowed Chair in Rheumatology
Professor of Medicine, Microbiology &
Immunology, and Pharmacology
Chief, Division of Rheumatology
Pennsylvania State University Milton S.
Hershey Medical Center
Hershey, Pennsylvania

Barbara E. Ostrov, MD
Professor of Pediatrics and Medicine
Pediatric Rheumatology and Rheumatology
Pennsylvania State University Milton S.
Hershey Medical Center
Hershey, Pennsylvania

Ann Ouyang, MB, BS
Professor of Medicine
Division of Gastroenterology and
Hepatology
Department of Medicine
Pennsylvania State University Milton S.
Hershey Medical Center
Hershey, Pennsylvania

Andrew Peters, DO
Resident
Department of Psychiatry
University of Maryland/Sheppard Pratt
Health Systems
Baltimore, Maryland

Michael A. Piskun, MD
Resident
Department of Surgery
Division of Urology
Pennsylvania State University Milton S.
Hershey Medical Center
Hershey, Pennsylvania

Min Pu, MD, PhD
Assistant Professor of Medicine
Pennsylvania State Heart and Vascular
Institute
Pennsylvania State University Milton S.
Hershey Medical Center
Hershey, Pennsylvania

David A. Quillen, MD
Chairman, Department of Ophthalmology
Professor of Ophthalmology
Pennsylvania State University
Hershey Medical Center
Hershey, Pennsylvania

Raymond K. Reichwein, MD
Assistant Professor of Neurology
Department of Neurology, M.C. H037
Pennsylvania State University Milton S.
Hershey Medical Center
Hershey, Pennsylvania

Nicholas Rider, DO
Chief Resident
Combined Internal Medicine/Pediatrics
Residency Program
Pennsylvania State University Milton S.
Hershey Medical Center
Hershey, Pennsylvania

Stephen C. Ross, MD
Director of Clinical Operations
Department of Neurology
Pennsylvania State University Milton S.
Hershey Medical Center
Hershey, Pennsylvania

Adam M. Rubin, MD
Fellow
Division of Nephrology
Department of Medicine
Pennsylvania State University Milton S.
Hershey Medical Center
Hershey, Pennsylvania

M. Najum Saqib, MD
Fellow
Division of Nephrology
Department of Medicine
Pennsylvania State University Milton S.
Hershey Medical Center
Hershey, Pennsylvania

Jennifer Sceppa, MD
Resident
Department of Dermatology
Pennsylvania State University Milton S.
Hershey Medical Center
Hershey, Pennsylvania

Pragnesh Shah, MD
Resident
Department of Medicine
Pennsylvania State University Milton S.
Hershey Medical Center
Hershey, Pennsylvania

Rohini Sharma, MD
Resident
Department of Medicine
Pinnacle Health System
Harrisburg, Pennsylvania

Steve Shearer, MD
Franklin Square Hospital Center
Baltimore, Maryland

Lisa L. Sherwood, MD
Resident
Department of Medicine
Pennsylvania State University Milton S.
Hershey Medical Center
Hershey, Pennsylvania

Lusine Simonyetsa, MD
Fellow
Pulmonary/Critical Care Medicine
Pennsylvania State University Milton S.
Hershey Medical Center
Hershey, Pennsylvania

Ellen G. Smith, MD, FAAFP
Heritage Family Medicine
Camp Hill, Pennsylvania

Kishori Somyreddy, MD
Resident, Combined Internal
Medicine/Pediatrics Residency Program
Pennsylvania State University Milton S.
Hershey Medical Center
Hershey, Pennsylvania

Monica Chadha Stiles, MD
Resident
Department of Medicine
Pennsylvania State University Milton S.
Hershey Medical Center
Hershey, Pennsylvania

Mehul Trivedi, MD
Resident
Department of Surgery
Pennsylvania State University Milton S.
Hershey Medical Center
Hershey, Pennsylvania

J.C. Trussell, MD
Assistant Professor
Department of Urology
Pennsylvania State University Milton S.
Hershey Medical Center
Hershey, Pennsylvania

Robert L. Vender, MD
Associate Professor of Medicine
Division of Pulmonary, Allergy, and
Critical Care Medicine
Pennsylvania State University Milton S.
Hershey Medical Center
Hershey, Pennsylvania

Navin Verma, MD
Assistant Professor
Division of Nephrology
Department of Medicine
Pennsylvania State University Milton S.
Hershey Medical Center
Hershey, Pennsylvania

Ronald J. Williams, MD, FAAP, FACP
Associate Professor of Pediatrics and
Medicine
Divisions of General Pediatrics and
General Internal Medicine
Director, Combined Internal
Medicine/Pediatrics Residency Program
Pennsylvania State University Milton S.
Hershey Medical Center
Hershey, Pennsylvania

Shern Willie, MD
Resident
Department of Medicine
Pennsylvania State University Milton S.
Hershey Medical Center
Hershey, Pennsylvania

Margaret M. Wojnar, MD
Associate Professor of Medicine
Department of Medicine
Division of Pulmonary, Allergy, and
Critical Care Medicine
Pennsylvania State University Milton S.
Hershey Medical Center
Hershey, Pennsylvania

Ali Zaidi, MD
Chief Resident
Department of Medicine
Pennsylvania State University Milton S.
Hershey Medical Center
Hershey, Pennsylvania

Crystal Zalonis, DO
Resident
Combined Internal Medicine/Pediatrics
Residency Program
Pennsylvania State University Milton S.
Hershey Medical Center
Hershey, Pennsylvania

Chapter Authors

Chapter Authors

SECTION 12: DERMATOLOGY

Pruritus—Soheil Chegini, MD

Urticaria (Hives)—Nicholas Rider, DO

Hyperhidrosis—Ellen G. Smith, MD

Dry Skin—Sonia Badreshia, MD, and Christine L. Mackley, MD

Acne Vulgaris—Sonia Badreshia, MD, and Christine L. Mackley, MD

Seborrheic Dermatitis—Emmy M. Fernandez, MD, and Christine L. Mackley, MD

Atopic Dermatitis—Merritt L. Fajt, MD, and Tim Craig, DO

Psoriasis—Catherine M. Headley, MD, and Christine L. Mackley, MD

Herpes Zoster—Anneli Fogelberg, MD, and Christine L. Mackley, MD

Warts—Gregory J. Fulchiero Jr., MD, and Christine L. Mackley, MD

Cellulitis—Elizabeth McIlmoyle, MD

Scabies—Jennifer Sceppa and Christine L. Mackley, MD

Skin Cancer—Gregory J. Fulchiero Jr., MD, and Christine L. Mackley, MD

SECTION 13: OPHTHALMOLOGY

Red Eye—Donald T. Hudak, MD, and Marcus Allan East, MD

Dry Eye—Marcus Allan East, MD, and Donald T. Hudak, MD

Visual Loss—Donald T. Hudak, MD, and Marcus Allan East, MD

Eye Pain—Donald T. Hudak, MD, and Marcus Allan East, MD

Glaucoma—Marcus Allan East, MD, and Donald T. Hudak, MD

Cataract—Marcus Allan East, MD, and Donald T. Hudak, MD

Macular Degeneration—Marcus Allan East, MD, and Donald T. Hudak, MD

Infectious Conjunctivitis—Donald T. Hudak, MD, and Marcus Allan East, MD

Hordeolum and Chalazion—Caryn M. Brenner-Williams, MD

Optic Neuritis—Donald T. Hudak, MD, and Marcus Allan East, MD

Iritis—Marcus Allan East, MD, and Donald T. Hudak, MD

Abbreviations

^{123}I	radioactive iodine
^{131}I	radioactive iodine
17-OH	17-hydroxy
ABG	arterial blood gas
Abs	antibodies
AC	acromioclavicular
ACE	angiotensin-converting enzyme
ACTH	adrenocorticotropic hormone
ADA	American Diabetes Association
AGUS	atypical glandular cells of undetermined significance
AIDS	acquired immunodeficiency syndrome
AIN	acute interstitial nephritis
ALS	amyotrophic lateral sclerosis
ALT	alanine aminotransferase (SGPT)
AMD	age-related macular degeneration
ANA	antinuclear antibody
Anti-SM	anti-Smith antigen antibody
ARB	angiotensin receptor blocker
AS	ankylosing spondylitis
ASC-H	atypical squamous cells, cannot exclude HSIL
ASC-US	atypical squamous cells of undetermined significance
ASO	antistreptolysin-O
AST	aspartate aminotransferase (SGOT)
AUB	abnormal uterine bleeding
AV	arteriovenous
AVM	arteriovenous malformation
BMI	body mass index
BP	blood pressure
BPH	benign prostatic hypertrophy
BRCA	breast cancer gene
BUN	blood urea nitrogen
C. trachomatis	Chlamydia trachomatis
C-ANCA	cytoplasmic–antineutrophil cytoplasmic antibody
CBC	complete blood count

cc	cubic centimeter
CDC	Centers for Disease Control and Prevention
CHF	congestive heart failure
CIN	cervical dysplasia severity classification (old)
CK	creatine kinase
CKD	chronic kidney disease
cm	centimeter
CMC	carpometacarpal joint
CMV	cytomegalovirus
CNS	central nervous system
CO_2	carbon dioxide
CRAO	central retinal artery occlusion
CRH	corticotrophin-releasing hormone
CRP	C-reactive protein
CRVO	central retinal vein occlusion
CT	computed tomography
CXR	chest X-ray
DES	diethylstilbestrol
DEXA	dual-energy X-ray absorptiometry
DHEA-S	dehydroepiandrosterone sulfate
DIP	distal intraphalangeal joint
DKA	diabetic ketoacidosis
dL	deciliter
DNA	deoxyribonucleic acid
DNase	deoxyribonuclease
DUB	dysfunctional uterine bleeding
E. coli	*Escherichia coli*
EBV	Epstein-Barr virus
ED	erectile dysfunction
EEG	electroencephalogram
EMG	electromyogram
ERG	electroretinogram
ESR	erythrocyte sedimentation rate
ESWL	extracorporeal shock wave lithotripsy
F_c	crystallizable fragment of immunoglobulin
FDA	Food and Drug Administration
FeNa	fractional excretion of sodium
FEV_1	forced expiratory volume in 1 second
FSGS	focal segmental glomerular sclerosis
FSH	follicle-stimulating hormone
FTA-ABS	fluorescent treponemal antibody
g	gram

GBM	glomerular basement membrane
GFR	glomerular filtration rate
GI	gastrointestinal
GIFT	gamete intrafallopian transfer
HGPRT	hypoxanthine-guanine phosphoribosyltransferase
HIV	human immunodeficiency virus
HLA	human leukocyte antigen
HPF	high-power field
HPV	human papilloma virus
HSIL	high-grade squamous intraepithelial lesion, or CIN II/III
HSV	herpes simplex virus
HUS	hemolytic uremic syndrome
ICU	intensive care unit
IFG	impaired fasting glucose
IgA	immunoglobulin A
IgG	immunoglobulin G
IgM	immunoglobulin M
IL	interleukin
IM	intramuscular
IV	intravenous
IVF	in vitro fertilization
IVIG	intravenous immunoglobulin
IVP	intravenous pyelogram
KOH	potassium hydroxide
KS	keratoconjunctivitis sicca
KUB	kidney urine bladder X-ray
LDH	lactate dehydrogenase
LE	leukocyte esterase
LGV	lymphogranuloma venereum
LH	luteinizing hormone
LSIL	low-grade squamous intraepithelial lesion, or CIN I
MAO	monoamine oxidase
MCP	metacarpophalangeal joint
MCV	mean corpuscular volume
MEN	multiple endocrine neoplasia
mEq	milli-equivalents
mg	milligram
MI	myocardial infarction
min	minute
mL	milliliter
mm	millimeter
MRI	magnetic resonance imaging

MTP	metatarsophalangeal
NAAT	nucleic acid amplification testing
ng	nanogram
NIH	National Institutes of Health
NSAID	nonsteroidal anti-inflammatory drug
P-ANCA	perinuclear–antineutrophil cytoplasmic antibody
Pap	Papanicolaou
pCO_2	partial pressure of carbon dioxide
PCOS	polycystic ovarian syndrome
P_{Cr}	plasma creatinine
pH	hydrogen ion concentration
PIP	proximal intraphalangeal joint
PMN	polymorphonuclear neutrophil
P_{Na}	plasma sodium
PPD	purified protein derivative (TB test)
PRPP	phosphoribosyl pyrophosphate
PSA	prostate-specific antigen
PTH	parathyroid hormone
PTK	phototherapeutic keratectomy
PTT	activated partial thromboplastin time
RA	rheumatoid arthritis
RBC	red blood cell
RPR	rapid plasma reagin
S. aureus	*Staphylococcus aureus*
S. saprophyticus	*Staphylococcus saprophyticus*
SLE	systemic lupus erythematosus
SS-A antibody	systemic sclerosis-A or (anti-Ro) antibody
SS-B antibody	systemic sclerosis-B or (anti-La) antibody
STD	sexually transmitted disease
T3	triiodothyronine
T4	thyroxine
TB	tuberculosis
TID	three times daily
TNF	tumor necrosis factor
TSH	thyroid-stimulating hormone
TURP	transurethral resection of the prostate
U	International Unit
U_{Cr}	urine creatinine
U_{Na}	urine sodium
URI	upper respiratory tract infection
UTI	urinary tract infection
UV	ultraviolet

VDRL	Venereal Disease Research Laboratory (test for syphilis)
VEP	visual evoked potentials
WBC	white blood cell
β-hCG	beta-human chorionic gonadotropin
μg	microgram

Behavioral

Insomnia

INTRODUCTION

- Insomnia is a common disorder of insufficient or poor-quality sleep that can result in adverse daytime consequences, such as fatigue, diminished energy, difficulty concentrating, memory impairment, low motivation, loss of productivity, irritability, interpersonal difficulties, increased worrying, anxiety, and depression
- It can present as trouble falling asleep, trouble staying asleep, or feelings of insufficient or nonrefreshing sleep
- Chronic sleep loss is a major risk factor for fatigue-related accidents, job loss, marital and social problems, major depression, impaired weight control, and heart disease

ETIOLOGY, EPIDEMIOLOGY, & RISK FACTORS

- Insomnia may be a primary disorder, or may occur secondary to another diseases
  - Primary insomnia is hypothesized to be a disorder of hyperarousal, either due to stress or lifestyle
  - Secondary insomnia may be caused by primary sleep disorders (e.g., restless legs syndrome, periodic limb movement disorder, sleep-related breathing disorder), medical comorbidities (e.g., sleep apnea, congestive heart failure, COPD, asthma, chronic pain syndromes, gastroesophageal reflux disease), or psychological disorders (e.g., depression, anxiety)
- Insomnia may be transient (e.g., related to stress, travel, or illness) or chronic (defined as occurring nightly for at least 6 months)
- One-third of the population has suffered from insomnia at some point in their lives
- Up to 20% of cases result in serious daytime consequences, which can include automobile accidents
- There is a higher prevalence in older persons; insomnia is the most common sleep disorder in persons older than 60

PATIENT PRESENTATION

- Inability to initiate or maintain effective sleep
- Many complain of excess daytime drowsiness and fatigue, sometimes to the point of falling asleep while driving or upon minimal stimulation (such as stopping at a red light or sitting down)
- Feelings of unrefreshing sleep, anxiousness, excessive worrying, or depression
- Question the patient and his/her bed partner about excessive snoring and periodic or sudden movements
- Review of symptoms for other medical, neurologic, or psychological diseases
- In cases of secondary insomnia, symptoms of the underlying disorder may be present (e.g., snoring and hypertension in patients with sleep apnea, rales and decreased exercise tolerance in patients with congestive heart failure, wheezing in patients with asthma, "heartburn" in patients with gastroesophageal reflux disease)

DIFFERENTIAL DX

- Mood disorder/depression
- Asthma or COPD
- Congestive heart failure
- Chronic pain
- Hyperthyroidism
- Gastroesophageal reflux disease
- Restless legs syndrome
- Obstructive sleep apnea
- Drugs (e.g., caffeine, alcohol, nonsedating cold medications, illicit drugs)
- Caretaker insomnia (i.e., presence of a newborn or ill family member)
- Circadian rhythm disruption (e.g., jet lag, shift work)
- Conditioned insomnia

DIAGNOSTIC EVALUATION

- Complete history and physical examination is necessary
  - History should be elicited from the patient and his/her bed partner, if possible
  - Pay careful attention to age of onset, predisposing factors and traits, precipitating events, duration, and specific characteristics (e.g., nightly vs. intermittent vs. situation-specific)
  - Review medications, with particular attention to stimulant medications (e.g., methylphenidate), over-the-counter drugs (e.g., caffeine, pseudoephedrine), and herbal or alternative agents (e.g., ephedra, nicotine)
  - Physical exam should pay attention to weight, body mass index, and examinations of the oropharynx, neck, heart and lungs
- Laboratory testing may include complete blood count, complete metabolic panel and thyroid studies
- Urine toxicology screen may be indicated to detect illicit use of stimulant drugs (e.g., amphetamines, cocaine)
- A sleep log or diary is useful to identify circadian rhythm disorders and determine the severity of the disorder
- Psychological screening (e.g., Beck Depression and Beck Anxiety Inventories) may identify the presence and severity of depression or other psychiatric disorders
- Polysomnography testing may be indicated to diagnose organic sleep disorders, such as obstructive sleep apnea, periodic limb movement disorders, or restless legs syndrome

TREATMENT & MANAGEMENT

- Treat underlying medical or psychiatric conditions as necessary
- Eliminate unnecessary stimulant medications, or move dosing to earlier in the day
- Educate patients on appropriate sleep hygiene
  - The bed should only be used for sleeping and sex
  - Sleep only in the bedroom, and avoid daytime naps
  - Keep regular bed times and wake at the same time every day
  - Leave the bedroom if awake for longer than 15-20 minutes and return only when sleepy
  - Avoid exercise prior to bedtime
  - Avoid alcohol as a sleep aid (alcohol limits deep, refreshing sleep)
  - Limit caffeine to the morning hours, if at all
- Relaxation training (e.g., progressive muscle relaxation, guided imagery, hypnosis, meditation, yoga, biofeedback) may be useful, especially in patients with excessive stress
- If necessary, short-acting hypnotics (e.g., zolpidem, zaleplon) can be used; longer acting medications (e.g., benzodiazepines, tricyclic antidepressants, doxepin, trazodone) should be used only for refractory cases and should be carefully monitored (especially in the elderly)
- Circadian rhythm disturbances often respond to bright morning light exposure; melatonin (0.5–3 mg) can shift the circadian rhythm in the opposite direction (i.e., when taken in the morning, it shifts rhythms later; when taken in the evening, it shifts rhythms earlier)
- Obstructive sleep apnea often responds to continuous positive airway pressure (CPAP)

PROGNOSIS & COMPLICATIONS

- Complications of chronic insomnia include excessive daytime somnolence with increased risk of accidents, mood disorders (including major depression), and worsening of medical conditions, such as congestive heart failure (due to chronic hypoxia) and hypertension
- Many patients will respond to nonpharmacologic behavioral approaches
- If medications are deemed necessary, short-acting hypnotics are preferable
- Referral to a certified sleep lab may be necessary for chronic or refractory cases

Tobacco Use and Cessation

INTRODUCTION

- Tobacco use is the single greatest cause of disease and premature death in the United States and is estimated to cause more than 400,000 deaths yearly
- Smoking is a powerful addiction; most smokers require at least several attempts at quitting before achieving success
- Physicians should approach tobacco use as a chronic disease with periods of remission and relapse
- Americans spend an estimated $50 billion annually on direct medical care for smoking-related illnesses, and another $47 billion is lost due to smoking-related disability

ETIOLOGY, EPIDEMIOLOGY, & RISK FACTORS

- Tobacco use increases the risk of many illnesses, including cancers, heart disease, peripheral vascular disease, chronic obstructive lung disease, respiratory infections, peptic ulcers, and osteoporosis
- Nicotine causes addiction; smoking cessation leads to typical withdrawal symptoms, including irritability, anger, impatience, restlessness, difficulty concentrating, insomnia, increased appetite, anxiety, and depressed mood
- Withdrawal symptoms begin a few hours after smoking the last cigarette, peak within 2-3 days, and then gradually subside after several weeks to months
- Smoking is also a learned behavior, adding psychological factors to the difficulty of quitting
- Nearly one-fourth of adult Americans currently smoke
- 3000 children and adolescents become regular users of tobacco daily
- 70% of smokers say they want to quit, and about 40% have tried quitting during the past year
- There is a decline in the excess risk of disease after smoking cessation; smokers who quit before the age of 50 have half the risk of dying within the next 15 years compared to those who continue to smoke

PATIENT PRESENTATION

- Psychological dependence may include the association of cigarette use with certain events, such as meals, sex, or partying, and the use of cigarettes to handle stress or negative emotions
- Stages of smoking cessation include precontemplation, contemplation, preparation, action, and maintenance
  - Precontemplation (40% of smokers): Patients in this stage have no plans to quit
  - Contemplation (40%): Patients in this stage are worried about the effects and risks of smoking, but are not yet ready to quit
  - Preparation (20%): Patients are ready to quit
  - Action: The act of quitting
  - Maintenance: Quit more than 6 months ago
- Physical withdrawal symptoms may include irritability, anger, impatience, restlessness, difficulty concentrating, insomnia, increased appetite, anxiety, and depressed mood

DIFFERENTIAL DX

- Coexistant substance abuse (e.g., marijuana, alcohol, prescription drugs, chewing tobacco)

DIAGNOSTIC EVALUATION

- Attempt to move each smoker from a lower stage to a higher one
- The five "A's" of assessment for people who want to quit:
  - Ask about current and past tobacco use
  - Advise and strongly urge all tobacco users to quit
  - Assess their willingness to quit
  - Assist the patient in quitting: set a quit date; inform friends and family of the quit date; anticipate challenges; remove tobacco products from the home, car, and workplace; set a quit plan with strategies on how to cope with withdrawal symptoms (e.g., exercise, behavioral modification, relaxation techniques), weight gain (e.g., eat low-calorie foods, exercise regularly), and relapses (e.g., reassess commitment, try again); dispense smoking cessation handouts, booklets, and instructions
  - Arrange for follow-up with primary care provider or a smoking cessation clinic
- In patients with comorbid conditions, medical testing may be indicated (e.g., electrocardiogram, lipid panel, chest X-ray)

TREATMENT & MANAGEMENT

- Nonpharmacologic interventions include counseling and group therapy
  - Hypnosis and acupuncture have been touted as useful but are unproven
- A combination of nonpharmacologic and pharmacologic treatments work best
- Nicotine-based pharmacotherapy includes nicotine gum (chew every 1-2 hours for 6-8 weeks, then wean), nicotine patches (21 mg per day for 4 weeks, followed by 14 mg per day for 2 weeks, followed by 7 mg per day for 2 weeks), nicotine oral inhaler (6-16 cartridges per day with continuous puffing [not inhaling] over 20 minutes for each cartridge), nicotine nasal spray (1 spray in each nostril 1-2 times per hour as needed), and nicotine lozenge (must be "parked" in cheek to absorb nicotine)
- Nonnicotine-based pharmacotherapy includes bupropion (start 2 weeks before quit date; contraindicated in patients with a history of seizures or at risk for seizures), nortriptyline (begin 10-28 days before quitting and continue for 3 months), and clonidine (more side effects); however, only bupropion is FDA approved for smoking cessation
- If the patient is not yet ready to quit, follow the 5 "R's" of motivation:
  - Relevance: ask the patient why quitting is important (e.g., effect on health, loved ones)
  - Risks: ask the patient to identify potential negative health risks
  - Rewards: ask the patient to identify the benefits of stopping
  - Roadblocks: ask the patient to identify barriers to quitting
  - Repetition: repeat a "quit offer" at every visit

PROGNOSIS & COMPLICATIONS

- A combination of nonpharmacologic and pharmacologic interventions results in quit rates of 40–50%, which is much higher than either alone
- Half of Americans who have ever been smokers have managed to quit
- Continuing to smoke significantly raises the risk of developing many serious health problems in both the patient and in those exposed to secondhand smoke
- Cough may increase during the first week after smoking cessation as the respiratory cilia can now effectively remove lung debris

Depression

INTRODUCTION

- Depression is characterized by a loss of interest or depressed mood that can interfere with work and personal relationships, as well as physical health (depleted motivation may contribute to poor self-care [nutrition, exercise], poor adherence to medical treatments, diminished social support, and possibly immunosuppression)
- Depression is estimated to be the 2nd leading cause of disability worldwide by 2020
- As few as 10% of patients who have an episode of major depression receive appropriate treatment (i.e., appropriate drug choice, dose, and duration; appropriate specialty referral)
- In primary care, two-thirds of patients stop antidepressants within 4 weeks; 20–50% will not accept a specialty referral (i.e., stigma of psychiatry)

ETIOLOGY, EPIDEMIOLOGY, & RISK FACTORS

- Depression is a heterogeneous category that subsumes multiple disorders and mechanisms
- The exact cause of depression is unknown; it is hypothesized to be due to both genetic vulnerability and emotional/environmental stressors
  - Postpartum depression appears to have a hormonal component
- Alterations of neurotransmitters have been postulated as potential causes
  - Serotonin is the primary neurotransmitter linked to depression, but remains unproven
  - Other neurotransmitters, in addition to serotonin, are also involved
  - The effectiveness of serotonin reuptake inhibitors may not be due to serotonergic actions
- Major depression typically develops gradually over weeks to months, often after a significant stressor (e.g., trauma, loss of a loved one, major life change)
- Depression is one of the most common chronic medical conditions
  - The lifetime prevalence of major depression is 20-25% in women and 7-12% in men
  - The point prevalence of major depression in primary care settings is 5-10%
- Risk factors include female gender, family history of affective disorder, postpartum period, problems in primary relationship, medical comorbidities (especially pain or disability), psychiatric comorbidities (e.g., anxiety, personality disorder, substance abuse), stressful life events, and neuroticism (e.g., insecurity, worry, brooding, pessimism)

PATIENT PRESENTATION

- Typical primary care presentations include fatigue, chronic pain, multiple somatic complaints, memory problems, weight changes, sleep problems, feeling stressed, angry outbursts, decreased libido, decreased concentration, frequent tearfulness, and cardiac-sounding symptoms (e.g., dyspnea, palpitations, chest pain)
- Any of the above should prompt screening for depression:
  - "During the past month, have you been bothered by feeling down, depressed, or hopeless?"
  - "Are you bothered by little interest or pleasure in doing things?"
  - If either is positive, proceed to diagnostic criteria

DIFFERENTIAL DX

- Thyroid disease
- Malignancy (especially pancreatic cancer)
- Diabetes mellitus
- Alcohol or drug use (e.g., betablockers, interferon, oral contraceptives, benzodiazepines reserpine, glucocorticoids)
- Stimulant withdrawal
- Vitamin B_6, vitamin B_{12}, or folate deficiency
- Normal bereavement
- Dementia (e.g., Alzheimer's disease, Parkinson's disease)
- Cushing's disease
- Neurologic disease or insult
- Cardiomyopathies
- Electrolyte abnormalities
- Systemic lupus erythematosus

DIAGNOSTIC EVALUATION

- A complete history and physical examination is necessary to rule out other causes
  - Assess personal and family history of affective disorders
  - Screen for comorbid anxiety and substance abuse disorders
  - Screen for suicide risk
  - Assess recent or ongoing stressors, especially bereavement and relationship problems
- Major depression is characterized by markedly decreased interest/pleasure or depressed mood for at least 2 weeks, accompanied by at least 3-4 additional symptoms (e.g., weight loss or gain, or increased or decreased appetite; insomnia or hypersomnia; overt psychomotor agitation or retardation; fatigue or diminished energy; feelings of worthlessness or inappropriate guilt; diminished thinking, concentration, or decisiveness; recurrent thoughts of death or suicide)
- Dysthymic disorder is characterized by depressed mood most of the time for at least 2 years, accompanied by at least 2 additional symptoms (e.g., poor appetite or overeating; insomnia or hypersomnia; low energy or fatigue; low self-esteem; poor concentration or indecisiveness; feelings of hopelessness)
- Screen for bipolarity by asking about history of manic or hypomanic symptoms (e.g., distinctly elevated or irritable mood, grandiosity, decreased need for sleep, pressured speech, racing thoughts, increased activity)
- Test for thyroid-stimulating hormone (TSH) and free T4 levels in women older than 65 or if signs of hypothyroidism are present

TREATMENT & MANAGEMENT

- For acute, mild-to-moderate depression, treatment may include lifestyle changes, stress reduction, relationship management, practical problem solving, or referral for counseling
- Persistent or severe depression should prompt evaluation for suicide risk, involvement of family, and need for specialty care, which may include hospitalization
- A combination of psychotherapy (cognitive-behavioral therapy, interpersonal therapy, or psychodynamic therapy) and antidepressant medications is most effective
- Selective serotonin reuptake inhibitors (SSRIs), escitalopram (in elderly), venlafaxine, mirtazapine, bupropion, and tricyclic antidepressants (TCAs) have established efficacy
  - No single drug has been proven more effective in treating depression; however, newer antidepressants (e.g., SSRIs) have fewer adverse effects
  - Drug selection can be based on previous responses, cost, frequency of dosing, potential for overdose, and anticipated side effects (most side effects are transient)
  - Dosing should be increased gradually to a target dose over approximately 10 days
  - If prominent fatigue or loss of energy, venlafaxine or bupropion may be most effective
  - Management of side effects (e.g., sedation, gastrointestinal symptoms, sexual effects, weight gain) and close follow-up are critical to adherence and treatment response
  - If there is no response after 4-6 weeks, consider switching to a different agent in same class or a different class; if partial response, consider raising the dose
- Electroconvulsive therapy is often effective for severe, intractable depression

PROGNOSIS & COMPLICATIONS

- Follow-up should be scheduled every 2 weeks during the initial 12 weeks of drug therapy
- Referral to psychiatry may be warranted if patient does not respond to medication, has a history of mania or psychosis, requires combination therapy, or is a suicide risk
- 50–60% of patients respond to an initial medication trial
- Recurrence is common, even with appropriate treatment
- Recurrence is less likely if multiple treatments are implemented (e.g., cognitive-behavioral therapy, mindfulness meditation, exercise program, stress management, couples counseling)
- Up to 20% will experience a chronic course that is largely refractory to treatment
- Lifetime suicide rates for major affective disorders approach 15%
- Monitor medication side effects and drug interactions; TCA overdose can be lethal

Section 2

Gastrointestinal

Nausea and Vomiting

INTRODUCTION

- Nausea is a feeling of sickness in the stomach characterized by an urge to vomit
- Vomiting denotes the forceful expulsion of gastric contents through the mouth
  - Distinguish vomiting from regurgitation (an effortless reflux of stomach contents) and rumination (purposeful regurgitation, chewing, and reswallowing of food after meals)
- Nausea and vomiting can occur as manifestations of a large group of disorders within and outside the gut, and as side effects of various drugs and numerous circulating toxins

ETIOLOGY, EPIDEMIOLOGY, & RISK FACTORS

- Vomiting is a complex, coordinated reflex orchestrated by neural mechanisms that originate in the chemoreceptor trigger zone and the vomiting center of the medulla
  - The chemoreceptor trigger zone, contained in the area postrema on the floor of the 4th ventricle, is particularly sensitive to chemical stimuli; it is readily accessible to emetic substances because the blood-brain barrier is poorly developed in this area
  - The vomiting center, located in the dorsolateral border of the reticular formation, coordinates the emetic response during the act of vomiting; it receives and integrates excitatory inputs from vagal sensory fibers in the gastrointestinal tract, the labyrinths, higher centers in the cortex, the chemoreceptor trigger zone, and intracranial pressure receptors
- During vomiting, gastric content is expelled following relaxation of the gastric and lower esophageal sphincter, retrograde contraction of the proximal small bowel and gastric antrum, abdominal muscle contraction, and cricopharyngeal contraction followed by relaxation
- Emesis provoked by noxious thoughts or smells originates in the cerebral cortex, where cranial nerves mediate vomiting after activation of the gag reflex; motion sickness and inner ear disorders act on the labyrinthine apparatus, while gastric irritants and emetogenic chemotherapy agents stimulate gastroduodenal vagal afferents; other stimuli (e.g., antibiotics, bacterial toxins, pregnancy, hypoxia, uremia) act on the chemoreceptor trigger zone

PATIENT PRESENTATION

- Onset: Acute onset suggests infection, ingestion of toxins or a new medication, pregnancy, head trauma, or acute bowel obstruction; chronic onset suggests partial obstruction, motility disturbance, metabolic, brain tumor, or psychogenic
- Timing and relation to meals: Early morning (prior to meals) suggests morning sickness of pregnancy, alcoholism, uremia, post nasal drip, or increased intracranial pressure; during meals suggests psychogenic or peptic ulcer disease
- Content of vomitus: Vomiting of undigested food suggests esophageal spasm, dysmotility, or diverticulum; the presence of old food in the vomitus suggests gastric outlet or high small bowel obstruction, or a gastric motility disorder; blood or coffee ground vomitus suggests upper GI bleed; bilious vomiting suggests distal bowel obstruction
- A feculent odor suggests ischemic gut, bacterial overgrowth, obstruction, gastrocolic fistula, or ileus

DIFFERENTIAL DX

- Intraperitoneal causes
  - Bowel obstruction
  - Infection
  - Inflammation (e.g., hepatitis, cholecystitis, pancreatitis)
  - Impaired motor function (e.g., gastroparesis, GERD)
  - Radiation treatment
- Extraperitoneal causes
  - Cardiopulmonary disease (e.g., myocardial infarction)
  - Labyrinthine disorders
  - Intracerebral disorders
  - Psychiatric disorders
  - Postoperative
  - Drugs and toxins
  - Endocrine/metabolic (e.g., pregnancy, uremia, thyroid disease, ketoacidosis)

DIAGNOSTIC EVALUATION

- The diagnostic workup should be directed by the history and physical examination
  - Assess the severity of the immediate complaint
  - Evaluate for useful "clues," such as fever, weight loss, jaundice, and dehydration
  - The abdominal exam should carefully evaluate for tenderness and bowel sounds
- Blood chemistries may reveal a metabolic disturbance (usually hypokalemic hypochloremic, metabolic alkalosis)
- Abdominal X-ray may reveal a mechanical obstruction
- Upper gastrointestinal X-ray series and endoscopy may be helpful when the history and physical examination suggest peptic ulcer disease or gastric outlet obstruction
- In patients with chronic nausea and vomiting who have normal findings on upper gastrointestinal series and endoscopy, a radionuclide or radio-opaque marker study to evaluate for gastric emptying should be considered

TREATMENT & MANAGEMENT

- Management involves restoration of normal fluid and electrolyte balance, specific treatment of identified underlying disorders, and antiemetic agents
- Neuroleptic agents (e.g., prochlorperazine, chlorpromazine) are effective in treating nausea and vomiting caused by drugs, radiation, or gastroenteritis
  - The most common side effect is sedation
  - Other potential side effects include blood dyscrasia, jaundice, and dystonia
- D2 receptor antagonists (e.g., metoclopramide, domperidone) are useful in treating vomiting caused by chemotherapy, gastroparesis, or pseudo-obstruction
  - Side effects range from mild anxiety and nervousness to dystonia or tardive dyskinesia
  - Domperidone does not readily cross the blood-brain barrier and causes fewer side effects
- Selective serotonin receptor antagonists (e.g., ondansetron) are very effective in controlling chemotherapy-induced emesis that is refractory to conventional agents
  - Adverse effects are minimal and include headache, constipation, diarrhea, and transient elevation of liver enzymes
- Prokinetic agents (e.g., erythromycin) may be useful to treat nausea or vomiting related to gastroparesis, gastroesophageal reflux disease, or pseudo-obstruction
  - Adverse effects include abdominal cramping, diarrhea

PROGNOSIS & COMPLICATIONS

- Medical complications resulting from persistent nausea and vomiting include weight loss, aspiration of vomit, electrolyte imbalance and dehydration, delayed oral therapy, and anxiety or depression leading to delayed further treatment
- Patients with refractory nausea and vomiting may pose significant treatment challenges; some of the newer therapies in such patients include somatostatin analogs (e.g., octreotide) for intestinal pseudo-obstruction, pyloric injections of botulinum or implantation of gastric electrical pacemakers and neurotransmitters for idiopathic vomiting or gastric gastroparesis, and surgical resection of the stomach in postvagotomy gastroparesis

Constipation

INTRODUCTION

- Constipation is the most common digestive complaint, leading to an estimated 2.5 million physician visits annually in the United States
- An estimated one-third of individuals with constipation seek health care
- Constipation can be difficult to assess because it is defined differently by patients and health care providers; a common definition is fewer than 3 stools per week; however, patient descriptions of constipation often include a myriad of complaints, including straining during defecation, hard stools, and a sensation of incomplete evacuation

ETIOLOGY, EPIDEMIOLOGY, & RISK FACTORS

- Successful defecation depends on normal colonic motility (peristalsis), rectal function, and coordination of the pelvic floor muscles, including the internal and external anal sphincters
  - Colonic peristalsis is regulated by neuronal excitation coupled with inhibition of contraction, which is mediated by the enteric nervous system and interstitial cells of Cajal; interference with this mediation, or decrease in the number of interstitial cells of Cajal, can lead to decreased colonic motility
  - Rectal function includes adaptation to increasing volumes of distension; altered rectal compliance can lead to enhanced or diminished rectal tone, including megarectum
  - The pelvic floor muscles and anal sphincters receive parasympathetic innervation from the sacral nerves; paradoxical contraction of the puborectalis muscles and anal sphincters during defecation or disruption of innervation may result in constipation
- Prevalence is higher in women and in the elderly and seems to increase as age advances
  - Prevalence is also higher in nonwhites and those with low income or low education level
- Risk factors include insufficient fluid intake, decreased mobility or inactivity, low calorie intake, diabetes mellitus, primary neurologic disease, and medications (often polypharmacy), including NSAIDs, opioids, diuretics, antihypertensives, antidepressants, antispasmodics, anticonvulsants, aluminum antacids, and calcium and iron supplementation

PATIENT PRESENTATION

- Patients may complain of infrequent defecation, straining, incomplete evacuation or anal blockage, small/hard stool, or a need for digital manipulation
- Patients may have evidence of anal fissures, rectocele, or abnormal anal sphincter tone
- The Rome II criteria suggest functional constipation if 2 or more criteria are present for at least 12 weeks during the past 12 months:
  - Straining in more than 1/4 of defecations
  - Lumpy/hard stool in more than 1/4 of defecations
  - Sensation of incomplete evacuation in more than 1/4 of defecations
  - Sensation of anorectal obstruction/blockage in more than 1/4 of defecations
  - Manual maneuvers needed to facilitate more than 1/4 of defecations
  - Fewer than 3 defecations per week
  - Absence of loose stool and insufficient criteria for irritable bowel syndrome

DIFFERENTIAL DX

- Idiopathic
- Decreased colonic transit
- Pelvic floor dysfunction
- Medication-induced
- Irritable bowel syndrome
- Metabolic/endocrine (e.g., diabetes mellitus, uremia, hypothyroidism, hypercalcemia)
- Myopathic (e.g., scleroderma, amyloidosis)
- Neurogenic (e.g., Parkinson's disease, Hirschsprung's disease, multiple sclerosis, spinal cord lesions)
- Mechanical obstruction (e.g., stricture, external compression, anismus, rectocele, anal fissure, colon cancer, megacolon, megarectum)

DIAGNOSTIC EVALUATION

- Detailed history and physical examination, including a thorough drug history (prescription and over-the-counter medications), neurologic exam, and rectal exam
- Laboratory studies include complete blood count, thyroid-stimulating hormone (TSH), serum calcium, and glucose
- Visualization of the colon will evaluate for anatomical lesions
  - Direct visualization by colonoscopy is preferable, especially for patients with hematochezia, heme-positive stools, anemia, weight loss, or advanced age (older than 50)
  - In patients under age 50 without alarming symptoms, a barium enema or flexible sigmoidoscopy may be considered as an alternative to colonoscopy
- Transit studies using radiopaque markers are useful to assess for delayed colonic transit
  - If the marker settles in the right colon, consider colonic inertia
  - If the marker settles in the sigmoid colon, consider outlet obstruction or pelvic floor dysfunction
- Defecography may be useful to evaluate the pelvic floor musculature and assess for the presence of a rectocele
  - Thick barium is introduced into the rectum; the patient then attempts to evacuate the barium under fluoroscopy
- Anorectal manometry is valuable for assessing rectal sensation and compliance of the internal and external anal sphincters and can rule out Hirschsprung's disease

TREATMENT & MANAGEMENT

- Correct any identifiable causes (e.g., medications, metabolic or endocrine disorders)
- Initial management should include patient education and dietary modification to achieve a gradual increase in fiber (target of 15-20 g per day) and fluid intake
  - Initiate bulk fiber supplementation, such as Citrucel
  - The addition of a daily stool softer may be helpful (e.g., docusate sodium)
- Use laxatives as necessary: Saline laxatives (e.g., milk of magnesia) act as hyperosmolar agents; stimulant laxatives (e.g., bisacodyl, senna) increase intestinal motility
- For patients who do not respond well to these recommendations, hyperosmolar agents (e.g., lactulose, sorbitol, polyethylene glycol) can be used
- Biofeedback and relaxation training are useful adjuncts to therapy for patients with pelvic floor dysfunction; suppositories may also be helpful
- Surgical management is typically reserved for patients who are refractory to medical therapy
  - Surgical repair of a rectocele or rectal prolapse can improve symptoms
  - Surgery is the treatment of choice for Hirschsprung's disease
  - Consider subtotal colectomy for refractory patients with delayed colonic transit

PROGNOSIS & COMPLICATIONS

- The prognosis for patients with constipation is generally good
- Most patients will respond to a stepwise approach, beginning with dietary modification and progressing with medical management
- Unfortunately, constipation may uncommonly be a symptom of colon cancer or an externally compressing mass with a poor prognosis
- Surgical treatment options have an increased risk of complications
- Complications of long-term constipation include decreased rectal sensation, megarectum, and, occasionally, fecal incontinence

Gastrointestinal Bleeding

INTRODUCTION

- Gastrointestinal (GI) bleeding is a common medical condition that results in high morbidity and medical costs
- Despite a broad range of etiologies, all gastrointestinal bleeds are characterized by blood loss at any location throughout the gastrointestinal tract
- Upper gastrointestinal bleeding is often defined as bleeding that occurs above the ligament of Treitz, whereas lower gastrointestinal bleeding occurs distal to the ligament of Treitz
- The clinical presentation varies depending on the location, volume, briskness, and duration of the bleeding

ETIOLOGY, EPIDEMIOLOGY, & RISK FACTORS

Upper GI bleeding
- Results in approximately 100 hospitalizations per 100,000 patients per year
- Peptic ulcer disease and gastritis are the most common causes of upper GI bleeding
  - These occur when there is disruption in the normal mucosal defense mechanism due to direct mucosal toxicity (e.g., NSAIDs, alcohol), reduced mucosal blood flow, inhibition of mucosal prostaglandin (e.g., NSAIDs), gastric metaplasia, altered gastric acid secretion, and reduced mucosal immune response
  - Incidence is twice as common in men and increases with age
  - Other risk factors include medications (e.g., NSAIDs, aspirin, steroids, anticoagulants, ginkgo biloba), *Helicobacter pylori* infection, GERD, coagulopathy, thrombocytopenia, chronic liver disease/portal hypertension, recurrent emesis, and chronic renal disease

Lower GI bleeding
- Diverticulosis is the most common cause, followed by colon polyps and angiodysplasia
- Other risk factors include increasing age, low-fiber diet, chronic constipation, prior radiation therapy, coagulopathy, thrombocytopenia, medications (NSAIDs, aspirin, steroids, anticoagulants, ginkgo biloba), recent colonic polypectomy, and renal failure

PATIENT PRESENTATION

- Upper GI bleeding can present with hematemesis (vomiting of reddish or coffee ground-colored blood), melena (black, tarry stools), occult blood loss, iron deficiency anemia, or abdominal pain
- Lower GI bleeding can present with hematochezia (passage of maroon/bright red blood or blood clots), melena (usually from an upper GI source or the cecum), bright red blood per rectum (refers to scant amount of blood found on anus or toilet paper, usually due to a rectal vault origin), occult blood loss, iron deficiency anemia, or abdominal pain
- If large amounts of blood have been lost, patients may present with hypotension or shock

DIFFERENTIAL DX

- Upper GI bleeding: Peptic ulcer disease, gastritis, varices, arteriovenous malformation, Mallory-Weiss tear, esophagitis, benign tumors (e.g., leiomyoma, polyp, lipoma), malignant tumors (e.g., gastric adenocarcinoma, lymphoma, leiomyosarcoma, Kaposi's sarcoma, carcinoid, melanoma)
  - Distinguish upper GI bleeding from hemoptysis and epistaxis
- Lower GI bleeding: Angiodysplasia, diverticular bleeding, hemorrhoids, ischemic colitis, radiation colitis, infectious colitis, inflammatory bowel disease, colonic polyposis

DIAGNOSTIC EVALUATION

- A thorough history and physical exam should be performed on all patients
  - Evaluate for the location, color, and quantity of blood loss; presence or absence of abdominal pain; recent changes in bowel habits; previous bleeding episodes; alcohol use; coagulation disorders; liver disease; drugs (e.g., NSAIDs, aspirin, steroids, anticoagulants)
  - Emesis preceding the bleeding may suggest a Mallory-Weiss tear
  - Pay particular attention to the hemodynamic assessment, including orthostatic blood pressure and pulse, and signs of anemia
  - Direct examination of stool obtained during the rectal examination
- Initial laboratory studies include complete blood count, coagulation studies, and complete metabolic profile (screen for renal or liver disease)
- Evaluate for the source of bleeding as appropriate
  - Nasogastric lavage and aspiration can diagnose upper GI bleeding
  - Anoscopy is useful to detect internal hemorrhoids
  - Esophagogastroduodenoscopy (EGD) is the diagnostic modality of choice for upper GI bleeding, will identify the bleeding site, and allows for intervention to stop the bleeding
  - Colonoscopy is the initial examination of choice for lower GI bleeding, will identify the bleeding site, and allows for biopsy and/or intervention to stop the bleeding
  - Radionuclide scanning (bleeding scan) is a highly sensitive test that can detect bleeding as slow as 0.1 mL per minute; however, it is relatively poor at localizing the site of bleeding
  - Angiography is usually reserved for uncontrolled bleeding to assess the need for surgery

TREATMENT & MANAGEMENT

- Many cases will cease spontaneously; the initial emphasis of treatment is supportive care and identification of patients at risk of massive or recurrent bleeding
  - Low-risk patients include younger, asymptomatic patients without comorbid conditions, with a single episode of self-limited bleeding
  - High-risk patients include those with hemodynamic instability, transfusion requirement, persistent bleeding, or comorbid conditions
- In patients who require hospitalization, ensure intravenous access (two 18-gauge or larger catheters), begin intravenous fluids, send for blood for type and cross, begin serial assessments of hemoglobin or hematocrit, and consider blood or platelet transfusions to correct coagulopathy, thrombocytopenia, or severe symptomatic anemia
- Emergent endoscopy or colonoscopy may be indicated for severe bleeding, and severe bleeding may require angiographic embolization or surgical intervention
- Discontinue medications that increase the risk of bleeding
- Treat underlying etiologies as appropriate (e.g., proton pump inhibitors and/or *H. pylori* antibiotic therapy for peptic ulcer disease, endoscopic or surgical treatment of diverticuli, octreotide or balloon tamponade for uncontrolled variceal bleeding)

PROGNOSIS & COMPLICATIONS

- Prognosis for recurrent bleeding varies widely depending on age, location of the bleed, endoscopic findings, ability to treat underlying cause, comorbid conditions, and the correction of predisposing factors
- Hospitalization may be indicated for hypotension, tachycardia, blood transfusion, active bleeding, severe anemia, thrombocytopenia, or coagulopathy
- Significant bleeding may lead to hypotenison, myocardial infarction, stroke, or death.

Jaundice & Abnormal Liver Function Tests

INTRODUCTION

- Jaundice in an adult patient can be benign or life threatening
- The classic definition of jaundice is yellow staining of the skin, sclera, and mucus membranes, which usually occurs when serum bilirubin exceeds 2.5-3 mg/dL
- Evaluation of jaundice generally requires a careful history and physical examination, as well as additional tests of liver injury, including AST, ALT, alkaline phosphatase, gamma-glutamyltransferase, and fractionated bilirubin
- Pseudojaundice can occur with excessive ingestion of foods rich in beta-carotene (e.g., carrots, squash, melons); in the case of pseudojaundice, hyperbilirubinemia is absent

ETIOLOGY, EPIDEMIOLOGY, & RISK FACTORS

- The differential diagnosis of jaundice and abnormal liver function tests is divided into prehepatic, intrahepatic, and posthepatic etiologies (see *Differential Dx* section)
- Prehepatic disease (hemolysis) is caused by excess heme release, which results in elevated conjugated (indirect) bilirubin
- Intrahepatic disease may be caused by:
  - Direct liver cell injury, which leads to elevated AST and ALT
  - Defective conjugation of bilirubin, which results in increased unconjugated bilirubin
  - Intrahepatic cholestasis, which results in elevated conjugated bilirubin
  - Infiltrative diseases, (e.g., sarcoidosis) which result in elevated alkaline phosphatase
- Posthepatic disease (extrahepatic cholestasis) results in elevated gamma-glutamyltransferase and conjugated bilirubin
  - Elevations of alkaline phosphatase are also seen in bone disorders and during pregnancy; however, concomitant increases in gamma-glutamyltransferase only occur in liver disease
- Risk factors for liver disease include alcohol use, blood transfusions prior to 1990, high-risk behavior for HIV or hepatitis, family history of liver disease, and high-risk travel
- Although acetaminophen toxicity often occurs in cases of drug overdose, it may also occur with therapeutic doses in patients with chronic liver disease or alcohol abuse

PATIENT PRESENTATION

- Yellowing of skin, sclerae, and mucous membranes
- Associated symptoms may include fever, chills, arthralgias, myalgias, anorexia, weight loss, pruritis, abdominal pain, fatigue, changes in urine and stool color, skin hyperpigmentation, xanthomas, and Kaiser-Fleischer rings
- Onset may be acute or chronic
- Signs of liver disease may include bruising, spider angiomas, testicular atrophy, palmar erythema, and ascites
- Because liver function tests are often obtained during routine screening, abnormal liver function is frequently detected in asymptomatic patients
- Be sure to review all medications (prescribed drugs, over-the-counter drugs, and herbal preparations) as possible causative agents

DIFFERENTIAL DX

- Prehepatic: Hemolysis
- Intrahepatic: Acute ischemic liver injury, hepatitis (e.g., viral, alcoholic, autoimmune), medications (e.g., NSAIDs, acetaminophen, antibiotics), Gilbert's syndrome, Crigler-Najjar syndrome, infiltration (fatty liver, tumors, sarcoidosis, fungal), hemochromatosis, Wilson's disease, primary biliary cirrhosis, $alpha_1$-antitrypsin deficiency, celiac sprue, muscle injury, pregnancy
- Posthepatic: choledocholithiasis, biliary tract tumors, primary sclerosing cholangitis, parasitic infections, ascending cholangitis

DIAGNOSTIC EVALUATION

- Assess liver function by measuring the aminotransferases (AST and ALT), alkaline phosphatase, gamma-glutamyltransferase, fractionated bilirubin, prothrombin time, albumin level, and serum ammonia
  - ATS and ALT are the most sensitive tests for acute hepatocellular injury; greatest elavations occur with viral hepatits and drun injury
  - Alkaline phosphotase is the best indicator for biliary obstruction
  - Bilirubin level corresponds to hepatic uptake, metabolic, and excretory functions
- The decision whether to further evaluate the etiology of abnormal liver function tests is based on the probability of underlying hepatobiliary disease
- If hepatocellular injury is suspected, obtain further serologic tests to further support or exclude likely diagnoses, which may include a complete blood count, viral hepatitis serologies, acetaminophen level, ceruloplasmin, serum iron and total iron-binding capacity, serum protein electrophoresis, antinuclear anti-smooth muscle antibody, liver-kidney microsomal antibody, $alpha_1$-antitrypsin level
- If intrahepatic or extrahepatic cholestasis is suspected, assess the biliary tree with a right upper quadrant ultrasound
- CT scan or endoscopic retrograde cholangiopancreatogram (ERCP) is often needed to identify the cause of a biliary obstruction
- Liver biopsy may be required for definitive diagnosis

TREATMENT & MANAGEMENT

- Medical emergencies include massive hemolysis, acetaminophen toxicity, acute liver failure, and ascending cholangitis
  - Treat the underlying cause of hemolysis (e.g., infection, medication toxicity, DIC); blood transfusion may be necessary
  - Acetaminophen toxicity is treated with activated charcoal and N-acetylcysteine (NAC); NAC reduces the production of toxic metabolites and acts as an anti-inflammatory and antioxidant agent
  - Ascending cholangitis is treated with broad-spectrum antibiotics and biliary drainage
  - Definitive treatment varies based on the underlying etiology (e.g., antiviral or immunosuppressive therapy for viral hepatitis)
- Further management should be aimed at controlling symptoms (e.g., ascites, portal hypertension) and preventing progression to cirrhosis or fulminant hepatic failure
- Patients with chronic liver disease (e.g., nonalcoholic fatty liver disease, chronic hepatitis C, alcoholic cirrhosis) should receive both hepatitis A and hepatitis B immunizations
- Liver transplantation may be necessary in severe cases when other treatment options have been exhausted
  - Contraindications to transplantation include active alcohol or drug use, HIV positivity, extrahepatic malignancy, extrabiliary infection, or advanced cardiopulmonary disease

PROGNOSIS & COMPLICATIONS

- Morbidity, mortality, and complications depend on the underlying disorder
- The leading cause of fulminant hepatic failure is acetaminophen toxicity, either from large ingestions or from therapeutic doses in those with chronic liver disease
- Liver function and prognosis is graded using the Child-Pugh system, which factors serum albumin, bilirubin, prothrombin time, and the presence of ascites or encephalopathy
- Hepatitis C virus causes 40% of cases of chronic liver disease and is the most common indication for liver transplantation
- The model for end-stage liver disease (MELD) score is a statistical model that uses serum bilirubin, creatinine, and International Normalized Ratio to predict 3-month survival in patients with cirrhosis; this aids in the timing and allocation of liver transplantation

Dysphagia

INTRODUCTION

- Difficulty swallowing occurs due to difficulty transferring a food bolus from the oropharynx to the upper esophagus (oropharyngeal or transfer dysphagia) or due to impaired transport of a food bolus through the body of the esophagus (esophageal or transport dysphagia)
- Dysphagia may occur independently, or with odynophagia, a sharp, substernal pain upon swallowing that reflects severe erosive disease and is most commonly seen with infectious esophagitis (caused by *Candida*, herpesviruses, or cytomegalovirus, especially in immuno-compromised patients) or corrosive injury

ETIOLOGY, EPIDEMIOLOGY, & RISK FACTORS

Transfer (oropharyngeal) dysphagia

- Neurologic: Stroke, brain mass, multiple sclerosis, ALS, dementia, tardive dyskinesia, pseudobulbar palsy, post polio, Guillain-Barré, Parkinson's or Huntington's disease
- Rheumatologic: Myopathy, polymyositis, oculopharyngeal dystrophy, Sjögren's syndrome
- Metabolic: Thyrotoxicosis, amyloidosis, Cushing's disease, Wilson's disease, medication side effect (e.g., anticholinergics, phenothiazines)
- Infectious: Polio, diphtheria, botulism, Lyme disease, syphilis, viral mucositis
- Structural: Zenker's diverticulum, cervical osteophytes, cricopharyngeal bar, esophageal webs, oropharyngeal tumor, postsurgical or radiation changes, pill-induced injury
- Motility disorders: Upper esophageal sphincter dysfunction

Transport (esophageal) dysphagia

- Mechanical obstruction: Schatzki's ring, peptic stricture, esophageal cancer
- Motility disorder: Achalasia, diffuse esophageal spasm, scleroderma

PATIENT PRESENTATION

- Oropharyngeal dysphagia is a difficulty of initiating swallows
  - May present with regurgitation of liquid through the nose, aspiration with swallowing, and an inability to propel food out of mouth
- Esophageal dysphagia results in a sensation of food "sticking" in the throat
  - May present with retrosternal fullness after swallowing and relief of symptoms upon regurgitation
- Mild weight loss may occur due to voluntary decrease in food intake; however, marked weight loss with anorexia suggests carcinoma or achalasia
- Difficulty with solids suggests an anatomic obstruction
- Difficulty with both solids and liquids suggests a motility problem

DIFFERENTIAL DX

- Gastroesophageal reflux
- Gastroparesis
- Esophageal spasm
- Systemic diseases (e.g., diabetes, myocardial infarction, thyroid disease, stroke, renal insufficiency)
- Ruptured aortic aneurysm
- Pregnancy
- Achalasia
- Oral or esophageal candidiasis
- Pancreatitis
- Cholecystitis
- Choledocholithiasis
- Intra-abdominal malignancy
- Gastric volvulus
- Paraesophageal hernia
- Esophageal rupture

DIAGNOSTIC EVALUATION

- History should include onset, duration, severity, dysphagia with liquid versus solids, past medical history including anxiety and other psychiatric illnesses, prior episodes of dysphagia or caustic substance exposure, and other head and neck problems
- Physical exam should include a thorough head, nose, mouth, neck/thyroid, and abdominal examination, including watching the patient swallow
- Barium swallow is often the first test indicated; it is less invasive than endoscopy and frequently sufficient for diagnosis
  - Identifies the area of the lesion
  - Differentiates motility disturbance from anatomic problems
- Endoscopy may be indicated as a complement to barium study
  - Allows better detection of mucosal lesions
  - Allows for biopsy and concomitant therapy (e.g., dilatation)
- Esophageal manometry may be indicated in patients with persistent dysphagia without a structural etiology
  - Evaluates motor function, measuring the strength, function, and coordination of the upper and lower esophageal sphincters, and the body of the esophagus in response to a swallow
- Esophageal 24-hour pH study may be indicated if suspect gastroesophageal reflux; provides a temporal correlation between symptoms and reflux
- Electromyography and nerve conduction studies may be indicated to rule out neurologic causes (e.g., myasthenia gravis, ALS)

TREATMENT & MANAGEMENT

- Speech therapy evaluation may be indicated for cases without an apparent etiology
- Treat the underlying causes as necessary
- Acute mechanical obstructions require urgent endoscopy to relieve the obstruction and prevent potential perforation
- Chronic mechanical obstruction from webs, rings, and strictures requires endoscopic treatment or thoracic surgery; balloon dilation may be considered
- Dysphagia due to gastroesophageal reflux disease can be minimized with antacid agents (e.g., proton pump inhibitors, H2 receptor antagonists) and lifestyle modifications
- Peptic ulcers may require therapy for *Helicobacter pylori* infection
- Lower esophageal spasm may improve with anticholinergic antispasmodics or the injection of botulinum toxin
- Some neurologic etiologies may require swallow precautions; if unsafe to swallow, a feeding tube or PEG tube may be indicated

PROGNOSIS & COMPLICATIONS

- Gastroenterology referral may be indicated for endoscopy
- Prognosis depends on the underlying etiology
- High risk for aspiration pneumonia in stroke patients
- Malnutrition may occur in patients with obstructions

Irritable Bowel Syndrome

INTRODUCTION

- Irritable bowel syndrome (IBS) is one of the most common conditions encountered in clinical practice but one of the least well understood; it is considered a functional gastrointestinal disorder characterized by abdominal pain and altered bowel habits in the absence of detectable structural abnormalities
- IBS can be diarrhea predominant, constipation predominant, or alternate between the two
- Affects as many as 15% of adults in the United States
- Women are diagnosed 3 times as often as men

ETIOLOGY, EPIDEMIOLOGY, & RISK FACTORS

- The pathophysiology is not completely understood, but the factors most commonly implicated are altered gastrointestinal motility, visceral hypersensitivity, central nervous system processing abnormalities, and psychosocial factors
- Rapid small bowel and colonic transit has been reported in patients with diarrhea-predominant IBS
- Patients with constipation-predominant IBS may have a component of disordered defecation, resulting in part from abnormal function of pelvic floor and anal sphincter muscle
- 40–60% of patients report psychiatric symptoms, such as depression, anxiety, or somatization; these may influence coping skills and illness-associated behaviors
  - A history of abuse (physical, sexual, emotional) has been associated with symptom severity
  - More than half of patients who are seen by a physician report stressful life events coinciding with or preceding the onset of symptoms
- IBS predominantly affects young populations; most patients present before age 45
- A history of stressful life events or a current distress often precedes the development of IBS

PATIENT PRESENTATION

- The hallmark of IBS is poorly localized abdominal pain; pain may occur after a meal, during stress, or during menses
- Altered bowel habits are common, including diarrhea, constipation, or alternating diarrhea and constipation
- Patients frequently report symptoms of other functional gastrointestinal disorders, including heartburn, nausea, dyspepsia, dysphagia, or a sensation of a lump in throat
- Symptoms may wax and wane for life and may be precipitated or exacerbated by stress
- Patients may have extraintestinal symptoms, including headache, sleep disturbances, myalgias, back pain, chronic pelvic pain, and temporomandibular joint pain
- Fibromyalgia occurs in up to one-third of patients

DIFFERENTIAL DX

- Diarrhea-predominant IBS:
- Bacterial overgrowth
- Celiac sprue
- Chronic mesenteric ischemia
- Drug effects
- Hyperthyroidism
- Infectious colitis
- Inflammatory bowel disease
- Lactose intolerance
- Secretory diarrhea
- Constipation-predominant IBS:
- Colon cancer
- Diverticulitis
- Drug effects
- Hypercalcemia
- Hypothyroidism
- Pain as predominant symptom:
- Acute intermittent porphyria
- Biliary colic or PUD

DIAGNOSTIC EVALUATION

- There are no diagnostic markers; all definitions of the disease are based on the clinical presentation
- The Rome II criteria have been designed to create a standardized system for diagnosis, but the utility of these criteria is not yet fully established
  - At least 12 weeks of continuous recurrent abdominal pain that is relieved by defecation, and/or associated with a change in the consistency of stool, and/or associated with a change in the frequency of stool
- Initial laboratory tests include complete blood count, chemistry panel, erythrocyte sedimentation rate, and stool test for occult blood
- Thyroid-stimulating hormone (TSH) is occasionally abnormal, but no studies have demonstrated improvement in symptoms if the abnormal thyroid function is corrected
- Stool testing for ova and parasites is generally of low yield
- Lactose malabsorption, celiac disease, and other malabsorption disorders should be considered in patients with diarrhea-predominant disease
- The presence of any of the following warrants evaluation for organic causes: Age greater than 50, unexplained weight loss, anemia, gastrointestinal bleeding, persistent or progressive symptoms, and family history of colon cancer

TREATMENT & MANAGEMENT

- Diarrhea-predominant IBS is often treated with fiber supplementation, antidiarrheal medications (e.g., Lomotil [atropine and diphenoxylate]), 5-hydroxytryptamine-3 (5-HT$_3$) receptor antagonists (e.g., alosetron), tricyclic antidepressants, and cognitive-behavioral therapy
- Constipation-predominant IBS is often treated with fiber supplementation
- Pain can be treated with anticholinergics, (e.g., dicyclomine, hyoscyamine) tricyclic antidepressants, or selective serotonin reuptake inhibitors (e.g., citalopram)
- Investigational drugs include agents that target visceral hypersensitivity, including 5-HT$_3$ antagonists, 5-HT$_2$ agonists (e.g., buspirone), opioid agonists (e.g., fedotozine), and alpha$_2$-adrenergic agonists (e.g., clonidine)

PROGNOSIS & COMPLICATIONS

- Patients should be assured that they do not have an increased risk of developing organic pathology (e.g., cancer)
- Symptoms are chronic and relapsing-remitting
- Life expectancy is similar to that of general population
- Symptoms tend to be stable; if new symptoms develop, a thorough workup should be done to evaluate for other diseases

Gastroesophageal Reflux Disease

- Gastroesophageal reflux disease (GERD) and associated esophagitis are important clinical disorders for 2 primary reasons: First, they are quite common (10–20% prevalence of GERD in Western countries; 7% of Americans experience GERD symptoms daily); second, they are often mistaken for life-threatening conditions (e.g., myocardial infarction, aortic aneurysm)
- Untreated GERD can result in Barrett's esophagus, strictures, recurrent pneumonitis, asthma, posterior laryngitis, chronic hoarseness, and laryngeal cancer
  - Patients with Barrett's esophagus have a 30-fold increased rate of adenocarcinoma
- GERD should be considered as an underlying etiology for chronic symptoms such as cough, hoarseness, difficulty sleeping, or chest pain

ETIOLOGY, EPIDEMIOLOGY, & RISK FACTORS

- Causes include motility defects (e.g., lower esophageal sphincter dysfunction, esophageal dysmotility), anatomic factors (e.g., hiatal hernia), mucosal factors (e.g., decreased mucosal gland output, decreased bicarbonate secretion, decreased saliva), noxious factors (e.g., severe hyperchlorhydria, duodenal bile acid reflux), and mucosal hypersensitivity (known as nonerosive reflux disease [NERD], which implies symptoms of GERD in the absence of esophagitis)
- The most common cause of GERD is dysfunction of the lower esophageal sphincter, which can be exacerbated by alcohol, caffeine, tobacco, fatty foods, pregnancy, chocolate, hiatal hernia, medications (e.g., anticholinergics, calcium channel blockers, theophylline, nitrates, meperidine, NSAIDs), prolonged gastric emptying (e.g., diabetes), and scleroderma
- In the general population, up to 40% of adults report reflux symptoms monthly, up to 20% report weekly symptoms, and up to 7% report daily symptoms
  - Up to 85% of asthmatic patients have symptoms of GERD
- Barrett's esophagus may occur over time secondary to chronic inflammation of the esophageal mucosa, resulting in replacement of squamous epithelium with precancerous intestinal columnar epithelium; 10–20% of GERD patients have evidence of Barrett's esophagus on esophagogastroduodenoscopy (EGD)

PATIENT PRESENTATION

- Burning, subxiphoid pain ("heartburn")
  - May radiate to back
  - Usually occurs 10–30 minutes after ingesting specific foods
  - Relieved by antacids or resolves spontaneously
  - Worsened by cough, bending, lifting, or laying down
- GERD is one of the most common causes of chronic cough
- Hoarseness may be a symptom of GERD, or it may herald a malignancy (e.g., lung cancer, laryngeal cancer)
- Regurgitation, hypersalivation, belching, and acid taste in mouth may occur
- GERD may mimic a cardiac syndrome (GERD is the most common cause of noncardiac chest pain)
- Atypical presentations include asthma, sinusitis, dental erosions, hoarseness, chronic cough, and otitis media

DIFFERENTIAL DX

- Esophageal disorders: Barrett's esophagus, peptic ulcer, pill esophagitis, acid brash, infectious esophagitis, stricture, esophageal malignancy, foreign body, dysmotility, scleroderma
- Laryngeal disorders: Vocal polyps, laryngopharyngeal reflux disease, hyperfunctional voice disorder, spasmodic dysphonia
- Atypical chest pain: Angina, myocardial infarction, diffuse esophageal spasm, pulmonary embolism
- Epigastric pain: Cholelithiasis or choledocholithiasis, hepatitis, acute pancreatitis, peptic ulcer disease, gastritis, pyelonephritis, mesenteric ischemia

DIAGNOSTIC EVALUATION

- Complete history and physical examination to identify risk factors, "red flag" symptoms, and evidence of extraesophageal manifestations
  - Rule out cardiac ischemia in appropriate patients
- A therapeutic trial of proton pump inhibitors can be diagnostic: The patient is administered a 2-week course of medications; if the pain resolves, GERD is the likely diagnosis
  - Has a sensitivity of 75% and a specificity of 80% if there is a 50% reduction in symptoms
- 24-hour pH monitoring can be used to measure the frequency and duration of acid reflux episodes, and it correlates esophageal pH to symptom onset
  - Indicated for diagnosis of atypical GERD, to document treatment failures, or to evaluate unsatisfactory response to a therapeutic trial
- Esophageal manometry is sometimes used but has low sensitivity for diagnosing GERD
  - It may be useful as a diagnostic test for achalasia or diffuse esophageal spasm
  - It may be useful to demonstrate normal esophageal motility, which is a necessary prerequisite for the fundoplication procedure
- Endoscopy (esophagogastroduodenoscopy [EGD]) is indicated for patients with severe or persistent GERD symptoms and in patients with Barrett's esophagus to monitor for progression to adenocarcinoma
- Swallowing study has low sensitivity for GERD (60%) but may be indicated if suspect aspiration during swallowing, strictures, webs, or diverticuli

TREATMENT & MANAGEMENT

- Lifestyle modifications are the initial therapy for mild disease (despite scant evidence of efficacy): Weight loss, dietary changes to eliminate predisposing foods (e.g., caffeinated drinks, carbonated drinks, fried and fatty foods, spicy foods, citrus fruits, tomatoes, onions, peppermint, chocolate), avoidance of alcohol and tobacco, avoidance of food within 4 hours of bedtime, and sleeping with the head of bed elevated (extra pillows are not sufficient)
  - Adjust the bed so the esophagus is higher than the stomach: Insert a firm foam wedge to raise the head of the mattress by 6-8 inches, or place blocks under the legs at the head of the bed; however, do not sleep on several pillows as it may increase intra-abdominal pressure and worsen the reflux
- Antiulcer or antacid medications are the mainstay of medical therapy
  - H2 receptor blockers are first-line therapy in mild disease
  - Proton pump inhibitors are used for more advanced disease; however, these can take 7-14 days until they become effective; should be continued indefinitely if the patient is found to have grade 2 or worse esophagitis by esophagogastroduodenoscopy (EGD)
- Antireflux surgery (laparoscopic or open fundoplication) provides a definitive treatment
  - Indications for surgery include presence of GERD complications (e.g., stricture), persistence of symptoms despite maximal medical therapy, and for patients who wish to avoid lifelong medical therapy
  - A motility study is indicated (surgery may lead to dysphagia if motility is abnormal)

PROGNOSIS & COMPLICATIONS

- The severity of symptoms does not necessarily correlate with degree of esophageal injury
- Proton pump inhibitor therapy heals more than 80% of cases of severe reflux; H2 receptor antagonists heal about 60% of cases
- A single endoscopy at age 50 for patients on continuous medical therapy for GERD is currently recommended; if Barrett's esophagus is not found, no further screening is currently recommended; the frequency of recommended follow-up for cases of Barrett's esophagus depends on the severity of the mucosal abnormalities
- "Red flag" symptoms that indicate a need for early endoscopy: Nausea/vomiting, heme-positive stools, weight loss, anemia, anorexia, dysphagia or odynophagia, long duration or new onset of symptoms (especially if older than 45 years), and noncardiac chest pain

Inflammatory Bowel Disease

INTRODUCTION

- Inflammatory bowel disease refers to Crohn's disease (CD) and ulcerative colitis (UC)
- Crohn's disease is a chronic, idiopathic disorder of the gastrointestinal tract characterized by transmural inflammation; it can affect almost any portion of the GI tract from mouth to anus (ileocolonic involvement is most common, followed by small bowel and colon)
- Ulcerative colitis is characterized by superficial inflammation of the colon that extends in a contiguous fashion beginning at the anal verge to involve all or part of the colon; the extent of disease is defined as: pancolitis (involves entire colon), extensive disease (extends beyond splenic flexure but not entire colon), left-sided disease (extends proximal to sigmoid but not beyond the splenic flexure), and proctitis or proctosigmoiditis

ETIOLOGY, EPIDEMIOLOGY, & RISK FACTORS

- The inflammatory processes of both Crohn's disease and ulcerative colitis are likely the result of a complex interaction of genetic susceptibility and numerous environmental influences
- Both disorders primarily affect persons in North America and Europe
- The incidence of ulcerative colitis has been stable, while that of Crohn's disease has increased 6-fold; both diseases have the greatest incidence in adolescents and young adults and a second, smaller peak between the fifth and eighth decades of life
- Males and females are affected equally in both diseases
- Common risk factors include Ashkenazi Jewish heritage, living in an urban area, living in northern climates, and higher socioeconomic class
- Smoking appears to be protective for ulcerative colitis but a risk factor for Crohn's disease (smokers are more than twice as likely to develop Crohn's disease compared with non-smokers)

PATIENT PRESENTATION

- Both diseases can present with weight loss, anorexia, fever, fatigue, and diarrhea
- Crohn's disease typically presents with right lower quadrant abdominal pain, while ulcerative colitis presents with cramping abdominal pain, tenesmus, or urgency
- Hematochezia occurs in ulcerative colitis
- The presence of intra-abdominal abscesses and perianal disease (e.g., perirectal abscess, anal fissure, perianal fistula, painful hemorrhoids) are invariably seen in Crohn's disease
- Extraintestinal manifestations that can occur during active inflammatory bowel disease include episcleritis, erythema nodosum, pyoderma gangrenosum, and reactive arthropathy of large joints; other extraintestinal manifestations that are generally not correlated with disease activity include sacroiliitis, scleritis, uveitis, and primary sclerosing cholangitis

DIFFERENTIAL DX

- Malabsorption syndromes (e.g., celiac sprue, microscopic colitis, ischemic colitis)
- Rectal bleeding (e.g., hemorrhoids, anal fissure)
- Neoplasm
- Colonic diverticuli
- Arteriovenous malformation
- Infections (*Clostridium difficile* colitis, *Salmonella*, *Shigella*, *E. coli*, *Campylobacter*, *Yersinia*, herpes simplex virus, *Cryptosporidium*, *Isospora*, cytomegalovirus)
- Colonic ischemia
- Radiation proctitis

DIAGNOSTIC EVALUATION

- History and physical examination, with attention to family history, tobacco use, recent travel, and sick contacts
- Laboratory testing includes complete blood count with differential, liver function tests, C-reactive protein, erythrocyte sedimentation rate, and albumin level
- Send stools for fecal leukocytes, *C. difficile* toxin, *Giardia* antigen, ova and parasites (O&P), and stool culture; if malabsorption is suspected, stool can also be sent for qualitative fecal fat (Sudan stain)
- Colonoscopy is helpful in diagnosing and determining the extent and severity of disease
- Contrast radiography of the small bowel is recommended to confirm the diagnosis of Crohn's disease and determine the extent and severity of disease
  - Contrast radiography has limited usefulness in the diagnosis of ulcerative colitis given the availability of flexible sigmoidoscopy and colonoscopy, which are more sensitive for detecting the disease
- Abdominal and pelvic CT scans can be helpful in evaluating for the presence of abscesses in Crohn's disease
- Capsule endoscopy has better sensitivity in detecting small bowel pathology compared with contrast radiography and may be helpful in the diagnosis of Crohn's disease
- Testing for P-ANCA and anti-*Saccharomyces cerevisiae* antibodies may be helpful in delineating Crohn's disease from ulcerative colitis

TREATMENT & MANAGEMENT

Crohn's disease
- Active disease is treated with oral mesalamine, sulfasalazine, or metronidazole
- Patients with moderate-to-severe disease or disease that is unresponsive to the above therapies can be treated with prednisone, budesonide, or infliximab
- Patients with severe, fulminant disease require hospitalization and treatment with IV hydrocortisone
- If abscesses are present, percutaneous or surgical drainage and IV antibiotics are indicated
- If intestinal obstruction occurs, surgical intervention is indicated
- Fistula formation may require surgical intervention
- Remission can be maintained with Imuran, 6-mercaptopurine, infliximab, or methotrexate; in addition, these agents are useful in disease that is refractory to steroids or for steroid-sparing therapy

Ulcerative colitis
- Mild-to-moderate left-sided colitis and proctosigmoiditis can be treated with mesalamine or hydrocortisone enemas or mesalamine suppository
  - Combinations of oral and topical mesalamines are most effective
- Corticosteroids should not be used as maintenance therapy in either disease
- Colectomy may be indicated for toxic megacolon or severe refractory disease

PROGNOSIS & COMPLICATIONS

- Crohn's disease has a high recurrence rate
- Complications of Crohn's disease include perforation, abscess, obstruction, fistula (to the bowel, bladder, or vagina), perianal fissures or abscesses, malabsorption syndromes, and cancers of the colon and small bowel
- Risk of colon cancer in ulcerative colitis becomes significant after 10 years
- Complications of ulcerative colitis include colorectal cancer, perforation, toxic megacolon, and obstruction; surgical complications can occur following colectomy
- Involvement of other organ systems occurs in 10% of patients, including skin (erythema nodosum), bones (osteoporosis), joints (enteropathic arthropathy), eyes (uveitis, iritis), liver (cholelithiasis, primary sclerosing cholangitis, pancreatitis), and lung (pulmonary embolus)

Chronic Abdominal Pain

INTRODUCTION

- Chronic abdominal pain is a common disorder that affects millions of Americans
- Pain can be continuous, intermittent, or recurrent, and may last longer than 3-6 months
- Diagnosis and treatment can be difficult, often resulting in unnecessary surgeries
- Complications from investigations and treatments can also lead to chronic pain
- Thoughtful workups, good physician-patient relationship, and defined, realistic expectations often lead to the best outcomes
- This chapter focuses on chronic abdominal pain without a known etiology, and although the underlying causes are vast, a select few will be discussed in detail

ETIOLOGY, EPIDEMIOLOGY, & RISK FACTORS

- The abdominal pain can be categorized into neurogenic, visceral, and psychiatric causes
- Neurogenic pain: Functional abdominal pain is multidimensional and involves psychological, genetic, and environmental factors; it can be thought of as dysregulation of the central nervous system and enteric nervous system, rather than dysmotility or visceral disease
  - Irritable bowel syndrome and abdominal migraine can also fit here
  - Referred pain: Pathology at different site (e.g., pelvic or back pain, radiculopathy, etc.)
- Visceral pain is related to direct disease or injury of the GI tract and encompasses a vast differential of which the key entities are listed below and in the *Differential Dx* section:
  - Peptic ulcer disease, GERD/gastritis, chronic infections, food allergy, lactose intolerance
  - Diabetes, cystic fibrosis, hypothyroidism, narcotic use or chronic laxative abuse can lead to gastroparesis, dysmotility, or constipation
  - Colon and gallbladder cancers; family history and obesity are risk factors
  - Atherosclerotic disease predisposes to mesenteric ischemia and intestinal angina
  - Abdominal wall: Trauma, fibromyalgia, painful rib syndrome, hernia (ventral, umbilical)
  - Some patients may have had an initial cause of pain that was investigated invasively, which may lead to chronic pain (e.g., scarring, adhesions, chronic pain syndrome)
- Psychiatric disease (e.g., somatization, malingering, Munchausen syndrome, depression)

PATIENT PRESENTATION

- Functional abdominal pain presents with years duration of generalized pain and is not influenced be eating or bowel movements
- Dull or cramping pain starting shortly after meals and lasting for hours is suggestive of chronic mesenteric ischemia/intestinal angina, gallbladder disease (usually right upper quadrant to flank or back), pancreatitis (usually right or left upper quadrant or back) and IBS (usually left side).
- Lactose intolerance can present as "gas" pain, dull ache, or bloating following eating and may persist intermittently throughout the day
- Chronic narcotic use may lead to constipation and pain
- Chronic pancreatitis is characterized by mid-epigastric pain radiating to back, nausea/vomiting
- Porphyria can be triggered by medications such as antibiotics (sulfonamide), anticonvulsants, and barbiturates

DIFFERENTIAL DX

- See etiology section above
- Medications (vast list)
- Inflammatory bowel disease
- Pancreatitis
- Gallstones
- Hiatal hernia
- Hepatitis
- Extra-abdominal causes:
  - Pelvic (e.g., ovarian cancer, endometriosis)
  - Musculoskeletal (e.g., vertebral nerve compression, costochondritis)
  - Cardiopulmonary etiologies (e.g., asthma, angina, mesenteric ischemia)
- Metabolic (porphyria, chronic renal failure, Addison's disease)
- Idiopathic

DIAGNOSTIC EVALUATION

- Complete history and physical examination
  - Note pain intensity, character, duration, location, exacerbating and relieving factors
- Note associated weight loss, change in stool pattern or caliber
- Include family history, travel history, psychosocial history, medication use, and alternative medicine or herbal remedies
- All females require a pelvic exam
  - Laboratory studies may include complete blood count, chemistries, liver function tests, erythrocyte sedimentation rate, thyroid studies, and stool occult blood testing
- A kidney-ureter-bladder X-ray may be useful
- Consider abdominal and pelvic CT scan with contrast (if renal function permits) and/or colonoscopy (especially in patients older than 50)
- Consider stool examination for ova and parasites
- Further testing and subspecialist referral may be indicated depending on the presumed etiology

TREATMENT & MANAGEMENT

- Treat the underlying cause, if identified
- Eliminate offending agents (e.g. medications, foods, etc.)
- Intractable cases may require a multidisciplinary approach, including gastroenterology, gynecology, pain specialists, and social workers
- Chronic narcotic use should be avoided to reduce impaired gastrointestinal motility and risk of addiction
- Tricyclic antidepressants and selective serotonin reuptake inhibitors (SSRIs) may improve function abdominal pain
- Mental health referral may be helpful
- Biofeedback and meditation may be helpful in reducing pain
- A cure may not be possible in all cases (e.g., metastatic cancers), but palliation should be sought; this may include pain-relieving surgery, analgesics, antidepressants, antiemetics, anxiolytics, meditation, and biofeedback

PROGNOSIS & COMPLICATIONS

- Complete resolution of functional abdominal pain is often difficult, but most patients can find improved quality of life; unfortunately, many end up with unnecessary surgeries and subsequent complications, such as abdominal adhesions
- Complications and prognosis are based on underlying problem and treatments

Cirrhosis

INTRODUCTION

- Cirrhosis is the end result of prolonged hepatocellular injury, resulting in irreversible destruction, fibrosis, and nodular regeneration of the liver
- This results in abnormal synthetic function of the liver cells, as well as abnormal metabolism of numerous enzymes, drugs, and hormones
- The prognosis is highly variable and does not necessarily correlate with the degree of histologic findings
- Complications of cirrhosis are numerous, including liver failure, encephalopathy, massive gastrointestinal bleeding, renal failure (hepatorenal syndrome), ascites, spontaneous bacterial peritonitis, hepatocellular carcinoma, and others

ETIOLOGY, EPIDEMIOLOGY, & RISK FACTORS

- Most cases are due to chronic alcohol abuse or viral hepatitis; however, any chronic liver disease (e.g., Wilson's disease, hemochromatosis, medications, primary sclerosing cholangitis) or massive acute injury (e.g., drug overdose) may result in cirrhosis
  - Most cases in the United States are due to chronic alcohol abuse and hepatitis C
  - Worldwide, the most common cause is schistosomiasis
  - Other etiologies include autoimmune hepatitis, primary or secondary biliary cirrhosis, primary sclerosing cholangitis, Wilson's disease, alpha$_1$-antitrypsin deficiency, granulomatous diseases (e.g., sarcoidosis), hemochromatosis, drug-induced (e.g., methotrexate), nonalcoholic steatohepatitis (NASH), and cystic fibrosis
- The clinical features and complications of cirrhosis result from hepatic cell dysfunction (e.g., decreased production of clotting factors and albumin), portal hypertension and portosystemic shunting (e.g., esophageal varices, splenomegaly, caput medusae), decreased metabolism of toxic substances (e.g., ammonia, which can result in hyperammonemia and hepatic encephalopathy), and destruction of bile flow (e.g., resulting in cholestasis, jaundice, elevated alkaline phosphatase)
- Cirrhosis is the 9th leading cause of death in the United States, accounting for about 30,000 deaths per year

PATIENT PRESENTATION

- The presentation is highly variable, ranging from an insidious onset of vague symptoms (e.g., fatigue, weakness, malaise, abdominal discomfort, weight loss, anorexia, nausea) to decompensated cirrhosis with coagulopathy, renal failure, hepatic encephalopathy, GI bleeding, or even sepsis
- Firm, nodular liver may be present
- Often, the presentations are the complications of cirrhosis:
  - Signs of liver failure include jaundice, spider angiomas, palmer erythema, gynecomastia, testicular atrophy, bruising, and hypocoagulation
  - Signs of portal hypertension include ascites (abdominal distension, dyspnea), esophageal varices (i.e., gastrointestinal bleeding), hepatosplenomegaly, and caput medusae
  - Signs of hepatic encephalopathy include lethargy, confusion, asterixis (flapping of hands when held out and flexed at the wrist), and coma

DIFFERENTIAL DX

- Primary biliary cirrhosis
- Secondary biliary cirrhosis
- Noncirrhotic hepatic fibrosis (due to congestive heart failure or constrictive pericarditis)
- Budd-Chiari syndrome (hepatic vein thrombosis)
- Congenital hepatic fibrosis
- Partial nodular transformation
- Portal vein thrombosis (e.g., post pancreatitis)

DIAGNOSTIC EVALUATION

- Complete history and physical examination
  - History is a key factor in diagnosis, with emphasis on alcohol use, exposure to drugs and toxins, viral infections, blood transfusions, risk factors for hepatitis, and family history
  - Physical examination should pay attention to skin abnormalities (e.g., spider angiomas, caput medusa), abdomen (e.g., ascites, hepatosplenomegaly), and breast or testicular exam (gynecomastia and small testes may occur in males)
- Initial laboratory testing is indicated to measure hepatic synthetic and enzymatic function, which includes complete blood count (may show thrombocytopenia due to spleen sequestration and portal hypertension), complete metabolic panel including liver function tests (often normal in late cirrhosis or mildly elevated in early cirrhosis), coagulation studies (often elevated), hepatitis panel, and albumin level (often decreased)
- Abdominal ultrasound and CT scan can provide evidence of abnormal liver architecture, ductal dilatation, hepatocellular carcinoma, and other abdominal pathology
- The gold standard for diagnosis is a liver biopsy; however, biopsy may not be necessary if clinical, laboratory, and radiologic evidence supports a diagnosis of cirrhosis
  - A biopsy may also shed light on the cause of cirrhosis (e.g., Wilson's disease, alpha$_1$-antitrypsin deficiency, hemochromatosis, NASH)
- Further testing as necessary (e.g., upper GI endoscopy if suspect esophageal varices, copper levels if suspect Wilson's disease)

TREATMENT & MANAGEMENT

- The goal of treatment is to remove or alleviate the underlying etiology, prevent further liver damage, prevent complications, and assess the appropriateness of liver transplantation
- Outpatient care with close follow-up is generally adequate, except for those who develop complications (e.g., variceal bleeding, encephalopathy, peritonitis, hepatorenal syndrome)
  - Variceal bleeding requires endoscopy to visualize and band the varices; in addition, prophylactic therapy to reduce portal hypertension with a beta-blocker can be effective
  - Hepatic encephalopathy is treated by avoidance of triggers (e.g., infections, dehydration, constipation, excess protein intake, narcotics, benzodiazepines) and lactulose (with or without neomycin) to decrease the ammonia level; surgical shunting may be necessary for advanced cases
  - Spontaneous bacterial peritonitis is an infection of ascitic fluid that is treated with IV antibiotics and paracentesis to remove the ascites; prophylactic oral antibiotic therapy may reduce the risk of future events
  - Hepatorenal syndrome is a feared consequence of ongoing cirrhosis; the only definitive treatment is liver transplantation
- Strict diet adherence is important: Avoid alcohol consumption; consume less than 2 grams per day of sodium to minimize ascites; consume minimal protein to avoid encephalopathy; and restrict fluid (1–1.5 L/d) to reduce the risk of hyponatremia
- Vaccinate against hepatitis A and B

PROGNOSIS & COMPLICATIONS

- The Child-Turcotte-Pugh classification is used to assess hepatic functional reserve: A score greater than 10 suggests a 50% mortality risk within 1 year

Variable	1 point	2 points	3 points
Total bilirubin	<2.0	2.0–3.0	>3.0
Albumin	>3.5	2.8–3.5	<2.8
Ascites	None	Controlled	Severe
Encephalopathy	None	Minimal	Coma
Prothrombin time	<4 sec	4–6 sec	>6 sec

Hemorrhoids

INTRODUCTION

- Hemorrhoids result from engorgement of the venous plexus of the rectum and anus
- Hemorrhoids become symptomatic when venous pressure is increased; over time, redundancy and enlargement of venous cushions occur, leading to hemorrhoidal bleeding or protrusion
- The dentate line defines the junction of the rectum (columnar epithelium) with the anus (squamous epithelium)
  - External hemorrhoids occur below the dentate line
- Internal hemorrhoids occur above the dentate line

ETIOLOGY, EPIDEMIOLOGY, & RISK FACTORS

- Increased hydrostatic pressure in the portal venous system leads to distention and engorgement of veins
- External hemorrhoids, when enlarged, can easily thrombose; the thrombus is usually at the level of sphincteric muscles, which often results in anal spasm
- As internal hemorrhoids enlarge, prolapse can occur through the anal canal, accompanied by edema and sphincter spasm
- Risk factors include constipation (e.g., low-fiber diet), straining with defecation, portal hypertension (e.g., cirrhosis), pregnancy, obesity, and sitting for long periods of time
- Internal hemorrhoids are classified by the degree of prolapse
  - First-degree hemorrhoids do not prolapse
  - Second-degree hemorrhoids prolapse with defecation but spontaneously reduce
  - Third-degree hemorrhoids are prolapsed and require manual reduction
  - Fourth-degree hemorrhoids are chronically prolapsed and cannot be reduced

PATIENT PRESENTATION

- Location of hemorrhoids (hemorrhoid quadrants) occur in the right anterolateral quadrant of the anus, the right posterolateral quadrant, and the left lateral quadrant
- Anal mass
- Bleeding (streaks of blood on toilet paper or bright red blood in toilet)
- Itching
- Internal hemorrhoids are usually painless, unless thrombosis occurs
- External hemorrhoids are typically painful
- Sudden onset of excruciating perirectal pain with a palpable mass usually suggests acute thrombosis of a hemorrhoid, which may appear as a tense, bluish, perianal, skin-covered nodule

DIFFERENTIAL DX

- Colorectal cancer
- Skin tag
- Rectal prolapse
- Perirectal abscess
- Anal fistula
- Ulcerative colitis
- Crohn's colitis
- Infectious proctitis
- Diverticular disease
- Papilloma (warts)
- Condyloma acuminatum (syphilis)

DIAGNOSTIC EVALUATION

- History and physical examination
  - Perianal exam will directly reveal external hemorrhoids; nonprolapsed internal hemorrhoids are not visible but may protrude through anus with gentle straining while the physician spreads the buttocks; prolapsed hemorrhoids appear as protuberant purple nodules covered by mucosa
  - The perianal region should also be inspected for fistulas, fissures, skin tags, and dermatitis
  - On digital exam, uncomplicated internal hemorrhoids will not be palpable or painful; pain on rectal exam implies proctitis and/or complicated hemorrhoidal disease
- Anoscopy, proctoscopy, or sigmoidoscopy provides optimal visualization of hemorrhoids
  - The colon mucosa should be well evaluated to rule out colitis and other mucosal diseases

TREATMENT & MANAGEMENT

- Treatment is initially conservative: High-fiber diet, stool softeners, appropriate anal hygiene, warm sitz baths, and topical steroids
- Surgical options may be indicated for internal hemorrhoids or large, refractory external hemorrhoids
  - Asymptomatic internal hemorrhoids should be left alone
  - Symptomatic hemorrhoids that do not respond to conservative treatment may be treated in an outpatient physician office by injuring the proximal mucosa with infrared coagulation or bipolar cautery, which causes fixation of the hemorrhoidal tissue to underlying connective tissue and reduces the blood supply
  - Third-degree hemorrhoids can be treated surgically with rubber band ligation
  - Fourth-degree hemorrhoids are treated with surgical excision
- Acute thrombosis of a hemorrhoid may require surgical drainage

PROGNOSIS & COMPLICATIONS

- Only 4% of cases are symptomatic
- Most cases respond to medical treatment
- Complications include thrombosis of hemorrhoid, infection, erosion of the overlying tissue, incontinence or sphincter incompetence, pelvic sepsis syndrome following band ligation (rare), or anemia due to chronic or profuse blood loss (rare)

Hepatitis

INTRODUCTION

- Inflammation of the liver can be caused by a multitude of etiologies, including infections (e.g., viral hepatitis), autoimmune disease, toxins (e.g., alcohol, *Amanita* mushrooms), ischemia (e.g., "shock" liver), and medications (e.g., isoniazid, methyldopa, ketoconazole, acetaminophen)
- Alcoholic and viral hepatitis are the most common causes in the United States
- Damage may be due to direct toxic effects, infiltration, or cholestasis
- Most cases are self-limited and relatively benign, but syndromes range from asymptomatic infection to fulminant hepatic failure (rapid deterioration of liver function within days) and may cause chronic infection that results in cirrhosis

ETIOLOGY, EPIDEMIOLOGY, & RISK FACTORS

- Drugs are among the most common etiologies, including drugs that act as direct hepatotoxins (acetaminophen, nevirapine), drugs that cause idiosyncratic reactions (isoniazid, NSAIDs, nitrofurantoin), drugs that cause allergic reactions (phenytoin, amoxicillin-clavulanate), drugs that cause cholestatic reactions (estrogens, rifampin, trimethoprim-sulfamethoxazole), drugs that cause a granulomatous reaction (methyldopa, sulfonamides), and drugs that cause microvesicular steatosis (tetracycline, nucleoside antiretrovirals)
- Viral hepatitis may be caused by the hepatitis viruses, Epstein-Barr virus, herpes simplex virus, cytomegalovirus, and others
  - Hepatitis A (HAV): Self-limited, rarely fatal, rarely result in chronic disease; fecal-oral transmission; common in children (day care) and developing countries
  - Hepatitis B (HBV): May result in cirrhosis or a chronic carrier state; transmitted parenterally (e.g., IV drug use, blood transfusions prior to screening) or by sexual contact
  - Hepatitis C (HCV): Mild acute disease, but up to 80% of patients will develop chronic disease and possible liver failure; spread parenterally (e.g., IV drug use, transfusion)
  - Hepatitis D (HDV): Requires coinfection with hepatitis B; results in fulminant liver failure
  - Hepatitis E (HEV): Requires coinfection with hepatitis C virus; generally self-limited, but infection may be severe in pregnancy

PATIENT PRESENTATION

- Acute hepatitis: Jaundice, hepatomegaly, fatigue, malaise, lethargy, right upper quadrant pain, nausea, vomiting, fever, and dark urine with light stools
- Patients with liver failure may present with ascites and peripheral edema due to hypoalbuminemia, hepatic encephalopathy (e.g., confusion, stupor, coma, rigidity, asterixis), and bleeding due to coagulation abnormalities
- Many patients are asymptomatic and are discovered by detection of transaminase elevations during routine laboratory studies

DIFFERENTIAL DX

- Fulminant hepatic failure
  - Viral hepatitis
  - Toxins (e.g., acetaminophen)
  - Vascular (portal vein thrombosis, Budd-Chiari)
  - Metabolic (Wilson's disease, pregnancy, Reye's syndrome)
  - Sepsis
  - Autoimmune hepatitis
- Alcoholic hepatitis
- Cholecystitis or cholangitis
- Nonalcoholic steatohepatitis
- Malignancy (hepatocellular carcinoma, lymphoma, liver metastases)
- Infections (HIV, tuberculosis, toxoplasmosis, leptospirosis, mononucleosis, measles, rubella, cytomegalovirus, malaria)

DIAGNOSTIC EVALUATION

- Thorough history and physical examination, including medications (prescribed medications, over-the-counter drugs, and herbal formulations); alcohol and drug use; medical history of autoimmune disease, malignancy, or inherited illnesses; and travel history
- Liver function tests (ALT, AST, direct and indirect bilirubin) are all elevated, with less significant elevation of alkaline phosphatase; check albumin level to assess synthetic function
- Coagulation studies are usually normal
  - Increased International Normalized Ratio (INR) may reflect severe liver damage and may indicate need for transplantation
- Ultrasound of the liver and biliary tree is indicated to rule out biliary obstruction
- Specific serologies for hepatitis viruses
  - Anti-HAV IgM reflects acute infection, IgG reflects past infection or vaccination
  - Hepatitis B surface antigens and anti-HBV core antigen IgM indicate acute infection; the presence of HBV e antigen (HBeAg) indicates active viral replication and infectivity, anti-HBeAg implies a more favorable prognosis, and HBsAb indicates past infection or vaccination
  - Anti-HCV, possibly with HCV viral load, if there is suspicion for hepatitis C infection
- Serologies for cytomegalovirus, Epstein-Barr virus, herpes simplex virus, and varicella-zoster virus in immunocompromised patients or when clinically indicated
- Antimitochondrial antibodies (AMA), anti-smooth muscle antibodies (ASMA), antinuclear antibodies (ANA), and ceruloplasmin if suspect noninfectious etiology

TREATMENT & MANAGEMENT

- Avoid causative drugs and toxins, and abstain from alcohol
- Indications for hospitalization include inability to tolerate oral intake, prolonged prothrombin time (PT) prolonged by > 3 seconds, absence of social support, or encephalopathy
- Supportive management includes intravenous fluids and electrolyte management
- Hepatotoxins should be strictly avoided, particularly alcohol and acetaminophen
- Monitor nutrition status and serum glucose; administer dextrose-containing solutions to maintain euglycemia
- Administer vitamin K to correct coagulation abnormalities if INR is elevated
- Encephalopathy and coagulopathy require immediate consultation with a gastroenterologist and consideration for liver transplantation
- Consider specific therapies for prophylaxis or acute infection:
  - Anti-HAV immunoglobulin for pre- and postexposure prophylaxis
  - Anti-HBV immunoglobulin for postexposure prophylaxis
  - Interferon-alfa with or without ribavirin for acute hepatitis C infection is investigational
- Consider specific therapies for chronic infections:
  - HBV: Lamivudine, interferon-alfa, interferon-gamma, adefovir, and entecavir
  - HCV: Pegylated interferon-alfa and ribavirin
- All patients with chronic HBV infection require vaccination for HAV
- All patients with chronic HCV infection require vaccination for HAV and HBV

PROGNOSIS & COMPLICATIONS

- Admit patients with any clinical or metabolic derangements (e.g., persistent nausea/vomiting, encephalopathy, renal failure, electrolyte disturbances) and patients who are pregnant or immunocompromised
- All patients with unexplained liver function test elevations must be evaluated by gastroenterology
- Chronic inflammation eventually scars the liver, producing cirrhosis with cellular dysfunction, portal hypertension, and portosystemic shunting of blood (see *Cirrhosis* entry)
- In patients who present with fulminant hepatic failure, the only therapy shown to improve outcome is liver transplantation

Peptic Ulcer Disease

INTRODUCTION

- The natural history of peptic ulcer disease (PUD) ranges from a benign course that resolves without intervention to a serious disorder with significant morbidity and mortality if bleeding and perforation occur
- The lifetime risk of developing peptic ulcer disease is 10–15% for persons infected with *Helicobacter pylori*
- Ulcers that occur due to nonsteroid anti-inflammatory drugs (NSAIDs) are more likely to bleed than ulcers that occur due to *H. pylori* infection
- Despite popular theories, personality type, dietary factors, and occupation are not significant factors in the development of peptic ulcer disease

ETIOLOGY, EPIDEMIOLOGY, & RISK FACTORS

- Erosion and ulceration of the gastric or duodenal mucosa occurs secondary to a disrupted balance between acid formation, production of mucous (to coat and protect the mucosa), and bicarbonate production (to buffer the acid) in the stomach
- *H. pylori* infection is the most common cause of peptic ulcer disease
  - *H. pylori* is a urease-producing, gram-negative rod that disrupts the mucosal protective barrier of the stomach
  - May be responsible for as many as 95% of duodenal ulcers and 85% of gastric ulcers
- Other causes of peptic ulcer disease include NSAIDs (they inhibit prostaglandin formation, thereby disrupting bicarbonate and mucous production), gastrin-secreting tumors (e.g., Zollinger-Ellison syndrome, gastrinoma), Crohn's disease of the stomach or duodenum, tobacco, steroid use, stress, family history, renal failure, and COPD
- Peptic ulcer disease accounts for more than $5 billion in health care expenditures yearly
- The complication rate has not been decreasing
- Risks factors for developing peptic ulcer disease or suffering bleeding or perforation include smoking (90% of all perforations occur in smokers), NSAID use, older age (50% of elderly ulcer patients will have a complication as their initial presentation), larger ulcers (because they heal slower), stress ulcers, and alcohol abuse (decreases healing)

PATIENT PRESENTATION

- Dyspepsia (a burning or gnawing epigastric pain) occurs in 80-90% of patients
  - Relieved by food, milk, or antacids
  - Often worse at night
  - Recurrent, rhythmic, or periodic pain
- Epigastric tenderness
- Vomiting, chest or back pain, and bloating may be present (nausea and belching are notably absent)
- Gastrointestinal bleeding may occur, resulting in guaiac-positive stool, melena, hemoptysis, hematochezia, and/or hypotension
- Perforation with peritoneal signs may occur

DIFFERENTIAL DX

- Acute gastritis
- Gastric cancer
- Pancreatitis
- Esophagitis
- Gastroesophageal reflux disease
- Esophageal motility disorder
- Nonulcer dyspepsia
- Biliary colic or cholecystitis
- Hepatitis
- Aortic dissection
- Abdominal aortic aneurysm
- Acute coronary syndrome
- Pneumonia
- Mesenteric ischemia
- Small bowel obstruction
- Pregnancy
- Diabetes mellitus gastroparesis
- Zellinger-Ellison syndrome

DIAGNOSTIC EVALUATION

- Patient evaluation is aimed at ruling out other potential causes of pain
  - Amylase and lipase levels to evaluate for pancreatitis
  - Liver function tests and abdominal ultrasound to evaluate for hepatic and biliary disease
  - Electrocardiogram and serial cardiac enzymes to evaluate for cardiac ischemia
  - Urine human chorionic gonadotropin testing for pregnancy
- Complete blood count may reveal anemia due to chronic blood loss
- Ulcer visualization by endoscopy or barium swallow (upper gastrointestinal X-ray series) is diagnostic, but may miss up to 30% of gastric ulcers
- *H. pylori* testing
  - IgG serology for *H. pylori* should be ordered in patients who were not previously treated for *H. pylori* infection (IgG remains positive even after appropriate therapy; thus, it is not useful in previously treated patients)
  - Previously treated patients require an outpatient urease breath test or endoscopic biopsy to determine whether active *H. pylori* is present
- In the case of gastric ulcers, it is also important to rule out gastric cancer via an endoscopic biopsy

TREATMENT & MANAGEMENT

- Treat *H. pylori*, if present, with triple drug therapy for 10–14 days
  - Bismuth subsalicylate, metronidazole, and tetracycline *or*
  - Ranitidine, tetracycline, and either clarithromycin or metronidazole *or*
  - Omeprazole, clarithromycin, and amoxicillin
- Antibiotic therapy is usually combined with a proton pump inhibitor or H2 receptor blocker to decrease healing time, especially in cases of large ulcers
  - Proton pump inhibitors offer a modest advantage over H2 receptor blockers in efficacy, but their high cost makes H2 blockers an excellent option in patients with limited financial resources
- Avoid aspirin, NSAIDs, and steroids (cyclo-oxygenase-2 inhibitors may be less ulcerogenic); if these medications cannot be avoided (e.g., aspirin for patients with coronary artery disease), administer a proton pump inhibitor
- Sucralfate (a mucosal protective agent that binds to the ulcer and forms a protective barrier against stomach acid) may also be used as an adjunct
- Indications for surgery include intractable bleeding, gastric outlet obstruction, perforation, and Zollinger-Ellison syndrome
- Consider long-term prophylaxis with an H2 receptor blocker or a proton pump inhibitor in patients with refractory disease, complicated disease (e.g., bleeding), and large ulcers (>2 cm)

PROGNOSIS & COMPLICATIONS

- Eradication of *H. pylori* infection decreases the rate of ulcer recurrence from 50-80% to less than 10%
- Patients who will be initiated on long-term NSAID therapy should be tested and treated for *H. pylori* infection
- Complications may include pancreatitis, perforation, gastric outlet obstruction, gastrointestinal bleeding, and gastric cancer
- Red flags that suggest a gastric malignancy include absence of extended ulcer history, no prior use of NSAIDs, very large ulcers (>2–3 cm), and certain ethnic groups raised in endemic areas (e.g., Latinos, Asians)
- Sucralfate may be a good choice for renal patients due to its ability to bind phosphorus

Acute Pancreatitis

INTRODUCTION

- Acute inflammation of the pancreas associated with severe upper abdominal pain and elevated serum pancreatic enzymes
- Disease varies from mild, self-limited illness to severe pancreatitis with multiorgan failure and death
- The diagnosis can be suspected clinically, but definitive diagnosis requires biochemical and radiologic verification given the nonspecific nature of the symptoms; indeed, diagnosis is often made only at autopsy, even in patients with severe disease
- 70–80% of cases of acute pancreatitis are mild; 20% of cases are severe, with systemic complications and mortality of approximately 40%

ETIOLOGY, EPIDEMIOLOGY, & RISK FACTORS

- Gallstones (gallstone pancreatitis) and chronic alcohol abuse (alcoholic pancreatitis) account for 75% of cases in the United States
- Other etiologies include drugs (e.g., azathioprine, NSAIDs, sulfonamides, didanosine, thiazides, valproic acid, and many others), hypercalcemia, hypertriglyceridemia, pregnancy, pancreas divisum, vascular disease, HIV, scorpion bites, genetic mutations (e.g., mutation of the trypsinogen gene), abdominal trauma, following endoscopic retrograde cholangiopancreatography (ERCP), and viruses (e.g., mumps, coxsackievirus, herpes simplex virus, Epstein-Barr virus, cytomegalovirus)
- The pathophysiology is still unclear; the leading theory is that autodigestion of the pancreas occurs secondary to intra-acinar activation of pancreatic enzymes
- In the United States, the incidence is roughly 0.03%
- There is a higher rate in African-Americans and HIV patients
- The etiology in men is often alcohol abuse; in women, the etiology is more likely to be gallstones
- 10% of alcoholics will develop pancreatitis
- Data suggest that a predisposition to pancreatitis may be inherited in an autosomal dominant or recessive fashion; there have also been gene mutations linked with the disease

PATIENT PRESENTATION

- Epigastric pain, generally abrupt in onset
  - Often exacerbated by eating, walking or lying supine
  - Improves upon sitting and leaning forward
  - Often radiates to the back, and may also be felt in the right or left upper quadrants
- Associated symptoms include nausea and vomiting, weakness, diaphoresis, and anxiety
- The abdomen is usually tender in epigastric area; peritoneal signs are usually absent
- Bowel sounds may be absent if a paralytic ileus has developed
- Biliary colic may also be a presenting feature
- Fever, hypotension, tachycardia, jaundice, pallor, clammy skin may occur in severe disease
- A mass (inflamed pancreas or pseudocyst) may be palpable
- Cullen's sign: bluish discoloration (hemorrhage) around the umbilicus
- Grey-Turner sign: bluish discoloration on flanks

DIFFERENTIAL DX

- Perforated viscus (e.g., peptic ulcer disease)
- Gastritis
- Acute cholecystitis
- Acute intestinal obstruction
- Mesenteric vascular occlusion
- Renal colic
- Myocardial infarction
- Aortic dissection
- Aortic abdominal aneurysm
- Connective tissue disorders with vasculitis
- Pneumonia
- Diabetic ketoacidosis
- Ectopic pregnancy

DIAGNOSTIC EVALUATION

- Diagnosis relies on careful clinical assessment in conjunction with laboratory and radiographic studies
- Elevated amylase is a cornerstone of diagnosis if presentation is within hours of onset; if not, an elevated amylase level can be nonspecific
- Elevated lipase has sensitivity of 85–100%, especially if presenting later in the course; however, elevated lipase can also be nonspecific
- In cases of gallstone pancreatitis, liver function tests (especially AST >150 U/dL), alkaline phosphatase, and bilirubin may be elevated
- Leukocytosis is common but nonspecific
- Abdominal X-ray may show gallstones, "sentinel loop" (localized small intestine ileus), "colon cutoff" sign (abrupt termination of gas within the proximal colon), or pleural effusion
- CT scan is the most important test for diagnosis and assessment of complications and severity; however, CT scan is not necessarily indicated in all patients
- MRI scan and magnetic resonance cholangiopancreatography (MRCP) have higher sensitivity than CT scan but are expensive and operator-dependent
- Ultrasound is the most sensitive and specific (100%) test to evaluate the biliary tract
- Endoscopic retrograde cholangiopancreatography (ERCP) may be necessary if gallstones are highly suspected but ultrasound is negative

TREATMENT & MANAGEMENT

- Treatment of mild disease is largely supportive: No oral intake, IV fluids, parenteral analgesia (e.g., morphine)
  - Note: Previous concerns that morphine use might cause sphincter of Oddi spasm have not been validated
- Nasogastric suction is appropriate for patients who have developed an ileus or severe vomiting; however, it does not increase pain relief or decrease the length of hospital stay
- Reverse the inciting agent, if possible (e.g., treat hypercalcemia and hypertriglyceridemia, eliminate drugs and alcohol)
- Severe pancreatitis requires aggressive treatment and may require intensive care unit admission to monitor for cardiopulmonary, renal, or septic complications
  - Aggressive fluid resuscitation; use urine output and cardiac filling pressures to monitor for adequate tissue perfusion
  - If CT scan shows more than 30% necrosis, consider initiating antibiotic therapy with broad-spectrum antibiotics that have adequate pancreatic tissue penetration; imipenem and piperacillin/tazobactam are good initial choices
  - General surgery should be consulted early if pancreatitis requires intensive care unit admission or a pseudocyst or abscess is suspected
- Gallstone pancreatitis may require removal of obstructing gallstones in the common bile duct by endoscopic retrograde cholangiopancreatography (ERCP)

PROGNOSIS & COMPLICATIONS

- Ranson's criteria may be used to estimate mortality risk: Mortality is less than 1% if fewer than 3 criteria are met, but nearly 100% if more than 6 criteria are met
  - Criteria on presentation: Age greater than 55, white blood cell count >16,000, blood glucose >200 mg/dL, serum LDH>350, AST >250
  - Criteria after 48 hours: Hematocrit decreased by >10%, BUN increased by >5 mg/dL, partial arterial pressure of oxygen (PaO_2) <60, fluid deficit >6 L, base deficit >4
- Complications include fat necrosis, pancreatic necrosis, pancreatic abscess or pseudocyst, pancreatic ascites, gastrointestinal hemorrhage, splenic vein thrombosis, acute renal failure, shock, disseminated intravascular coagulation, and acute respiratory distress syndrome

Cardiovascular

Chest Pain

INTRODUCTION

- Chest pain represents one of the most challenging entities encountered in the outpatient setting; although most cases of chest pain are due to benign etiologies, such as mild gastroesophageal reflux or a muscle strain, life-threatening etiologies must be considered and treated immediately, if present
- The goal of the physician in the outpatient setting is to quickly and accurately separate the emergent cases from the rest, urgently seeking care for serious etiologies and minimizing unnecessary testing and hospitalization for benign etiologies

ETIOLOGY, EPIDEMIOLOGY, & RISK FACTORS

- There are 5 primary etiologies of acute, life-threatening chest pain: Aortic dissection, myocardial infarction, esophageal rupture, tension pneumothorax, and pulmonary embolism (PE)
- Certain risk factors help to evaluate the etiology of chest pain:
  - Coronary artery disease: Tobacco use, hyperlipidemia, hypertension, family history of premature coronary artery disease, history of cocaine use, older age
  - Aortic dissection: Hypertension, history of vasculitis, collagen vascular diseases, recent cardiac surgery
  - Pericarditis: Recent infection or myocardial infarction, trauma, cardiac surgery, medications (especially isoniazid, hydralazine, or procainamide), history of radiation exposure

PATIENT PRESENTATION

- Coronary artery disease: Chest discomfort that is exacerbated by physical or emotional stress and relieved by rest; it lasts up to 20 minutes and may radiate to the shoulder, neck, jaw, or arm; may be associated with diaphoresis, palpitations, dyspnea, nausea, and vomiting
- Aortic dissection: Severe, "tearing" chest pain
- Pericarditis: Sudden onset of anterior chest pain that increases upon inspiration and is relieved by sitting upright and leaning forward
- GERD: Squeezing or burning chest pain ("heartburn") that lasts minutes to hours; may be associated with burning in the throat and dyspepsia
- Musculoskeletal: Localized, sharp pain that is worse with changes in position, palpation, and/or movements of arm
- Pneumonia: Fever, chills, cough, dyspnea
- Zoster: Pain and rash along a dermatome
- PE: Dyspnea, hemoptysis, and sharp chest pain

DIFFERENTIAL DX

- Cardiac: Coronary artery disease, aortic dissection, pericarditis, valvular heart disease, myocarditis
- Pulmonary: Pulmonary embolus, pneumothorax, pleuritis, pneumonia, lung cancer, sarcoidosis, pleuritis
- Gastrointestinal: GERD, peptic ulcer disease, esophageal dysmotility/spasm, esophagitis, pancreatitis, cholecystitis
- Musculoskeletal: Trauma, rib fracture, costochondritis, muscle strain, arthropathy, fibromyalgia, Tietze's syndrome
- Skin: Herpes zoster
- Psychiatric: Panic or anxiety disorder, factitious disorder

DIAGNOSTIC EVALUATION

- A complete, accurate, and systematic history and physical examination is key
  - Immediately obtain vital signs, including pulse oximetry (and fingerstick, if applicable)
  - Note onset, duration, location, radiation, type of pain, and exacerbating/alleviating factors
  - Cardiovascular evaluation includes assessment of heart sounds, murmurs, gallops or rubs, and carotid bruit
  - Lung exam may reveal crackles at bases (CHF) or absent breath sounds (pneumothorax)
  - Chest wall exam to rule out musculoskeletal etiologies
  - Abdominal exam to evaluate for GERD, cholecystitis, and pancreatitis
- Electrocardiogram may reveal ischemia (e.g., new bundle branch block, ST segment or T-wave changes) or arrhythmias; widespread ST elevations suggest pericarditis
- If acute ischemia cannot be ruled out in the office, the patient should be transported to the emergency department for further evaluation and management
- Patients with suspected coronary artery disease may require stress testing, echocardiogram, and/or cardiac catheterization

TREATMENT & MANAGEMENT

- If suspect myocardial infarction, response time is key
  - Immediately administer aspirin, supplemental oxygen, and nitroglycerin
  - Call Emergency Medical Services for transfer to an emergency room; monitor vitals frequently
  - An automated external defibrillator (AED) should be available in any office setting and ready for use if an arrhythmia occurs
  - Further intervention at the emergency room may include anticoagulation (e.g., heparin or low molecular weight heparin), beta-blockers, ACE inhibitors, clopidogrel, glycoprotein IIb/IIIa inhibitors (e.g., tirofiban), thrombolysis, or cardiac catheterization
- Assess for other emergent etiologies (e.g., aortic dissection, pneumothorax, pulmonary embolus, esophageal rupture); if suspected, initiate care and transfer to the nearest hospital
- Treat other etiologies as appropriate
  - Pericarditis: Treat with NSAIDs and schedule a nonurgent echocardiography to assess for pericardial effusion or hemodynamic compromise
  - GERD: Educate the patient on lifestyle changes (see *GERD* entry), and consider therapeutic challenge with proton pump inhibitors; however, note that clinical improvement following the use of antacids does not rule out the possibility of a cardiac etiology
  - Treat musculoskeletal pain with NSAIDs, stretching, and physical therapy

PROGNOSIS & COMPLICATIONS

- Approximately 1.1 million Americans have a new or recurrent myocardial infarction per year, and 220,000 nonhospitalized patients die of myocardial infarction per year
- The speed of response and the availability of early thrombolysis or angioplasty in patients with acute myocardial infarction is key to reducing mortality
- Complications of myocardial infarction include ventricular wall rupture, ventricular septal defect, left ventricular aneurysm, postinfarction ischemia, papillary muscle dysfunction, acute mitral regurgitation, pericarditis, mural thrombus, heart failure, arrhythmias, hypotension, shock, and sudden death
- Proper training and use of automated external defibrillators (AED) by physicians and non-physicians alike has led to a reduction in sudden cardiac death in the community

Palpitations

INTRODUCTION

- Palpitations are subjective sensations that the heart is beating rapidly, strongly, or irregularly; it often means that a rapid heart rate is occurring, but palpitations can also be seen even when the heart rate is normal, such as in anxious patients
- Palpitations are a very common complaint among outpatients, accounting for as many as 16% of ambulatory visits
- The differential diagnosis is vast, but a specific cause is determined in more than 85% of cases

ETIOLOGY, EPIDEMIOLOGY, & RISK FACTORS

- A wide variety of etiologies can cause palpitations; etiologies are generally divided into intrinsic causes (cardiac or psychiatric) or extrinsic causes (medications)
- Psychiatric: Anxiety is a common cause of rapid or forceful heartbeats secondary to fear; this is the diagnosis in as many as 30% of cases; patients most commonly present to the office
- Cardiac: There are many benign and malignant conduction abnormalities that cause palpitations; some are congenital, some are related to prior injury, and some are normal variants (e.g., premature ventricular contractions); cardiac etiologies are the diagnosis in as many as 45% of cases; patients more commonly present to the emergency department
- Catecholamine excess: Often related to medications (including caffeine); however, other conditions (e.g., thyrotoxicosis, anemia, mastocytosis) must be ruled out
- Young people are more likely to have benign conditions related to anxiety or other psychiatric causes; if ventricular tachycardia is documented in a younger person, evaluation for prolonged QT interval should be done
- Risk factors for a cardiac etiology include male gender, irregular heartbeat, history of heart disease, and duration greater than 5 minutes (patients with 3 of these predictors have 70% probability that the palpitations are of cardiac origin)
- Drug use (e.g., cocaine) can cause malignant arrhythmia and palpitations that lead to MI

PATIENT PRESENTATION

- The sensation of palpitations can be described in many ways, and may be a clue to the etiology:
  - "Flip-flopping" in the chest: Supraventricular tachycardia, premature atrial or ventricular contractions
  - Forceful contraction after a pause: Premature ventricular contractions
  - Rapid fluttering: Supraventricular tachycardia, sinus tachycardia, atrial fibrillation
  - "Pounding" in the neck: AV dissociation
  - "Irregular heartbeat": Atrial fibrillation, heart block, premature ventricular contractions
- Palpitations associated with syncope or presyncope may be malignant or benign
- Complaints of episodic or random palpitations may represent premature ventricular contractions; a longer duration of palpitations should raise concern for a cardiac etiology

DIFFERENTIAL DX

- Arrhythmias (e.g., premature ventricular or atrial contractions, sinus tachycardia, atrial fibrillation, paroxysmal atrial tachycardia, and others)
- Valvular disease (e.g., mitral valve prolapse)
- Myocardial ischemia
- Catecholamine excess (e.g., caffeine, tobacco, cocaine, cold medicine [pseudoephedrine, ephedrine], bronchodilators, theophylline, amphetamines, herbs [ma huang])
- Anxiety
- Thyrotoxicosis
- Dehydration
- Pheochromocytoma
- Anemia

DIAGNOSTIC EVALUATION

- History and physical examination
  - Note duration, frequency, and precipitating factors
  - May be associated with chest pain, dyspnea, diaphoresis, or lightheadedness/syncope
  - Heart rhythm may be regular or irregular
  - The patient should be questioned about the palpitations; they should be asked to "tap" the speed and rhythm of the palpitation sensation; additionally, teaching the patient to measure his or her pulse during the palpitations may give further clues to the etiology
  - May have family history of prolonged QT syndrome, hypertrophic cardiomyopathy, syncope, arrhythmias, or sudden death
- Electrocardiogram (EKG) is indicated in all patients
- If no abnormality is found on EKG, laboratory studies may be done to rule out organic causes (e.g., anemia, hyperthyroidism); these tests may include complete blood count, electrolytes, glucose, and thyroid-stimulating hormone
- If the diagnosis is still unclear and the patient is intolerant of the palpitations or there are concerning risk factors, ambulatory monitoring is indicated (e.g., Holter monitoring)
- If there is concern for a malignant arrhythmia, electrophysiology testing can be performed; however, this is only recommended for those with a high pretest probability of a serious arrhythmia (i.e., sustained palpitations and history of heart disease)

TREATMENT & MANAGEMENT

- Eliminate causative medications, if possible
- Psychiatric causes may require a combination of anxiolytics (e.g., lorazepam, buspirone) and behavioral interventions
- Cardiac arrhythmias can be managed in variety of ways, which may include medications (e.g., beta-blockers, calcium channel blockers, other antiarrhythmics) or invasive ablation therapy; in general, if a cardiac etiology is suspected, referral to a cardiologist is indicated
  - Malignant arrhythmias or those associated with heart disease may require placement of an implantable cardioverter-defibrillator
- Sinus tachycardia is usually benign but requires investigation as to the cause (e.g., fever, anxiety, pain, anemia, hypoxia)

PROGNOSIS & COMPLICATIONS

- Prognosis is directly linked to the etiology of the palpitations
- If the etiology can be ascertained and treated (e.g., removal of an offending drug, treatment of an arrhythmia), the morbidity and mortality are extremely low
- Nonsustained ventricular tachycardia or atrial fibrillation in the setting of coronary artery disease can result in myocardial infarction and death

Peripheral Vascular Disease

INTRODUCTION

- Atherosclerosis is a generalized systemic process that affects multiple vascular beds, including the cerebral, coronary, renal, and peripheral arteries
- Peripheral vascular disease (PVD) is an atherosclerotic obstructive disease of the arteries of the lower extremities and, less often, of the upper extremities
- PVD is a strong marker for cardiovascular disease and stroke
  - Over a 10-year period, PVD has been shown to be associated with a 6-fold increased risk of death due to cardiovascular disease
- Affects 5% of the 50- to 70-year-old population and 10% of people >70 years old (approximately 10 million people in the United States)

ETIOLOGY, EPIDEMIOLOGY, & RISK FACTORS

- Atherosclerotic plaque formation is a complex interaction involving lipid-laden macrophages (foam cells), smooth muscle proliferation, growth factors, impairment of endothelium-dependent vasodilatation (endothelial dysfunction), and arterial lumen narrowing, leading to impaired blood flow
- Progressive stenosis leads to ischemia, resulting in claudication of affected extremities
- Arteries involved may include the carotids, vertebral, subclavian, innominate, renal, aorta, iliac, femoral, popliteal, tibial, and peroneal
- Diabetic peripheral vascular disease accounts for more than 60% of leg amputations in the United States
- Risk factors include coronary atherosclerosis, diabetes mellitus, tobacco use, hyperlipidemia, hypertension, elevated homocysteine levels, obesity, and family history

PATIENT PRESENTATION

- Claudication is the characteristic symptom, resulting from ischemia of muscles (usually the calf muscles)
  - Lower extremity discomfort with exercise (pain, tightness, cramping)
  - May be unilateral or bilateral
  - Presents at relatively constant walking distance
  - Symptoms disappear upon resting
  - May continue even at rest in severe disease
- Decreased or absent peripheral pulses
- Arterial bruits
- Pallor of feet upon exercise or elevation
- Muscle atrophy, hair loss, thickened toenails, skin fissures, shiny skin
- Severe disease results in ulceration, tissue necrosis, and gangrene
- Subclavian or innominate stenosis may result in arm claudication or subclavian steal syndrome
- Renal artery stenosis may result in hypertension

DIFFERENTIAL DX

- Lumbar spinal stenosis: "Pseudoclaudication" (usually bilateral pain and paresthesias in the lower extremities upon walking or standing; symptoms abate with sitting or bending forward)
- Thromboangiitis obliterans (Buerger's disease)
- Popliteal artery entrapment
- Deep venous thrombosis
- Radiculopathy
- Peripheral neuropathy
- Baker's cyst
- Vasculitis
- Muscle strain or trauma

DIAGNOSTIC EVALUATION

- History and physical exam (diagnosis is usually made clinically)
- Fontaine classification may be used to characterize the degree of disease:
  - Stage I: Asymptomatic
  - Stage II: Intermittent claudication
  - Stage III: Pain at rest and nocturnal pain
  - Stage IV: Necrosis, gangrene
- Ankle:brachial index (ABI) with or without exercise is used to evaluate the severity
  - ABI of 0.8–0.9 at rest or 0.5–1.0 with exercise signifies mild disease
  - ABI of 0.5–0.8 at rest or 0.2–0.5 with exercise signifies moderate disease
  - ABI <0.5 at rest or <0.2 with exercise signifies severe disease
  - ABI and segmental pressures may be inaccurate in diabetic patients with severe calcific atherosclerosis
- Noninvasive testing may include segmental leg pressures, duplex ultrasound, magnetic resonance angiography, or CT angiography
- Peripheral angiography is a highly accurate, although invasive, method of testing; used if surgical or percutaneous intervention is planned

TREATMENT & MANAGEMENT

- Initial treatment includes risk factor modification: Smoking cessation, tight glycemic control, lipid lowering (target low-density lipoprotein [LDL] <100), antihypertensive therapy, dietary modifications, and a supervised walking program
- Consider elevating the head of the bed by 4-6 inches to allow for improved distal circulation
- Antiplatelet agents (e.g., aspirin, clopidogrel, ticlopidine) are commonly used
- Specific treatment for intermittent claudication includes cilostazol (phosphodiesterase inhibitor resulting in vasodilation and inhibition of platelet aggregation) and pentoxifylline (results in vasodilation, decreased platelet aggregation, and decreased blood viscosity)
- Percutaneous revascularization of blockages with angioplasty and stent placement may be indicated for severe disease
- Surgical revascularization (bypass) of blockages may be indicated for ischemia, peripheral emboli, impotence, and in patients with lifestyle-limiting symptoms

PROGNOSIS & COMPLICATIONS

- Patients with peripheral vascular disease have an increased risk of angina, nonfatal and fatal myocardial infarction, CHF, and stroke
- Peripheral vascular disease is a marker of atherosclerotic disease; affected patients have a high incidence of coronary artery and cerebrovascular disease
  - 5- and 10-year mortality rates are directly related to coronary and cerebral disease
- 75% of patients with claudication improve with conservative therapy
- 30% 5-year mortality rate in patients with claudication
- Severity of disease predicts mortality
  - ABI >0.85 has 75% 10-year survival rate
  - ABI of 0.4–0.85 has 55% 10-year survival rate
  - ABI <0.4 has 35% 10-year survival rate
- Operative mortality rate is 1-3%, with most deaths due to cardiac events

Bradycardia and AV Block

INTRODUCTION

- Sinus bradycardia is identified by sinus rhythm with a rate less than 60 beats/min
  - P waves have normal contour and occur before each QRS complex; PR interval is constant
- AV block is a failure of appropriate conduction of atrial impulse to the ventricles; the atrial impulse is delayed or is not conducted at all to the ventricles
  - 1st-degree AV block: Prolonged PR interval that remains constant
  - 2nd-degree Mobitz I AV block: Progressive prolongation of the PR interval until a P wave fails to conduct, AV conduction recovers, then repeats
  - 2nd-degree Mobitz II: Intermittent nonconducted P waves without preceding PR delay
  - 3rd-degree AV block: Complete failure of conduction from the atria to the ventricles

ETIOLOGY, EPIDEMIOLOGY, & RISK FACTORS

- Bradycardia may be caused by intrinsic cardiac dysfunction or be secondary to the influence of extrinsic, noncardiac factors
- Etiologies intrinsic to the heart include idiopathic degeneration (occurs in the elderly due to fibrosis of the conduction system), acute myocardial ischemia or infarction, congenital heart disease, paravalvular abscess, surgical trauma including valve replacement (due to edema of the conduction system), infiltrative diseases (e.g., sarcoidosis, amyloidosis, hemochromatosis), and infectious diseases (e.g., Chagas disease, Lyme disease, endocarditis, myocarditis)
- Extrinsic etiologies include autonomically mediated syndromes (e.g., neurocardiogenic syncope, carotid artery hypersensitivity, coughing, micturition, defecation), medications and antiarrhythmic agents (e.g., beta-blockers, calcium channel blockers, digoxin, clonidine, lithium), hypothyroidism, myxedema, hypothermia, electrolyte disturbances (e.g., hypo- or hyperkalemia), collagen vascular disease (e.g., SLE, rheumatoid arthritis, scleroderma), neuromuscular disease (e.g., muscular dystrophy), tumors (intracranial, cervical, mediastinal), and trauma (e.g., myocardial contusion)
- Bradycardia is a normal finding in well-trained athletes

PATIENT PRESENTATION

- May be asymptomatic
- Symptoms may include palpitations, dyspnea, dizziness, presyncope or syncope, chest pain, and mental status changes
- Physical exam may reveal irregular heartbeat, jugular venous distension, S4 gallop, variable intensity of carotid upstrokes, hypotension, or signs of heart failure
- Atrial fibrillation with complete heart block and resulting bradycardia is pathognomonic for digitalis toxicity
- The classical syncopal episode caused by a bradyarrhythmia is a *Stokes-Adams* attack
  - Sudden-onset immediate collapse with loss of consciousness
  - Patients appear pale and still as if dead for up to 1–2 minutes and then have rapid recovery
- Obstructive sleep apnea could lead to severe nocturnal bradycardia

DIFFERENTIAL DX

- 1st-degree AV block
- 2nd-degree AV block
- 3rd-degree AV block
- Atrial fibrillation
- Atrial flutter with variable conduction
- Normal athletic heart
- Symptomatic bradycardia can manifest with a variety of nonspecific complaints (e.g., dizziness, syncope, fatigue) that may mimic numerous conditions

DIAGNOSTIC EVALUATION

- Complete history and physical examination with close attention to medications
- Electrocardiogram (EKG) is often diagnostic
  - 1st-degree AV block: Prolonged PR interval ($>$200 ms); each P wave followed by a QRS
  - Mobitz I: Progressive prolongation of PR interval and progressive shortening of the RR interval until a P wave is not conducted, usually associated with narrow QRS complex
  - Mobitz II: Regular sinus or atrial rhythm with intermittent nonconducted P waves; QRS complex is usually wide; PR interval remains fixed
  - 3rd-degree AV block: Atrial impulses consistently fail to reach the ventricles; atrial and ventricular rhythms are independent of each other; PR interval varies; PP and RR intervals are constant; atrial rate exceeds ventricular rate (maintained by junctional or escape rhythm)
- Laboratory studies may include thyroid function tests, electrolytes, calcium, magnesium, glucose, and toxicology screen
- 24- to 48-hour ambulatory EKG monitoring (e.g., Holter or event monitor, telemetry) may be useful
- Electrophysiologic testing may be indicated if the mechanism for bradycardia remains uncertain
- Exercise stress testing may be useful to evaluate for sinus node disease

TREATMENT & MANAGEMENT

- Asymptomatic bradycardia (sinus bradycardia, 1st-degree AV block, Mobitz I) may not require therapy
- Emergent treatment is indicated for symptomatic bradycardia
  - Atropine increases sinoatrial (SA) and AV nodal conduction and is indicated for asystole, symptomatic bradycardia, or symptomatic AV block
  - Epinephrine is indicated for asystole and refractory symptomatic bradycardia
  - Emergency transvenous cardiac pacing is indicated for asystole, symptomatic bradycardia, and patients at high risk of progression to asystole (e.g., Mobitz II or 3rd-degree heart block)
  - Dopamine infusion may also be used to increase the heart rate
- Bradycardia induced by beta-blockers or calcium channel blockers is treated with IV calcium and glucagon, which increases chronotropy and inotropy
- Bradycardia due to digoxin toxicity may be treated with Digibind (digoxin-specific antibody fragments) in cases of life-threatening toxicity
- Permanent pacemaker implantation may be indicated for symptomatic and irreversible bradyarrhythmias

PROGNOSIS & COMPLICATIONS

- 1st-degree block is benign in the absence of QRS widening, but may worsen heart failure
- 2nd-degree Mobitz I AV block is generally benign; Mobitz II often progresses to complete heart block, thus requiring permanent pacing
- 3rd-degree AV block can be life threatening and often requires permanent pacing
- Overall, prognosis is variable and depends on underlying heart disease
- Patients with AV block have a worse prognosis than those with sinus node dysfunction, probably because the former have greater degrees of structural heart disease
- 5-15% of acute MIs are complicated by complete heart block and may require permanent pacemaker insertion
- Lyme disease may cause AV conduction disturbances, which usually have good prognoses

Syncope

INTRODUCTION

- A sudden, brief loss of consciousness and postural tone with spontaneous recovery that is caused by a transient decrease in cerebral blood flow
- Etiologies include neurocardiogenic (i.e., vasovagal), cardiac, neurologic, orthostatic, and others
- No cause identified in up to 50% of cases
- Syncope accounts for about 5% of hospital admissions and 3% of emergency department visits
- In children, breath holding may result in syncope

ETIOLOGY, EPIDEMIOLOGY, & RISK FACTORS

- **Neurocardiogenic (vasovagal) syncope** (35% of cases) is the most common etiology
  - This is a reflex syncope associated with an inappropriate decrease in sympathetic tone along with increased parasympathetic (vagal) tone
  - Results in bradycardia and hypotension
  - Causes include carotid sinus massage (pressure on the internal carotid artery leads to slowing of the sinoatrial [SA] node rate and impaired AV node conduction), micturition, Valsalva, and strong emotional responses
- Cardiac syncope (20% of cases) results from inadequate cardiac output
  - Etiologies leading to decreased cardiac output include arrhythmias, left ventricular dysfunction, heart block, volume depletion, aortic and mitral valve disease, hypertrophic cardiomyopathy, pulmonary embolism, cardiac tamponade, and pulmonary hypertension
- Orthostatic syncope (10% of cases) results from venous pooling of blood upon moving from a supine to upright position; most common in the elderly
- Syncope is common in the elderly (annual incidence of 5% in individuals older than 75)
  - Risk factors in the elderly include multiple comorbidities, medications that cause volume depletion (e.g., diuretics) or altered vascular tone (e.g., beta-blockers), and physiologic impairments (e.g., impaired thirst, baroreceptor sensitivity, decreased cerebral blood flow)

PATIENT PRESENTATION

- Loss of consciousness (seconds to minutes)
- Prodromal symptoms are often present (e.g., lightheadedness, dizziness, nausea, weakness, vision changes, pallor, diaphoresis)
- Incontinence and brief clonic movements may occasionally occur
- Mental status is at baseline following the syncopal episode
- Symptoms due to specific etiologies may be present (e.g., palpitations, slow heart rate, angina, headache, murmurs, carotid bruit)
- Syncope without prodrome or with associated trauma suggests a cardiac etiology
- Determinants of a serious underlying cardiac cause may include syncope while supine, cardiac symptoms, old age, incontinence, prolonged loss of consciousness, tongue biting, trauma following syncope (signifies lack of warning), headache or neurologic symptoms, or no prodromal symptoms

DIFFERENTIAL DX

- Seizure
- Psychiatric disorder (anxiety, hysteria)
- Hypoglycemia
- Hyperventilation
- Vertigo
- Vertebrobasilar insufficiency
- Complicated migraine
- Subarachnoid hemorrhage
- Arrhythmias
- Orthostatic hypotension
- Aortic stenosis
- Myocardial infarction
- Stroke or transient ischemic attack
- Medications

DIAGNOSTIC EVALUATION

- History and physical examination may be diagnostic
  - A history consistent with vasovagal syncope typically does not require further evaluation
  - Orthostatic blood pressures should be assessed
  - Review medications that may result in vasodilation (e.g., anticholinergics, tricyclic antide-pressants, phenothiazines, antihypertensives)
- Electrocardiogram (EKG) should be evaluated in all patients
  - EKG is abnormal in 50% of patients but is not usually diagnostic of the underlying cause
  - Evaluate for prolongation of the QT interval, arrhythmias, or acute ischemia patterns
- Testing for cardiogenic etiologies may include cardiac enzymes if EKG and history suggest ischemia; echocardiography to identify structural cardiac abnormalities and valvular disease; ambulatory EKG monitoring (e.g., 24-hour Holter monitor, event recorder, implantable loop recorder) to detect transient arrhythmias; stress testing; or electrophysiologic testing
- Carotid sinus massage or tilt-table testing may be useful to reproduce neurocardiogenic syncope
- Neurologic studies (e.g., EEG, neuroimaging, carotid Doppler scan) are generally of low yield and should only be considered if the patient has neurologic symptoms or signs of transient ischemia

TREATMENT & MANAGEMENT

- Vasovagal syncope can be avoided by patient education
  - Instruct patients to assume a recumbent position when presyncopal symptoms occur
  - Avoid prolonged standing, heat, large meals, fasting, lack of sleep, alcohol, and dehydration
- Discontinue medications that may provoke postural hypotension
- Hypovolemia may respond to fluids, salt, and volume expanders
- Patients with orthostatic and reflex-mediated syncope should avoid the precipitating factors, should increase fluid and salt intake, and may benefit from pharmacologic therapy (e.g., beta-blockers, selective serotonin reuptake inhibitors, midodrine, fludrocortisone)
- Carotid-sinus hypersensitivity may require cardiac pacing
- Cardiac arrhythmias may require medical or invasive therapies
  - Bradyarrhythmias generally require a cardiac pacemaker
  - Tachyarrhythmias may be treated with drug therapy (beta-blockers, calcium channel blockers, or other antiarrhythmics) and/or implantable cardioverter-defibrillators

PROGNOSIS & COMPLICATIONS

- Prognosis depends on the etiology
- Vasovagal syncope is more common in the young and may resolve over time
- Patients with cardiac syncope have a high mortality if specific treatment is not instituted; however, cardiogenic syncope should resolve once cardiac output is maintained
- Predictors of severe cardiac arrhythmias or death within the first year after syncope include age older than 45, history of heart failure or ventricular arrhythmias, and abnormal EKG
- Complications are related to injuries that may occur at the time of the fall

Congestive Heart Failure

INTRODUCTION

- Congestive heart failure is a clinical syndrome in which the heart is unable to maintain adequate cardiac output to meet the needs of the body
- Symptomatic left ventricular systolic dysfunction (symptoms including fatigue, volume overload, reduced exercise tolerance) is considered congestive heart failure
  - Left ventricular systolic dysfunction is defined as reduced left ventricular ejection fraction secondary to loss of myocardial contractility
- The New York Heart Association (NYHA) system classifies the degree of heart failure based on functional capacity (see *Diagnostic Evaluation* section); this classification is used to describe patients' baseline status but does not apply to acute exacerbations

ETIOLOGY, EPIDEMIOLOGY, & RISK FACTORS

- The most common etiologies are coronary artery disease and hypertension
  - Pericardial etiologies: Pericardial constriction or tamponade
  - Endocardial (valvular) etiologies: Valvular stenosis, valvular insufficiency, or rupture (especially severe aortic and mitral regurgitation, and severe aortic stenosis)
  - Myocardial etiologies: Ischemia or infarction, cardiomyopathy, arrhythmias
- Classified as systolic (inability to eject blood) or diastolic (inability to fill with blood)
  - Systolic dysfunction is more common: Decreased myocardial contractility and ejection fraction; most commonly due to coronary artery disease, hypertension, dilated cardiomyopathy, and valvular disease
  - Diastolic dysfunction: Impaired myocardial relaxation, resulting in decreased ventricular filling (ejection fraction may be normal); most commonly due to hypertension, hypertrophic obstructive cardiomyopathy, and restrictive cardiomyopathy
- High-output heart failure: Inability to meet high tissue demands (e.g., thyrotoxicosis, sepsis, anemia) despite a normal heart (however, many also have heart disease)
- Nearly 3 million Americans have documented congestive heart failure, and there are more than 400,000 new cases in the U.S. yearly, resulting in nearly 200,000 deaths every year
- Accounts for at least 20% of all hospitalizations in patients older than 65

PATIENT PRESENTATION

- May be symptomatic or asymptomatic; onset of symptoms is usually gradual, unless secondary to a catastrophic event such as a myocardial infarction
- Left-sided heart failure primarily results in pulmonary symptoms
  - Dyspnea (ranges from exertional dyspnea to severe dyspnea at rest)
  - Symptoms of volume overload: Orthopnea, paroxysmal nocturnal dyspnea, peripheral edema
  - Fatigue, weakness, decreased exercise tolerance
  - Tachypnea, tachycardia
  - S3 may be present
  - Rales (crackles)
  - Laterally displaced apical impulse
- Right-sided failure causes peripheral symptoms
  - Jugular venous distention
  - Hepatomegaly, hepatojugular reflux
  - Ascites and abdominal fullness
  - Peripheral edema, weight gain

DIFFERENTIAL DX

- Cardiovascular: Coronary artery disease, valvular disease, aortic dissection, arrhythmias, endocarditis, myocarditis, hypertensive emergency, infiltrative disorders (e.g., sarcoid, amyloid)
- Pulmonary: COPD, asthma, interstitial fibrosis, pulmonary hypertension, pneumonia, pulmonary embolism
- Symptomatic anemia
- Thyrotoxicosis
- Hepatic failure
- Renal failure
- Hypoalbuminemia
- Toxins (e.g., NSAIDs, alcohol, cocaine, doxorubicin)
- Deconditioning

DIAGNOSTIC EVALUATION

- Diagnosis is largely based on history and physical exam; focus on compliance with medical therapy, dietary changes, weight change, chest pain, changes in exercise tolerance
- The New York Heart Association classification is used to assess function capacity:
  - Class I: No symptoms with normal activity
  - Class II: Comfortable at rest, but symptoms (angina, dyspnea) occur on moderate exertion
  - Class III: Comfortable at rest, but symptoms occur with mild physical activity
  - Class IV: Symptoms occur at rest; any degree of physical activity causes symptoms
- Initial laboratory tests include CBC, chemistries (hypo- or hyperkalemia may occur due to medications), and liver function tests (may be elevated due to hepatic congestion)
- B-type natriuretic peptide (BNP) $<$100 pg/mL generally rules out congestive heart failure; elevated BNP is nonspecific, but BNP $>$500 pg/mL suggests CHF
- Cardiac enzymes are positive in 30% of patients with acute congestive heart failure
- Chest X-ray may show cardiomegaly, increased pulmonary vasculature (e.g., cephalization, hilar fullness, Kerley B lines), interstitial edema, and pleural effusions
- Electrocardiogram (EKG) may show evidence of coronary artery disease, left ventricular hypertrophy, arrhythmias, or changes suggestive of acute ischemia
- Echocardiography is universally indicated because it can assess ejection fraction, left ventricular size, wall thickness, diastolic dysfunction, and valvular function
- All patients with newly diagnosed left ventricular dysfunction should be evaluated for coronary artery disease with stress testing or coronary angiography (left heart catheterization)

TREATMENT & MANAGEMENT

- Treatment involves correction of the underlying cause and control of CHF symptoms
- Supplemental oxygen may be necessary to maintain oxygen saturation $>$90%
- The goal of therapy is to decrease preload (by venodilation) and afterload (by arteriodilation and volume reduction) in order to improve forward blood flow
  - ACE inhibitors (e.g., enalapril) are the mainstay of afterload reduction and have been shown to improve mortality; they should be used cautiously in patients with renal failure
  - Nitrates decrease preload and afterload, resulting in increased stroke volume and decreased ventricular systolic wall stress; use with caution in hypotensive patients (systolic BP $<$100)
  - Hydralazine reduces afterload but requires thrice-daily dosing
  - Loop diuretics are the treatment of choice once the diagnosis of CHF is certain; however, they may *increase* mortality in patients with COPD and pneumonia
  - β-blockers (e.g., carvedilol, metoprolol) are used in both systolic and diastolic failure and have been shown to improve mortality; however, they should be avoided during acute CHF
  - Aldosterone antagonists (spironolactone) are indicated for class III/IV heart failure
- Patients with coronary artery disease should be treated as appropriate, including beta-blockers, aspirin, ACE inhibitors, and possibly coronary revascularization
- Implantable cardiac defibrillator may be necessary if ejection fraction is $<$30%
- End-stage heart failure may require a left ventricular assist device and/or cardiac transplantation

PROGNOSIS & COMPLICATIONS

- Despite advances in care, mortality from CHF has been increasing
- Left ventricular ejection fraction and severity of symptoms are strong predictors of survival
- Untreated asymptomatic patients have a 25% 4-year mortality rate
- Patients with left ventricular ejection fraction $<$30% are candidates for chronic anticoagulation due to risk of mural thrombus and may benefit from an implantable defibrillator
- Patients who have hypertension prior to a myocardial infarction are much more likely to develop heart failure when cardiac remodeling occurs following the infarction
- There is a mortality benefit from spironolactone in patients with class III/IV heart failure

Atrial Fibrillation

INTRODUCTION

- Atrial fibrillation (afib) is an irregularly irregular rhythm arising from disorganized atrial activity; it results in irregular impulse conduction through the AV node to the ventricles
- It is the most common sustained arrhythmia
- Can occur in individuals with normal hearts or those with underlying heart disease
- Defined as *paroxysmal* if it spontaneously remits (episodes generally last less than 24 hours or up to a several days), *persistent* if it has to be cardioverted, or *permanent* if it cannot be cardioverted
- *Lone atrial fibrillation* is defined as afib in the absence of structural heart disease
- Patients with paroxysmal afib may be asymptomatic and unaware of their condition

ETIOLOGY, EPIDEMIOLOGY, & RISK FACTORS

- As the atria contract rapidly and irregularly at rates of 400-600 beats/min, the AV node is rapidly stimulated by the excessive electrical activity and blocks many of these signals from passing to the ventricles (only 1 or 2 of every 3 beats passes through); this results in a rapid ventricular response (ventricular rate of 110-180 beats/min), which may lead to left ventricular (LV) dysfunction, decreased cardiac output, and congestive heart failure
  - In contrast, atrial flutter has an atrial rate of 250-350 beats/min, and conduction to the ventricles is often regular, with every second or third atrial contraction being conducted
- Major complications of afib are emboli (due to blood stagnation) and heart failure
  - May allow clots to form in the atria, which can embolize to cause stroke (3% risk/year)
  - Risk of clot formation and stroke increase after 24 hours of sustained arrhythmia
- Risk factors include hypertension, coronary artery disease, sick sinus syndrome, valve disease, cardiomyopathy, cardiac surgery, myocarditis, pericarditis, thyrotoxicosis, alcohol use, Wolff-Parkinson-White syndrome, sepsis, and pulmonary disease
  - Any medication that causes a decrease in vagal tone can cause afib (e.g., theophylline, adenosine, digitalis)
- Affects nearly 1% of the population, and is more common as age increases: Less than 1% risk if younger than age 60; greater than 6% risk if older than 80

PATIENT PRESENTATION

- Patients may be asymptomatic, especially if the ventricular rate is controlled
- Common symptoms include palpitations, light-headedness or presyncope, dyspnea, fatigue, decreased exercise tolerance, and angina
- Heart rate is often tachycardic but may be normal or even bradycardic
- A small number of patients present after an embolic event (e.g., transient ischemic attack or stroke) or right-sided heart failure (weight gain, ascites, peripheral edema)
- Polyuria is a common complaint secondary to the release of atrial natriuretic peptide
- Exam shows an irregularly irregular pulse, irregular jugular venous pulsations, a variable S1, and no S4

DIFFERENTIAL DX

- Narrow QRS complex with irregular rhythm: Sinus rhythm with frequent premature atrial contractions, atrial flutter, multifocal atrial tachycardia
- Wide QRS complex with irregular rhythm: Pre-excited afib, afib or atrial flutter with aberrancy
- Narrow QRS complex with regular rhythm: Atrial flutter, afib with complete heart block (rates will be 40–60 beats/min), other supraventricular tachycardias
- Wide QRS complex with regular rhythm: Atrial flutter, supraventricular tachycardia with aberrancy

DIAGNOSTIC EVALUATION

- Electrocardiogram (EKG) is diagnostic in most cases
  - Atrial fibrillation: P waves are absent, EKG baseline has fine irregular fibrillation waves at 300–600 per min, and QRS complexes are irregularly irregular
  - Atrial flutter: P waves are absent, EKG baseline shows regular "sawtooth" flutter waves at about 300/min, and QRS conduction is usually 1:2 (150/min and regular)
  - Atrial fibrillation (i.e., no P waves) with a regularly occurring QRS complex (regular RR interval) is pathognomonic for digitalis toxicity
- Continuous EKG monitoring (e.g., event monitoring or Holter monitoring) may detect paroxysms of arrhythmia
- IV adenosine may be necessary to slow AV conduction for easier rhythm interpretation
- Evaluate for acute causes of afib, including alcoholic "holiday" heart, hyperthyroidism, pericarditis, myocarditis, myocardial infarction, surgery, pulmonary embolism, other pulmonary diseases, and medications that decrease vagal tone or increase sympathetic tone
- Echocardiogram should be considered to evaluate left ventricular size and function, underlying valvular disease, etiology of congestive heart failure, atrial size, left ventricular hypertrophy, and pericardial diseases
  - Transesophageal echocardiogram may be necessary to evaluate for left atrial thrombus if cardioversion is needed prior to a period of adequate anticoagulation

TREATMENT & MANAGEMENT

- The initial goal of treatment is rate control: This can be achieved with β-blockers or non-dihydropyridine calcium channel blockers; digoxin is used if decreased LV ejection fraction
  - Contraindicated in patients with pre-excited afib (antiarrhythmic drugs are needed)
  - AV node ablation with pacemaker implantation is a last resort for rate control
  - Guidelines recommend target rates of 60-80 bpm at rest and 90-115 bpm with exertion
- The second goal of therapy is stroke prevention: Patients <60 without risk factors for stroke are treated with aspirin prophylaxis; patients with risk factors or age 60–75 are treated with coumadin with INR goal of 2.0-3.0; high-risk patients (e.g., rheumatic heart disease, prosthetic valves, prior TIA or stroke) require coumadin therapy with INR goal of 2.5–3.5
- Patients who are asymptomatic after rate control and stroke prophylaxis and are in permanent or persistent afib do not require more aggressive therapy
- Symptomatic patients may require electrical or medical cardioversion
  - Flecainide and propafenone can be considered in lone afib or atrial flutter
  - All other cases are restricted to sotalol, amiodarone, or dofetilide
  - Direct current cardioversion may be indicated for patients with new-onset afib of less than 48 hours duration; to perform cardioversion if duration of afib is longer than 48 hours or unknown, cardiac thrombi must by ruled out by transesophageal echocardiogram or the patient must be anticoagulated for 3 weeks before and 4 weeks after the cardioversion
  - Hemodynamically unstable patients require immediate electrical cardioversion

PROGNOSIS & COMPLICATIONS

- Rates of ischemic stroke are 5-7% in nonrheumatic and nonvalvular afib
  - The risk is 5 times higher in the setting of rheumatic heart disease
  - Stroke risk is present even in patients with paroxysmal afib
  - However, patients with lone afib have a risk close to the general population
- Mortality rates are doubled in patients with afib secondary to underlying coronary artery disease
- Uncontrolled ventricular rates can lead to tachycardia-induced cardiomyopathy and CHF
- Afib or flutter in the setting of a rapidly conducting accessory pathway can lead to excessive ventricular rates, causing ventricular fibrillation and sudden cardiac death

Hypertension

INTRODUCTION

- Hypertension is the most common primary diagnosis in the United States, accounting for 35 million office visits
- Optimal blood pressure is less than 120/80 (based on the mean of 2 or more readings at separate office visits)
  - Stage 1 hypertension: Systolic pressure 140-159 mmHg or diastolic pressure 90–99 mmHg
  - Stage 2 hypertension: Systolic >160 mmHg or diastolic >100 mmHg
- 95% of cases are idiopathic (essential hypertension)
- More than half of the elderly population has hypertension, and the number of patients with hypertension is likely to grow as the population ages

ETIOLOGY, EPIDEMIOLOGY, & RISK FACTORS

- Essential hypertension is twice as common in individuals with hypertensive parents and is associated with excessive alcohol intake, obesity, and African-American race
- Etiologies of secondary hypertension include chronic kidney disease, renovascular disease (e.g., renal artery atherosclerosis, fibromuscular dysplasia), Cushing's syndrome and chronic steroid use, pheochromocytoma, primary hyperaldosteronism, hyper- and hypothyroidism, hyperparathyroidism, coarctation of the aorta, and oral contraceptive use
- The prevalence of hypertension has increased from 25% in 1988 to 29% in 2000, affecting 50 million individuals in United States and approximately 1 billion people worldwide
- Hypertension is an independent risk factor for cardiovascular disease and is the second most common cause of end-stage renal disease

PATIENT PRESENTATION

- The majority of cases are asymptomatic, with elevated blood pressure an incidental finding during routine physical exam
- In cases of hypertensive crisis or long-term uncontrolled hypertension, target organ damage may be apparent
  - Retinal vessels (e.g., papilledema, retinal hemorrhages, exudates)
  - Hypertensive encephalopathy (e.g., headache, nausea, vomiting, mental status change, focal neurologic deficits, seizures)
  - Renal failure
  - Cardiac ischemia
  - Congestive heart failure may be present

DIFFERENTIAL DX

- Essential hypertension
- Secondary hypertension
- "White coat" hypertension
- Elevated blood pressure associated with pain, stress (e.g., surgery, emotional), or exercise
- Extracellular volume overload (e.g., excess sodium intake, inadequate diuretic therapy, fluid retention due to kidney disease)
- Excessive alcohol intake
- Drug-induced (e.g., NSAIDs, sympathomimetics, steroids, oral contraceptives, cyclosporine, erythropoietin, cocaine)
- Improper measurement

DIAGNOSTIC EVALUATION

- History and physical examination
  - Preferably use a mercury sphygmomanometer that is properly calibrated and validated; ensure proper cuff size and cuff bladder encircling 80% of the arm; the patient should be comfortably seated for at least 5 minutes prior to measurement
  - Assess risk factors (e.g., history of diabetes, family history of heart disease, smoking, elevated cholesterol, drug use, stress, pain, obesity, body mass index)
  - Evaluate for target organ disease
- Initial laboratory testing may include urinalysis, basic metabolic panel (electrolytes, glucose, BUN/creatinine, calcium,) lipids, electrocardiogram (EKG), echocardiogram, glomerular filtration rate, and urinary albumin (albumin:creatinine ratio)
- Consider secondary causes of hypertension if sudden onset of hypertension, significant hypertension (>180/110), abnormally young (<30) or old (>50) patient, presence of target organ symptoms, or poor response to treatment (not controlled with 3 medications)
  - Elevated creatinine suggests renal parenchymal disease
  - Abdominal bruits and hypokalemia suggest renal vascular disease
  - Cushing's syndrome is associated with osteoporosis, obesity, muscle weakness, moon facies, hirsutism, elevated lipids and sugar, and low potassium
  - Pheochromocytoma is associated with extremely labile blood pressure (episodic or paroxysmal hypertension), headaches, palpitations, and diaphoresis
  - Primary hyperaldosteronism is associated with isolated low potassium

TREATMENT & MANAGEMENT

- Lifestyle changes (e.g., smoking cessation, dietary changes, exercise, moderate alcohol) are usually the initial intervention for essential hypertension
  - Patients should be counseled to lower salt and increase potassium and calcium in the diet
- Pharmacologic therapy usually begins with a diuretic, beta-blocker, and/or ACE inhibitor
  - Diuretics are first-line agents, especially in CHF, diabetes, and coronary artery disease (CAD)
  - Use ACE inhibitors in patients with CHF, CAD, renal disease, and diabetes
  - Use beta-blockers in CAD, recent MI, CHF, atrial fibrillation, migraines, hyperthyroidism
  - Additional drugs may include angiotensin receptor blockers (especially in patients who experience cough when using ACE inhibitors), calcium channel blockers, and alpha-blockers
  - Preferred drugs in pregnancy include methyldopa, beta-blockers, and vasodilators (avoid ACE inhibitors and angiotensin receptor blockers during pregnancy)
- Self-monitoring of blood pressure at home may be recommended
- After starting therapy, patients should be followed up on a monthly basis to encourage lifestyle changes and ensure optimal medication dosing
  - Once blood pressure goal is attained, follow-up can be at 3- to 6-month intervals
- Monitor serum potassium and creatinine at least 1-2 times per year
  - If hyperkalemia develops, attempt dietary changes before stopping medications
  - A rise in creatinine of less than 25% above baseline is acceptable

PROGNOSIS & COMPLICATIONS

- Antihypertensive therapy is associated with a 35–40% reduction in incidence of stroke, 20–25% reduction in incidence of MI, and 50% reduction in incidence of heart failure
- Left ventricular hypertrophy is common and is associated with increased morbidity and mortality and increased incidence of CHF, MI, arrhythmias, and sudden cardiac death
- Hypertension is one of the most important and common risk factors for stroke, cerebral hemorrhage, and chronic kidney disease

Deep Venous Thrombosis

INTRODUCTION

- Deep venous thrombosis (DVT) and pulmonary embolism (PE) are part of the continuum of the disease process known as venous thromboembolism, which most often arises from the veins of the lower extremities but can also occur in the veins of the upper extremities or pelvis
- Venous thromboembolism is diagnosed in 260,000 patients each year in the United States, but the actual incidence is closer to 600,000 because most cases are clinically unsuspected; presentation can be subtle, atypical, or obscured by other disease, leading to underdiagnosis, delayed therapy, and excess morbidity and mortality
- PE usually results from a lower extremity DVT, within or proximal to the popliteal vein

ETIOLOGY, EPIDEMIOLOGY, & RISK FACTORS

- In 1856, Rudolf Virchow described three factors leading to intravascular coagulation (Virchow's triad): 1) trauma to the vessel wall; 2) venous stasis; and 3) hypercoagulability
  - Damage to the vessel wall disrupts endothelial function and prevents normal inhibition of coagulation and fibrinolysis
  - Venous stasis due to obstruction or immobilization (e.g., hospitalization, prolonged bed rest) decreases dilution and clearance of activated clotting factors
  - Acquired or congenital thrombophilias promote hypercoagulability
- Deep vein thrombosis usually begins in the venous sinuses of the calf muscles; normally, these calf thrombi will spontaneously lyse, but in about 25% of cases, they propagate proximally to the popliteal and femoral veins; of these more proximal thrombi, 50% will embolize to the pulmonary circulation, though many remain asymptomatic
- DVT is suspected to occur in 20–70% of hospitalized patients
- Common risk factors include recent surgery (especially orthopedic surgeries), immobilization, obesity, lower extremity trauma, malignancy, use of oral contraceptives or hormone replacement therapy, pregnancy, and history of a prior DVT
  - Less common risk factors include thrombophilias (protein C/S deficiency, factor V Leiden mutation, prothrombin mutation) and myeloproliferative disorders (polycythemia vera)

PATIENT PRESENTATION

- DVT is most commonly associated with lower extremity symptoms (e.g., erythema, warmth, pain, swelling, tenderness); however, repeated clinical studies demonstrate these findings lack sufficient sensitivity and specificity for accurate diagnosis
- Homan's sign (increased calf pain upon dorsiflexion of the foot) is also unreliable (sensitivity, 13–48%; specificity, 39-84%)
- Patients with DVT may present with signs and symptoms of pulmonary embolism (e.g., pleuritic chest pain, dyspnea) in the absence of typical DVT symptoms

DIFFERENTIAL DX

- Cellulitis
- Lymphedema
- Lymphangitis
- Acute arterial ischemia
- Ruptured popliteal (Baker's) cyst
- Chronic venous insufficiency (the most common cause of unilateral leg edema)
- Ruptured calf muscle
- Achilles tendonitis
- Lower extremity trauma
- Drug-related edema
- Superficial thrombophlebitis

DIAGNOSTIC EVALUATION

- The evaluation begins with a thorough history and physical, including identification of any risk factors or possible precipitating events
  - Perform a thorough family history (e.g., history of thromboembolism, miscarriage, or malignancy) and medication history (e.g., oral contraceptives, estrogen replacement, ginkgo)
- Laboratory evaluation should include complete blood count, basic chemistries, coagulation studies, liver function tests, urinalysis, and a D-dimer assay
- The gold standard for diagnosis is contrast venography (sensitivity of 100%); however, this is an invasive study with inherent risks and is rarely used anymore
- Compression ultrasonography is the noninvasive test of choice and is generally available in most institutions
  - Sensitivity and specificity exceed 95% for DVTs proximal to the knee
  - The examination can be limited by pain, obesity, edema, or immobilization devices (e.g., casts)
- Impedance plethysmography is an acceptable alternative to ultrasound and may be better than ultrasound for detecting recurrent DVTs; however, it is not always readily available
- D-dimer assays have a high negative predictive value when less than 500 ng/mL; however, values above 500 ng/mL are nonspecific
  - D-dimer is best used in conjunction with other noninvasive studies or as a screening test
- Testing for pulmonary embolism may be indicated (see *Pulmonary Embolism* entry)
- Testing for thrombophilia is controversial; consider in young patients with recurrent DVT

TREATMENT & MANAGEMENT

- The best treatment is prevention: Patients at high risk (e.g., hospitalization, immobility, hypercoagulability) should ambulate as much as possible, wear compression stockings, and consider anticoagulation therapy
  - Moderate-risk patients are generally treated with low molecular weight heparin (LMWH) or unfractionated subcutaneous heparin; in patients at risk for bleeding in whom anticoagulation is contraindicated, intermittent pneumatic compression can be used
  - High-risk patients (e.g., post hip or knee surgery) are treated with LMWH or oral anticoagulants (e.g., warfarin), preferably starting prior to the date of surgery
- Patients with acute DVTs should be treated immediately to prevent clot extension and PE
- Treatment consists of anticoagulation with unfractionated heparin or LMWH, with concomitant warfarin dosing after the first 24 hours of heparin therapy
- Optimal duration of warfarin therapy is controversial
  - Those with a major transient risk factor for thrombosis have a 3% per year risk of recurrent thrombosis after 3 months of anticoagulation
  - Those with an idiopathic DVT treated for 6 months versus 3 months have a lower risk of recurrence 1 year after stopping anticoagulation (10% vs. 10–30%)
  - Patients with continuing risk factors (cancer, inherited thrombophilia, recurrent DVT) may require indefinite therapy
- Inferior vena cava filter may be indicated if there are contraindications to anticoagulation

PROGNOSIS & COMPLICATIONS

- Postphlebitic syndrome is the most common long-term complication of DVT
- A workup for underlying malignancy or hypercoagulable state should be pursued in patients without an obvious cause for DVT, particularly after the second or third episode
  - Ensure that all patients are up to date on all recommended malignancy screenings for his/her age (e.g., colonoscopy, Pap smears, mammogram, prostate-specific antigen)
- Most patients with DVT do not require hospitalization
- Screening for underlying risk factors is undertaken on an individual basis
- Consideration for an inferior vena cava (IVC) filter should be given to patients who cannot take warfarin therapy (i.e., history of GI bleeding) or who have failed warfarin therapy

Hyperlipidemia

INTRODUCTION

- Cholesterol is an essential nutrient; it is a precursor for many hormones, a major component of bile, and a central component of cell membranes, among other vital functions
- However, excessively elevated cholesterol and lipid levels are strongly correlated with diseases of atherosclerosis, including coronary artery disease, cerebrovascular disease, and peripheral vascular disease
- Lifestyle changes and medical therapies to lower cholesterol and lipid levels are central aspects of primary and secondary prevention of the diseases of atherosclerosis, particularly coronary artery disease

ETIOLOGY, EPIDEMIOLOGY, & RISK FACTORS

- Serum lipids consist of very low-density lipoproteins (VLDL), low-density lipoproteins (LDL), high-density lipoproteins (HDL), and triglycerides (TG)
  - LDL becomes deposited in arterial walls, where it is oxidized and accumulates in macrophages turned "foam cells"; continual excessive deposition can lead to a progressive growth of atherosclerotic plaques and narrowing of the arterial lumen; an inflammatory cascade is a central part of this process and, ultimately, may be responsible for the tendency for plaques to rupture, resulting in thrombosis and possible occlusion of the artery
  - HDL serves as a reverse transporter, removing cholesterol from atherosclerotic plaques and transporting it back to the liver for processing and excretion; low levels of HDL are a strong risk factor for the atherosclerotic diseases
  - High levels of VLDL and TG also contribute to the development of atherosclerosis, but their exact roles are not as clear
- Only about one-third of U.S. patients who have had a coronary event are on lipid-lowering therapy, and nearly 50% of patients with documented coronary artery disease do not achieve the National Cholesterol Education Program III (NCEP III) goals for lipid levels
- In addition to hyperlipidemia, other classical risk factors for atherosclerotic diseases include tobacco use, hypertension, diabetes mellitus, metabolic syndrome, and family history

PATIENT PRESENTATION

- Most patients with hyperlipidemia are asymptomatic
- Severely elevated lipids may cause eruptive xanthomas, lipemia retinalis, tendon xanthomas, xanthelasma, or tuberous xanthomas
- High triglycerides may lead to pancreatitis
- Hyperlipidemia is strongly associated with the development of atherosclerosis
- The serum of patients with high lipid levels may have a creamy or lipemic layer

DIFFERENTIAL DX

- Primary (nonfamilial) hypercholesterolemia
- Familial hyperlipidemia (types I, IIa, IIb, III, IV, V)
- Metabolic syndrome/obesity
- Diabetes
- Hypothyroidism
- Chronic liver disease
- Kidney disease/nephrotic syndrome
- Medications that alter lipid levels (e.g., antiretroviral drugs, cyclosporine)
- Alcohol

DIAGNOSTIC EVALUATION

- Complete history and physical examination, including family history of early coronary disease and other risk factors
- Laboratory testing includes fasting lipid profile with measurement of total cholesterol, LDL, HDL, and triglycerides; other labs may include TSH, blood glucose, electrolytes, and liver function tests
- Several nontraditional risk factors [e.g., C-reactive protein, homocysteine, lipoprotein (a), fibrinogen] may be used to help risk stratify patients with borderline lipid levels
- A global risk score using data from the Framingham Study can be calculated based on risk factors of age, LDL, HDL, hypertension, diabetes, and smoking
  - A score of 3 or lower indicates less than 1% 10-year risk of developing heart disease, whereas a score of greater than 14 conveys nearly a 60% 10-year risk
- NCEP III Guidelines for initiating therapy:
  - Low risk (>10% 10-year risk, >2 risk factors): LDL >160
  - Moderate risk (10-20% risk, <2 risk factors): LDL >130
  - High risk (<20% risk, CAD, diabetes, PVD): LDL >100
  - Very high risk (CAD with diabetes, peripheral vascular disease): LDL >70

TREATMENT & MANAGEMENT

- The initial intervention in most patients is lifestyle modifications, including smoking cessation, dietary changes, weight reduction, and exercise
  - Some dietary suggestions include reduced saturated fat intake to <7% of calories, reduced cholesterol intake to <200 mg/day, increased fiber intake, and increased consumption of fish or a fish oil supplement
- When medical therapy is necessary, statins are generally the preferred drug
  - Side effects include myositis and elevated transaminases
  - Rhabdomyolysis and liver failure is rarely reported
- Ezetimibe inhibits absorption of lipids from the GI tract; it may be used as single agent, but it is most effective if used in combination with a statin
- Niacin is one of the few agents that raise HDL cholesterol; however, poor tolerability (flushing, decreased glucose intolerance) limits its use
  - Taking 325–650 mg of aspirin 15–30 minutes before the dose may decrease flushing
- Fibric acid derivatives (gemfibrozil, fenofibrate) may be effective to lower TG and raise HDL; however, combined use with statins may raise the risk of myositis
- Bile acid-binding resins (cholestyramine, colesevelam) lower cholesterol levels by binding bile acids and cholesterol in the intestinal tract and increasing their excretion
- Recheck fasting lipid levels 3–4 months after intervention

PROGNOSIS & COMPLICATIONS

- Hyperlipidemia is a strong risk factor for atherosclerosis
- Reducing LDL cholesterol is useful in both primary and secondary prevention of coronary arterial disease
- Lifestyle changes, in addition to drug therapy, are extremely important in the management of hyperlipidemia
- When starting a statin, liver function tests should be monitored at initiation and 3 months thereafter

Coronary Artery Disease

INTRODUCTION

- Coronary artery disease (CAD) is the most common and most life-threatening illness in the United States, causing more deaths and economic costs than any other condition
- It has become the most common cause of death worldwide
- Classically occurs secondary to atherosclerotic plaque formation, which results in artery narrowing and decreased myocardial oxygen supply
- Other causes are rare but include infection (e.g., syphilis), inflammatory disorders (e.g., rheumatic vasculitis), congenital anomalies, and coronary artery aneurysm

ETIOLOGY, EPIDEMIOLOGY, & RISK FACTORS

- Myocardial ischemia is due to an imbalance between oxygen supply and demand
  - Decreased oxygen supply may occur due to decreased arterial oxygen content, decreased coronary blood flow, decreased cardiac output, arterial stenosis, arterial vasospasm, arterial thrombi, endothelial dysfunction, and decreased diastolic perfusion pressure
  - Increased oxygen demand/consumption is due to increased myocardial workload and may be caused by increased ventricular wall tension and increased heart rate or contractility
- Major risk factors include personal or family history of CAD, older age, diabetes mellitus, hypertension, tobacco use, male sex, and hyperlipidemia
- Nonconventional risk factors include elevated small, dense LDL particles, lipoprotein (a), homocysteine, C-reactive protein, fibrinogen, and others
- Atherosclerotic plaque formation is a complex interaction involving lipid-laden macrophages (foam cells), smooth muscle proliferation, and growth factors
  - Initiation of atherosclerosis involves accumulation of lipoprotein particles in the intimal layer of arteries and is associated with inflammatory processes, foam cell formation, and smooth muscle cell proliferation
  - Impairment of endothelium-dependent vasodilatation (endothelial dysfunction) and arterial lumen narrowing results, leading to impaired coronary blood flow

PATIENT PRESENTATION

- May be asymptomatic, especially in diabetics, women, and the elderly
- Chest pain is the most common presenting symptom
  - Usually left-sided
  - May radiate to arms, neck, jaw, shoulders, or back
  - Pain is often characterized as "crushing" or a "pressure"
- Dyspnea is another common symptom, especially in women
- Other associating symptoms may include nausea, vomiting, diaphoresis, lightheadedness, or fatigue
- Physical exam is generally not useful (may have S3, S4, systolic murmur, or CHF)
- Hypertension or hypotension may be present
- Arrhythmias may occur

DIFFERENTIAL DX

- Stable angina
- Unstable angina
- Non-ST elevation MI
- ST elevation MI
- Noncardiac atherosclerotic disease
  - Carotid artery disease
  - Stroke or transient ischemic attack
  - Peripheral vascular disease
  - Renal artery disease
  - Aortic aneurysm
  - Arteritis
- Sudden cardiac death

DIAGNOSTIC EVALUATION

- History is an important component in the evaluation for CAD
- EKG may be abnormal, including ST segment changes, T-wave abnormalities, and/or presence of Q waves
- Echocardiography is indicated to evaluate left ventricular systolic and diastolic function and valves
- Stress testing is used to evaluate the extent of CAD and the risk for MI in symptomatic patients
  - Exercise stress testing is the preferred method
  - Pharmacologic stress testing is used in patients who cannot exercise (e.g., arthritic disease, peripheral vascular disease, pulmonary disease)
  - Imaging (thallium, technetium, or echocardiography) is generally used with stress testing to increase the sensitivity and specificity of the stress test
- Coronary angiography is the gold standard to document significant CAD and assess the need for revascularization; it should be considered if the diagnosis is uncertain and in high-risk patients
- Electron beam CT scan or CT angiography may have a role in detecting and determining the extent of coronary artery disease

TREATMENT & MANAGEMENT

- Patients with unstable symptoms require immediate evaluation and treatment
  - Attention to airway, breathing, and circulation
  - Have the patient chew an aspirin (unless contraindicated)
- Risk factor modification is an important initial component of treatment, including diet, exercise, smoking cessation, strict control of diabetes and hypertension, and treatment of hyperlipidemia
- Medical therapy is indicated in patients with known CAD
  - Aspirin: Inhibits platelet aggregation
  - Beta-blockers: Decrease myocardial oxygen demand
  - ACE inhibitors: Control hypertension by afterload reduction
  - Nitrates: Increase coronary blood flow and reduce preload
  - Lipid-lowering agents: Have been shown to reduce myocardial events
- Interventional treatments are indicated for significant CAD to provide symptomatic relief; however, they have not been proven to reduce the risk of subsequent myocardial infarction
  - Angioplasty (with or without stenting) is indicated to relieve angina in patients with significant coronary disease (>70% occlusion of an epicardial coronary vessel)
  - Coronary artery bypass grafting: Has only been shown to be beneficial for left main disease, proximal left anterior descending artery disease, triple vessel disease, left ventricular dysfunction, and severe myocardial ischemia

PROGNOSIS & COMPLICATIONS

- Prognostic factors include left ventricular ejection fraction, severity of CAD and ischemia, and functional status
- Aggressive primary and secondary prevention is crucial to lower morbidity and mortality
- 14% of patients with newly diagnosed angina pectoris progress to unstable angina, MI, or death within 1 year
- Cardiac rehabilitation decreases hospitalization rate but has not been shown to improve mortality
- Other sequelae include congestive heart failure, valvular heart disease, and arrhythmias

Orthostatic Hypotension

INTRODUCTION

- Orthostatic hypotension is usually defined as:
  - Decrease in systolic blood pressure of at least 20 mmHg
  - Decrease in diastolic pressure of at least 10 mmHg
  - Signs of cerebral hypoperfusion when adjusting to an upright position
- May be asymptomatic
- Causes significant disability in the elderly

ETIOLOGY, EPIDEMIOLOGY, & RISK FACTORS

- Blood pressure can be altered by many variables; in orthostatic hypotension, blood pressure is altered by decreased effective venous volume/return
- Causes of decreased venous return can be categorized into two groups:
  - Decreased circulatory volume (e.g., bleeding, dehydration, third space losses)
  - Decreased vasomotor tone (e.g., autonomic nervous system failure, vasodilation due to sepsis, adrenal insufficiency, vasodilator drugs)
- Autonomic dysfunction, severe reduction in circulatory volume, or profound vasodilation beyond the ability of the autonomic nervous system to compensate causes orthostatic hypotension and cerebral hypoperfusion, which leads to dizziness and syncope
- It is believed that as many as 20% of patients over 65 have postural hypotension
- The most common cause in the elderly is antihypertensive medications
- Other etiologies include volume depletion, anemia, adrenal insufficiency, and hypothyroidism

PATIENT PRESENTATION

- Lightheadedness, dizziness
- Dimming or loss of vision
- Diaphoresis
- Diminished hearing
- Pallor
- Weakness
- Frank syncope may occur
- Aggravation of orthostatic hypotension may occur by autonomic stresses, such as meals, hot baths, and exercise

DIFFERENTIAL DX

- Medications (e.g., diuretics, antihypertensives, tranquilizers)
- Alcohol use
- Various medical disorders (e.g., diabetes, amyloidosis, renal failure)
- Metabolic diseases (e.g., vitamin B_{12} deficiency, porphyria, Fabry's disease, Tangenier disease)
- Primary disorders of the autonomic nervous system (e.g., Shy-Drager syndrome), Parkinson's disease
- Secondary neurogenic disorders (e.g., aging, Guillain-Barré syndrome, rheumatoid arthritis, SLE, Eaton-Lambert syndrome, multiple sclerosis)

DIAGNOSTIC EVALUATION

- History and physical examination
  - Review medications, over-the-counter drugs, and alternative medicines
  - Assess for orthostasis; some data suggest that the clinical definition of orthostasis (decline in systolic blood pressure of at least 20 mmHg within 3 minutes of standing) may not be as appropriate as a 1-minute value, particularly for older persons
  - Consider using the Hallpike-Dix maneuvers of head and neck rotation to elicit symptoms and nystagmus
  - Evaluate for bleeding, diarrhea, prolonged vomiting, careful drug history, diabetes, neurologic diseases (e.g., Parkinson's disease), family history of pertinent differential diagnoses, prior episodes of syncope, valvular heart disease, and others
  - Perform a complete physical exam of the heart and peripheral vessels, neurologic system, and pupils
- Laboratory studies may include complete blood count, electrolytes, urinalysis, blood culture, blood type and cross for possible transfusion, and adrenal evaluation
- Consider tilt table testing in equivocal cases

TREATMENT & MANAGEMENT

- Discontinue offending drugs, if possible
- Replete fluids and electrolytes, as necessary
  - Consider a high-salt diet (10–20 g/day) in patients with inadequate blood volume
- Elastic pressure stockings and elevation of the head of the bed may be useful
- Fludrocortisone and hydrocortisone in adrenal insufficiency
  - Potassium supplement is necessary with chronic fludrocortisone use
- Administer sympathomimetic medications in patients with autonomic failure
  - Midodrine is a prodrug that is converted in the body to desglymidodrine; both are active on the arterioles and venules
  - Unlike ephedrine and methylphenidate and other amphetamines, midodrine does not cross the blood-brain barrier and does not provoke CNS side effects
  - The most common side effects of midodrine are piloerection, scalp pruritus, and paresthesias; other side effects include urinary retention, chills, and supine hypertension

PROGNOSIS & COMPLICATIONS

- Orthostatic hypotension and syncope are among the most common causes of falls in elderly
- May result in hypoperfusion and ischemic organ damage (e.g., ischemic stroke, MI)

Bacterial Endocarditis

INTRODUCTION

- Infective endocarditis is usually of bacterial etiology, it but can also be caused by infections with chlamydia, rickettsia, mycoplasmas, and fungi
- Bacterial endocarditis is an infection of the endocardium that has 4 primary components:
  - Cardiac involvement (murmur, abscess, congestive heart failure)
  - Systemic inflammation (fever, fatigue, rheumatologic symptoms)
  - Embolic phenomenon (stroke, mycotic aneurysms, renal and splenic emboli)
  - Immune complex disease (glomerulonephritis, Osler nodes, Roth spots)
- Annual incidence is 2-6 cases per 100,000 patients per year; however, the incidence in patients with mitral valve prolapse is 100 cases per 100,000 patients per year

ETIOLOGY, EPIDEMIOLOGY, & RISK FACTORS

- Native valve endocarditis (NVE): >70% of cases are caused by streptococci and *S. aureus*
  - Although rheumatic fever was historically considered a major predisposing factor, currently, mitral valve prolapse, aortic sclerosis, and bicuspid aortic valve are the most frequent underlying causes of NVE in the United States
  - Less common bacterial causes are the HACEK group (*Haemophilus, Actinobacillus, Corynebacterium, Eikenella, Kingella*), other gram-negative aerobic bacilli, enterococci, meningococci, and gonococci
- Prosthetic valve endocarditis (PVE): >50% caused by *S. aureus* and *S. epidermidis*
  - Infection within 2 months of surgery is classified as early PVE: gram-negative bacilli and *Corynebacterium* (diphtheroids) account for about one-third of early PVE cases
  - Infection after 2 months of surgery is considered late PVE: *S. aureus* and *S. epidermidis* account for less than half of late PVE cases; streptococci cause about 25%
- *S. aureus* is the most common cause in IV drug users (>50% of cases); the next most common pathogens are streptococci and enterococci
  - The tricuspid valve is more frequently affected
  - Septic pulmonary emboli are common (occurs in 3/4 of patients with tricuspid involvement)
- Median age has recently increased from 30–40 years to 50–69 years

PATIENT PRESENTATION

- Fever is present in more than 95% of cases
- Nonspecific symptoms (e.g., weakness, weight loss, night sweats)
- Audible heart murmur occurs in more than 85% of cases
- Splenomegaly (25–60% of cases)
- Petechiae (20–40%)
- Neurologic deficits (25–35%)
- Osler nodes (10–25%)
- Splinter hemorrhages (10–30%)
- Musculoskeletal manifestations (25–45%)
- Major embolic episodes (>30%)
- Roth spots (<5%)
- Janeway lesions (<5%)
- Clubbing (10–20%)

DIFFERENTIAL DX

- Atrial myxoma
- Infection elsewhere (e.g., abscess, osteomyelitis) with unrelated heart murmur
- Vasculitis
- Immune complex disease
- Serum sickness
- Drug allergy
- Infected intravascular device
- Pericarditis and myocarditis
- Nonbacterial thrombotic endocarditis

DIAGNOSTIC EVALUATION

- Echocardiography is necessary to evaluate cardiac valves and identify vegetations
  - Transesophageal echocardiogram offers higher sensitivity and specificity compared with transthoracic echocardiogram
- Laboratory testing includes blood cultures, complete blood count, erythrocyte sedimentation rate (ESR), urinalysis, chest X-ray, and electrocardiogram (EKG)
  - Take 2–3 blood cultures from separate sites
  - Duke Criteria for diagnosis: Probable diagnosis requires 2 major criteria OR 1 major criterion and 3 minor criteria OR 5 minor criteria; possible diagnosis requires 1 major criterion and 1 minor criterion OR 3 minor criteria
- Major criteria: Typical micro-organism from 2 separate blood cultures (e.g., *S. viridans*, *S. bovis*, HACEK group, community-acquired *S. aureus*, *Enterococcus*) or persistently positive blood cultures for any micro-organism; evidence of endocardial involvement; vegetation on echocardiogram; oscillating intracardiac mass on valve or supporting structures or in the path of regurgitant jets; perivalvular abscess; new valvular regurgitation
- Minor criteria: Predisposing heart condition; IV drug use; fever; vascular phenomena (e.g., arterial embolism, septic pulmonary infarcts, mycotic aneurysm, Janeway lesions); immunologic phenomena (e.g., Osler nodes, Roth spots, glomerulonephritis, rheumatoid factor), echocardiogram findings not meeting major criterion, microbiologic evidence (e.g., positive blood culture but not meeting major criterion above)

TREATMENT & MANAGEMENT

- Hospitalization is usually required for initial treatment with IV antibiotics
- Begin organism-specific antibiotics as soon as cultures and sensitivities are available
  - IV antibiotics are recommended over oral drugs
  - Antibiotic combinations may produce a more rapid clearance of bacteremia but do not affect overall mortality
  - Selection of antibiotics should be based on susceptibility tests, and treatment should be monitored clinically and by antimicrobial blood levels
  - The penicillins, often in combination with gentamicin, remain cornerstones for therapy of NVE due to susceptible streptococci (use vancomycin for patients with penicillin allergy)
  - Most regimens are continued for 4–6 weeks
- Obtain blood cultures during the early phase of therapy to ensure eradication
- In patients with mechanical valves, anticoagulation may be indicated
- Aspirin may decrease the growth of vegetative lesions and prevent cerebral emboli
- Cardiac surgery may be required if infection cannot be controlled medically

PROGNOSIS & COMPLICATIONS

- Untreated bacterial endocarditis is uniformly fatal
- Despite successful treatment, sterile emboli or even valve rupture can occur up to 1 year later
- Relapse following treatment usually occurs within 4–8 weeks
- Recurrence of endocarditis after 6 weeks in patients with native valves usually represents a new infection rather than a relapse
- Outcomes are determined by organism involved, amount of valvular destruction, size of vegetations and potential for embolization, and the length of treatment and choice of antibiotics
- Time to blood culture negativity takes 3–7 days in most cases

Respiratory

Cough

INTRODUCTION

- Cough is the most common symptom for which patients visit primary care physicians
- Coughing is an important defense mechanism that protects the airway from aspiration of excessive secretions and foreign material
  - It is generally reflexive but can be initiated (and sometimes suppressed) voluntarily
- Cough can be a symptom of a variety of underlying conditions
- Categorized as acute (lasting less than 3 weeks) or chronic (lasting more than 8 weeks)
  - Acute cough is most frequently due to the common cold
  - Chronic cough is often simultaneously due to more than one condition; the most common causes are postnasal drip syndrome, asthma, and gastroesophageal reflux disease (GERD)

ETIOLOGY, EPIDEMIOLOGY, & RISK FACTORS

- Cough involves a complex reflex arc that begins with the stimulation of airway receptors
  - The afferent limb involves receptors in the large- to medium-sized airways and pharynx, which can be triggered by mechanical, chemical, and thermal stimuli
  - The vagus nerve transmits signals to a discrete cough center in the medulla and initiates the efferent limb via the vagus, phrenic, and spinal motor nerves to the expiratory, laryngeal, and pharyngeal muscles
- Cough begins with a deep inspiration followed by a compressive phase of high intrathoracic pressure, contraction of expiratory muscles, and closure of the glottis
- Abrupt opening of the glottis results in rapid airflow and sudden expulsion of air, which results in removal of debris and secretions from the airway
- Associated symptoms may include nasal discharge, malaise, fever, chills, night sweats, sputum production, congestion, headache or facial pain, or a recent history of upper respiratory infection
- Triggers include cold air, dust, smoke, upper respiratory infections, and allergens

PATIENT PRESENTATION

- Note time course (i.e., acute vs. chronic)
- Note quality (productive vs. dry; barking, honking, or brassy)
- Note general appearance (cyanosis or pallor)
- Note signs of respiratory distress (tachypnea or accessory muscle use)
- Barrel chest
- Nasal polyps
- Tracheal deviation
- Signs of atopic disease
- Sinus tenderness, purulent posterior pharyngeal drainage, and halitosis
- Decreased breath sounds
- Prolonged expiratory phase/wheezing
- Crackles, rales, and rhonchi
- Clubbing
- Evidence of congestive heart failure
- Diffuse and displaced cardiac impulse
- Lower extremity edema

DIFFERENTIAL DX

Acute cough
- Upper respiratory infection
- Bronchitis or pneumonia
- Sinusitis
- Pharyngitis or laryngitis
- Reactive airway disease
- Irritation or allergy
- Foreign body

Chronic cough
- Asthma, bronchitis, sinusitis
- GERD
- Postinfectious
- Bronchiectasis/cystic fibrosis
- Vocal cord dysfunction
- Medications (e.g., captopril)
- Aspiration/foreign body
- Tuberculosis
- Lung or upper airway tumor

DIAGNOSTIC EVALUATION

- Chest X-ray may be indicated if there are concerning symptoms
  - Infiltrates suggest pneumonia, pneumonitis, or tuberculosis
  - Bronchiectasis suggests cystic fibrosis, immunodeficiency, ciliary dyskinesia, or chronic aspiration
  - Volume loss may indicate aspiration of a foreign body
  - Hyperinflation suggests asthma or chronic obstructive pulmonary disease (COPD)
  - Mediastinal lymphadenopathy suggests tuberculosis, fungal infection, or malignancy
- Testing for tuberculosis (e.g., purified protein derivative [PPD]) as indicated
- Consider pulmonary function testing
- Blood testing may include complete blood count or blood cultures
- Consider sputum gram stain and culture
  - Eosinophils suggest asthma or a hypersensitivity reaction
  - Polymorphonuclear cells suggest acute infection
  - Routine or special cultures may be indicated based on likely pathogens
- Consider testing for GERD
- Consider sweat chloride test if suspect cystic fibrosis
- Consider bronchoscopy to identify subtle pulmonary etiologies

TREATMENT & MANAGEMENT

- Emergency management, including possible intubation, may be necessary if signs or symptoms of respiratory distress are present
- The key to success is to rule out serious causes and to identify the etiology of the cough
- Treat the underlying cause of cough rather than the cough itself
- Treatment is often empiric and based on history
- An empiric therapeutic trial for asthma, GERD, postnasal drip, sinusitis, or bronchitis may be advisable
- Speech therapy is very helpful for vocal cord dysfunction or habit cough
- Cough suppression medication should generally be avoided but may assist with sleep
- Over-the-counter therapies are of little value
- Smoking cessation

PROGNOSIS & COMPLICATIONS

- Complete resolution is achieved in 80–90% of cases
- A persistent, nonproductive cough caused by ACE inhibitors (e.g., captopril) must not be overlooked because it is both concerning and annoying to the patient and can be remedied by adjusting the medication regimen

Hemoptysis

INTRODUCTION

- Hemoptysis is the expectoration of blood or blood-tinged sputum from the lower respiratory tract (i.e., below the vocal cords)
- Distinguish hemoptysis from other sites of bleeding (nose, mouth, throat, GI tract)
  - It can be particularly difficult to discern hemoptysis from hematemesis
- Massive hemoptysis (expectoration of >100–600 mL within 24 hours), though uncommon, is a medical emergency that may be fatal due to asphyxiation or respiratory failure
- Although the mortality of patients who present with acute hemoptysis is low, the amount of blood expectorated is a major determinant of morbidity, while the underlying etiology remains an important determinant of long-term survival

ETIOLOGY, EPIDEMIOLOGY, & RISK FACTORS

- The lungs have a dual blood supply from the pulmonary and bronchial arteries
  - The pulmonary arterial circulation is a high-compliance, low-pressure system that is responsible for gas exchange; the bronchial arteries (branches of the aorta) are a high-pressure system that provide nutrients to the lung parenchyma and major airways
  - Most cases of hemoptysis are caused by disruptions of the bronchial arterial tree
- The most common etiologies include bronchitis, lung cancer, pneumonia, tuberculosis, bronchiectasis, and cryptogenic
  - Tuberculosis is a leading cause in developing countries and should be considered in immigrants from countries with a high prevalence
  - Even after careful investigation, as many as 30% of cases may not have an identified cause; these cases are classified as cryptogenic hemoptysis

PATIENT PRESENTATION

- Blood-streaked sputum
- Gross blood in absence of any sputum
- Stridor or wheezing may indicate a foreign body, endobronchial tumor, or tracheolaryngeal obstruction
- Associated hematuria may suggest a pulmonary-renal syndrome
- Pleuritic chest pain
- Dyspnea may suggest congestive heart failure due to mitral stenosis
- Weight loss may suggest a neoplasm
- Petechiae or bleeding from other sites may suggest hematologic disease
- Fever suggests infection

DIFFERENTIAL DX

- Infectious: Bronchitis, pneumonia, lung abscess, fungal/ parasitic infection, tuberculosis
- Bronchiectasis
- Neoplasms: Primary lung cancer, bronchial adenoma, metastatic lung cancer
- Cardiovascular: Pulmonary embolus, mitral stenosis, arteriovenous malformation
- Vasculitis: Behçet's disease, Wegener's granulomatosis, Goodpasture syndrome, SLE, antiphospholipid syndrome
- Hematologic
- Traumatic
- Cryptogenic
- Freebase cocaine use
- Cystic fibrosis

DIAGNOSTIC EVALUATION

- Establish that the source of expectorated blood originates from the lower respiratory tract, rather than the upper gastrointestinal tract (hematemesis) or upper respiratory tract (epistaxis)
- History and physical examination should investigate for underlying pulmonary or cardiovascular disease, risk factors for lung cancer, bleeding tendencies or anticoagulant therapy, recent trauma, and occupational exposures
- Laboratory studies include a complete blood count, coagulation studies, urinalysis and renal function tests
  - Consider sputum culture for acid-fast bacillus and cytology, if clinically indicated
- A standard chest X-ray should be obtained in all patients with hemoptysis
- Nonsmokers who present with mild hemoptysis and symptoms of an upper respiratory infection may not require further workup
- Bronchoscopy and/or chest CT scan may be indicated, particularly if the chest X-ray is abnormal, if hemoptysis persists longer than 1–2 weeks or the volume of hemoptysis increases, and in smokers older than 40
  - Bronchoscopy allows direct visualization of the airways, lateralization of bleed, and collection of samples for histology and microbiology
  - Chest CT scan is helpful to assess malignant lesions and bronchiectasis

TREATMENT & MANAGEMENT

- Mild hemoptysis associated with an acute respiratory tract infection and a normal chest X-ray may be treated with outpatient antibiotic therapy, inhaled bronchodilators, and/or antitussives
- Massive hemoptysis may require stabilization of the airway, monitoring of oxygenation, intubation for acute respiratory failure, correction of coagulopathy or thrombocytopenia, and/or volume resuscitation
  - Once the patient is stabilized, find and control the bleeding site
  - Protect the nonbleeding lung by placing the bleeding lung in a dependent position (i.e., prevent spillage of blood into the nonbleeding lung by placing the patient on his or her side)
- Bronchoscopy can be used to visualize and treat the source of hemoptysis via balloon tamponade, lavage with iced saline, application of topical therapies, or coagulating laser phototherapy
- Arteriographic embolization can be used as treatment or as a bridge to surgery
- Surgery is an option for patients with refractory bleeding with adequate pulmonary reserve

PROGNOSIS & COMPLICATIONS

- Hemoptysis is usually a self-limited process with a benign etiology
- Massive hemoptysis is responsible for less than 5% of all cases, but mortality may be as high as 85%
- Morbidity and mortality is significantly greater when emergent surgery for persistent massive bleeding is necessary
- Arteriographic embolization can achieve control of bleeding in approximately 90% of patients, with a relapse rate of approximately 20%
- The majority of patients with cryptogenic hemoptysis have a good prognosis and experience resolution of symptoms within 6 months

Dyspnea

INTRODUCTION

- Dyspnea is one of the most common symptoms encountered in clinical practice
- It is a subjective awareness of breathing discomfort
- It is one of the cardinal symptoms of cardiac and pulmonary disease but may also result from abnormalities of the chest wall, neurologic disorders, and anxiety
- A marked acute change in the severity of dyspnea should be taken seriously as this may be a manifestation of a life-threatening underlying condition
- Dyspnea may be acute, chronic, or acute-on-chronic; this entry focuses on chronic dyspnea

ETIOLOGY, EPIDEMIOLOGY, & RISK FACTORS

- The mechanism of dyspnea is poorly and incompletely understood
  - There is no single neural pathway or brain center for dyspnea; it is believed to arise from multiple receptors (muscle and joint receptors, chemoreceptors, vagal afferents, and others)
- Increasing exercise intensifies dyspnea
- There is no precise data on the prevalence of dyspnea
- In the Framingham Study, the prevalence of dyspnea in an adult population was 6-27%, depending on gender and age groups
- Many disorders can result in dyspnea: In a study of patients who presented to pulmonary clinics with chronic dyspnea, 75% had respiratory disease (primarily lower respiratory tract etiologies), 10% cardiac, 5% gastroesophageal reflux disease (GERD), 5% deconditioning, and 5% psychogenic
  - Among the respiratory diseases, 40% of patients had asthma, 18% had chronic obstructive pulmonary disease (COPD), 18% had interstitial lung disease, and 3% had bronchiectasis

PATIENT PRESENTATION

- Determine the duration of dyspnea (acute or chronic) and rapidity of onset
- Note whether symptoms occur on a regular basis (e.g., COPD, interstitial lung disease, pulmonary hypertension) or are intermittent (e.g., asthma, congestive heart failure)
- Assess the rate of progression over the past months or years to determine workup and management
- Note associated symptoms of left heart failure (paroxysmal nocturnal dyspnea, orthopnea, S3, S4), right heart failure (loud P2, peripheral edema, jugular venous distension, hepatomegaly), bronchiectasis (purulent sputum, weight loss), obstructive airway disease (wheezing, chest tightness, recurrent bronchitis), pulmonary thromboembolism (acute dyspnea, pleuritic chest pain, hemoptysis, DVT), neuromuscular weakness, or rheumatologic symptoms (arthritis, skin rash)

DIFFERENTIAL DX

- Obstructive pulmonary disease: Asthma, COPD, bronchiectasis, pneumonia
- Restrictive pulmonary disease: Interstitial lung diseases, neuromuscular disease, myopathies, obesity, kyphoscoliosis
- Cardiac disease: Left heart failure, valvular disease, pericardial disease, acute coronary syndrome
- Pulmonary vascular disease: Acute or chronic pulmonary embolism, pulmonary hypertension
- Gastroesophageal reflux disease
- Psychogenic
- Malignancy

DIAGNOSTIC EVALUATION

- After a thorough history and physical examination, a chest X-ray is indicated in almost all patients
- Consider pulmonary function tests if lung disease is suspected to differentiate between obstructive and restrictive disease
  - Asthma is a common diagnosis; more than 20% improvement in forced expiratory volume in 1 second (FEV1) upon acute administration of bronchodilators generally indicates a diagnosis of asthma
- If suspect cardiac ischemia, consider electrocardiogram (EKG), stress test, or coronary angiography
- In patients with normal pulmonary function testing, normal chest X-ray, and no heart disease:
  - Consider echocardiogram to evaluate for pulmonary vascular disease (e.g., pulmonary hypertension, chronic pulmonary thromboembolism); further testing may include right heart catheterization, ventilation/perfusion (V/Q) scan, or pulmonary angiography
  - Consider neurology evaluation if suspect neuromuscular disease
- A 6-minute walk test is a simple but useful test to determine the need for oxygen supplementation or to assess response to therapy or disease progression

TREATMENT & MANAGEMENT

- Attention to airway, breathing, and circulation; administer supplemental oxygen as needed
- Treatment depends on the underlying condition
- If patient continues to experience dyspnea despite optimal treatment of the underlying disease, consider energy-conservation strategies (e.g., walk more slowly to be able to walk for a longer time), breathing techniques (e.g., pursed-lip breathing in COPD to reduce early airways closure), strengthening exercises for the respiratory muscles, and appropriate nutrition in cachectic patients
- Anxiolytics and narcotics to alleviate dyspnea is still controversial, except in very advanced disease where they are used as palliative measures; these drugs should only be used as a last resort and with extreme caution, as they may precipitate hypercapnic respiratory failure and hypotension

PROGNOSIS & COMPLICATIONS

- The prognosis depends on the underlying disease condition
- For many diseases (e.g., congestive heart failure, COPD, pulmonary hypertension) there are convincing studies that patients with more severe dyspnea (as determined by history, 6-minute walk test, or cardiopulmonary exercise test) have a worse prognosis
- Consider referral to specialists when necessary

Solitary Pulmonary Nodule

INTRODUCTION

- A solitary pulmonary nodule, also called a "coin lesion," is a lesion seen on chest X-ray or CT scan that measures less than 3 cm in its smallest diameter (as opposed to a mass, which measures larger than 3 cm) and is surrounded by normal lung tissue
- This is one of the common radiographic abnormalities and is typically discovered as an incidental finding
- Malignant, isolated pulmonary nodules without spread to lymph nodes or distant sites (i.e., $T_1N_0M_0$) have a 75% 5-year survival with surgical excision (overall 5-year survival rate for lung cancer is just 15%); thus, appropriate workup and treatment is essential

ETIOLOGY, EPIDEMIOLOGY, & RISK FACTORS

- The three most common etiologies are malignant neoplasm (e.g., primary lung cancer), granuloma (e.g., lung infection), and benign lesions (e.g., hamartoma)
- Nodules measure 5–8 mm before they become noticeable on a chest X-ray; depending on its growth, 10 years or more may ensue before the nodule becomes clinically apparent
- Growth of the nodule depends on the etiology: Bronchial carcinoid has one of the slowest doubling times (400 days), and oat cell carcinoma has the fastest (30 days); adenocarcinoma, the most common malignant cause, has a doubling time of 180 days; infectious lesions can double in less than 20 days
- Approximately 150,000 cases are detected on chest X-rays or CT scans every year; of these, less than 50% are malignant; however, the frequency of major diagnoses varies significantly depending on the population
- Risk factors for malignant lesions include older age (less than 3% of all patients diagnosed with lung cancer are younger than 39; 50% are over 60) and a history of tobacco use (90% of lung cancer patients are smokers)
- Occupational exposures to asbestos or radon are additional risk factors
- There is a much higher proportion of benign nodules in areas where certain infections (e.g., fungal, tuberculosis, parasitic diseases) are endemic

PATIENT PRESENTATION

- Most nodules are detected incidentally
- Cough or hemoptysis may be associated with a solitary pulmonary nodule; however, hypoxemia, hypercapnia, shortness of breath, or any significant physiologic derangement should prompt evaluation for an alternative etiology
- Evaluate potential risk factors for malignancy (e.g., smoking, older age, personal or family history of malignancy) and cancer screening status (e.g., Pap smear, mammogram, testicular examination, colonoscopy)
- Hemoptysis may suggest tuberculosis, malignancy, or arteriovenous malformation
- Review exposure to asbestos, tuberculosis, endemic fungi, or parasitic diseases
- A complete physical examination should include evaluation for finger clubbing, lymphadenopathy, focal neurologic signs, or ascites

DIFFERENTIAL DX

- Primary lung cancer
  - Adenocarcinoma
  - Squamous cell carcinoma
- Metastatic lung cancer (usually present with multiple nodules)
- Carcinoid
- Infectious granuloma (e.g., tuberculosis, nocardiosis, *Aspergillus*, blastomycosis, histoplasmosis, coccidioidomycosis, parasitic)
- Hamartoma
- Lipoma
- Fibroma
- Arteriovenous malformation

DIAGNOSTIC EVALUATION

- Compare chest X-rays or CT scan with prior films to determine if the lesion has grown
  - The lesion is unlikely to be malignant if the doubling time is less than 20 days or more than 2 years
- Most patients require a chest CT scan
  - Unless contraindicated, contrast should be used for better visualization of mediastinal lymph nodes, vascular structures, pleural anatomy, and enhancement characteristics
  - High-resolution CT scan should not be performed, as this may miss small nodules
  - Whenever possible, three-dimensional volume reconstruction or thin cuts through the nodule should be used to follow-up smaller nodules
  - Positron emission tomography (PET) with ^{18}F-fluorodeoxyglucose (FDG) can be used as an additional tool for risk stratification; in patients with high clinical risk for lung cancer, it has sensitivity of nearly 97% and specificity of nearly 80%
- Radiographic features of malignancy include larger size, spiculation, location in the upper lobe, and absent, stippled, or eccentric calcification
- Lab studies are nonspecific
  - Severe anemia or ESR above 100 may indicate malignancy
  - No serologic markers are available for clinical purpose
  - Sputum cytology generally has low yield and is not used in clinical practice
  - Be sure to obtain baseline spirometry measurements

TREATMENT & MANAGEMENT

- In patients without risk factors, observation with serial CT scans is acceptable; if the lesion changes at all on subsequent radiographs, aggressive workup is indicated
- Resection of the lesion is indicated if it is noncalcified, fast growing, of suspicious morphology, or of large size AND the patient is a good operative candidate; otherwise, biopsy via fine needle or bronchoscopy should be attempted first (but this does not rule out cancer)
- Resection techniques include:
  - Video-assisted thoracoscopic surgery (VATS): As good as open thoracotomy for peripheral lesions; can be extended to open thoracotomy if necessary
  - Minithoracotomy
  - Thoracotomy: Allows for mediastinal and lymph node exploration
- There should be a low threshold for surgery; a malignant lesion could be deadly, and surgery is relatively benign in good surgical candidates

PROGNOSIS & COMPLICATIONS

- Most cases are benign
- While survival in lung cancer is dismal (overall 5-year survival rate is just 15%), an early-stage tumor smaller than 3 cm and without spread to lymph nodes or a distant site (i.e., $T_1N_0M_0$), is associated with a greater than 70% survival rate
- The majority of solitary pulmonary nodules larger than 2 cm are malignant; 50% of those measuring less than 2 cm are benign
- Follow-up CT scans done at 3, 6, 12, and 24 months with absence of growth over 2 years suggest a benign lesion, but the negative predictive value of such follow-up may be as low as 65%; serial CT scans for a total of 5 years may be more sensitive

COPD

INTRODUCTION

- Chronic obstructive pulmonary disease (COPD) is a progressive, irreversible airway obstruction that is usually caused by tobacco smoking
- Presents as one of two pathologic conditions: chronic bronchitis and emphysema
  - Chronic obstructive bronchitis is a disease of the conducting airways and terminal bronchioles; it is defined clinically as a productive cough lasting for 3 months per year for 2 consecutive years plus evidence of airway obstruction on pulmonary function testing
  - Emphysema is defined pathologically as the permanent enlargement of airspaces distal to the terminal bronchioles and destruction of parenchyma causing closure of small airways and loss of lung elasticity

ETIOLOGY, EPIDEMIOLOGY, & RISK FACTORS

- Pathologically, COPD affects the entirety of the respiratory tract
  - In the conducting airways, chronic bronchitis results from the irritant effects of smoke-induced expansion of the mucus-secreting glands
  - In the terminal bronchioles, there is increased airway resistance caused by smoke-induced lymphocytic airway wall inflammation
  - In the lung parenchyma, there is smoke-induced emphysematous lung destruction attributed to an imbalance of neutrophil, macrophage, and interstitial proteolytic enzymes that act on elastin and collagen in the gas exchange units
- Lung dysfunction results from airflow limitation (loss of elastic recoil, increased collapsibility, and narrowing of small airways) and impaired gas exchange (V/Q mismatch, alveolar destruction, increased dead space resulting in hypercarbia)
- Risk factors include cigarette smoking (accounts for more than 90% of cases), air pollution, occupational inhalation, and alpha$_1$-antitrypsin deficiency
- Not all smokers get COPD (only about 15%); there are genetic predispositions
- COPD is the 4th leading cause of death in the U.S., and the incidence and mortality rate are increasing; it is the 6th most common cause of death worldwide and increasing
- Causes 250,000 hospitalizations yearly

PATIENT PRESENTATION

- Patients usually have a combination of chronic bronchitis and emphysematous symptoms
  - Symptoms of bronchitis ("blue bloaters") include productive cough, dyspnea, fatigue, rhonchi, wheezes, cyanosis, hypoxia, obesity
  - Symptoms of emphysema include severe dyspnea, minimal cough, increased work of breathing, decreased air movement, prolonged expiration, accessory muscle use, barrel chest, pursed lip breathing, weight loss, "tripod" sitting, hyperresonance, minimal hypoxemia
- The course is frequently complicated by acute deteriorations in respiratory status, usually due to an acute respiratory irritant (e.g., viral or bacterial infection, environmental exposure)
  - Known as "acute exacerbation of COPD"
  - Defined clinically by increased cough, change in sputum quantity/quality, or worsening dyspnea

DIFFERENTIAL DX

- Congestive heart failure
- Asthma
- Bronchiectasis
- Pneumonia
- Pulmonary embolism
- Pulmonary vascular disease
- Bronchiolitis
- Toxic inhalations
- Cystic fibrosis
- Pneumothorax
- Gastroesophageal reflux disease

DIAGNOSTIC EVALUATION

- Pulmonary function testing showing an obstructive pattern is the gold standard for diagnosis
  - Decreased forced expiratory volume in 1 second (FEV1)/forced vital capacity (FVC) ratio (<70% predicted) is the best indicator of obstruction
  - Increased lung volumes (functional residual capacity [FRC], residual volume [RV], RV/total lung capacity [TLC] ratio) may occur due to airway obstruction, resulting in air trapping and hyperinflation
  - Decreased diffusing capacity is especially common in emphysema
- Chest X-ray may reveal flattened diaphragms, hyperinflation, bullae, increased lucency in the lungs, and a small heart; however, radiographic appearance does not correlate with the degree of lung dysfunction
- Arterial blood gas (ABG) analysis may reveal hypoxia (due to V/Q mismatch) and hypercarbia
- Complete blood count may reveal polycythemia secondary to chronic hypoxia
- Chest CT scan may reveal centrilobular emphysema and bullae
- In atypical presentations (e.g., young age), consider measuring alpha$_1$-antitrypsin levels

TREATMENT & MANAGEMENT

- Avoidance of cigarette smoking is the only way to slow disease progression
- Administer appropriate immunizations (pneumovax and yearly influenza vaccine)
- Medical management includes:
  - Bronchodilators: Anticholinergics are the preferred agents; long-acting beta-agonists decrease infections and improve symptoms
  - Oxygen: Continual or nighttime oxygen improves mortality and quality of life in patients with chronic hypoxemia
  - Antibiotics: Beneficial in exacerbations but not as prophylaxis
  - Corticosteroids: The role of inhaled steroids is unclear; few patients show improvement; systemic steroids are useful in acute exacerbations
  - Theophylline: Causes improvement in 20% of patients
  - Noninvasive positive pressure ventilation (biPAP) decreases the need for mechanical ventilation in acute exacerbations
- Lung volume reduction surgery and lung transplantation may benefit selected patients with end-stage disease

PROGNOSIS & COMPLICATIONS

- COPD causes significant morbidity in a large number of patients; however, the majority of deaths occur in patients with severe cases
- In most clinical situations, COPD is a manageable but not curable disease; lost lung function is rarely recoverable
- Inpatient hospitalization for acute exacerbations has 5-10% mortality rate
- Intubation and the need for mechanical ventilation increase mortality to above 20%
- Because of the concomitant risk factor of cigarette smoking, patients with COPD have an increased risk for lung cancer; studies are in progress to assess the potential benefits of various screening modalities (e.g., chest CT scan) to identify early-stage and potentially curable cancers, but so far, no validated screening recommendations have been made

Asthma

INTRODUCTION

- Asthma is a chronic inflammatory disorder of the airways characterized by 3 elements: Chronic airway inflammation, bronchial hyperreactivity to common triggers, and reversible airway obstruction
- Airway inflammation leads to symptoms of cough, wheezing, chest tightness, and shortness of breath, particularly at night or in the early morning
- Asthma remains one of a few diseases in the United States that is increasing in incidence in children and adults despite scientific advances in understanding and treatment
- Mortality has also been increasing, perhaps due to overreliance on bronchodilator drugs

ETIOLOGY, EPIDEMIOLOGY, & RISK FACTORS

- Asthma is considered a complex inflammatory disease of multifactorial origin
- Pathologic findings include a patchy loss of bronchial epithelium usually associated with eosinophil infiltration, contraction and hypertrophy of bronchial smooth muscles, bronchial mucosa edema and increased blood flow, bronchial gland hyperplasia with excessive secretion of thick mucus, and basement membrane thickening
- Numerous inflammatory cells work in conjunction in the pathogenesis of asthma; these include lymphocytes, mast cells, macrophages, eosinophils, and neutrophils
- Asthma can be categorized as extrinsic or intrinsic
  - Extrinsic asthma: Hypersensitivity to an allergen (e.g., pollen, dust mites)
  - Intrinsic asthma: Airway reactivity to a nonimmune trigger (e.g., exercise, cold air, aspirin, NSAIDs, beta-blockers, sulfites, irritant dusts, pollutants, infection, stress)
- Affects 5–10% of the population
- The cost of asthma is associated with both direct costs (e.g., medical care treatment) and indirect costs (e.g., missed days of work or school) and is estimated to exceed $12 billion yearly in the United States
- Half of cases have onset before age 10, but asthma can develop at any age
- Affected individuals often have a family history of asthma or atopic diseases

PATIENT PRESENTATION

- Cough
- Shortness of breath
- Chest tightness
- Expiratory wheezing or prolonged expirations
- Sputum production (mucorrhea)
- Nocturnal awakenings
- Lung overinflation with air, mucus, debris
- Sleep disturbance
- Tachycardia or tachypnea during episodes
- Severe acute exacerbations: Accessory muscle use, inability to speak in full sentences, decreased air movement, hyperinflation (increased anteroposterior diameter of the thorax), altered mental status (secondary to hypoxia), and pulsus paradoxus (fall in systolic blood pressure by 10 mmHg or more during inspiration)

DIFFERENTIAL DX

- COPD
- Congestive heart failure
- Pulmonary edema
- Laryngeal or vocal cord dysfunction
- Upper airway obstruction (e.g., tumor, croup, edema, foreign body)
- Drug-induced cough (e.g., ACE inhibitors)
- GERD
- Bronchiectasis
- Cystic fibrosis
- Pulmonary embolus
- Anaphylaxis/allergic reaction
- Bronchiolitis
- Upper airway disease (e.g., allergic rhinitis)
- Vascular ring, laryngeal web

DIAGNOSTIC EVALUATION

- Complete history and physical examination should be performed; most often, individuals presenting with symptoms consistent with asthma have a normal respiratory examination; occupational history should be carefully examined to explore possible workplace exposure
- Pulmonary function tests showing airway obstruction are the most objective diagnostic findings
  - Often reveals decreased FEV1 and FEV1/forced vital capacity (FVC) ratio, increased total lung capacity (TLC), and increased residual volume (RV)
  - FEV1 increases by at least 15% following bronchodilator therapy
- Peak expiratory flow rate (PEFR) measurements can be used to follow the course and severity of disease
  - 400–600 is normal; 100–300 is moderate exacerbation; <100 is severe exacerbation
- Chest X-ray may reveal hyperinflation or atelectasis
- Arterial blood gas (ABG) measurement may reveal respiratory alkalosis in mild exacerbations; as the patient tires from hyperventilation during severe attacks, the impending respiratory failure causes pCO_2 to progress to normal and then above normal
  - Hypoxemia and metabolic acidosis are signs of severe disease (due to poor oxygenation and ventilation/perfusion [V/Q] mismatching)
- Sputum culture may reveal increased eosinophils and secondary infection
- Measurement of bronchial hyperreactivity via a methacholine or exercise challenge test can be performed to diagnose questionable cases of asthma

TREATMENT & MANAGEMENT

- Avoid potential triggers
- Administer supplemental oxygen during acute attacks
- Mild, intermittent asthma (symptoms <2 times/week, peak flow >80% of normal, nocturnal symptoms <2 times/month): Treat with a short-acting, inhaled beta-agonist (albuterol) as needed
- Mild, persistent asthma (symptoms >2 times/week, peak flow 70-80% of normal), nocturnal symptoms 3-4 times/month): Treat with inhaled, low-dose corticosteroids (or leukotriene antagonist) and beta agonist inhaler as needed.
- Moderate, persistent asthma (daily symptoms, peak flow 60-70% of normal), nocturnal symptoms > once per week): Treat with inhaled steroids, leukotriene antagonists, and beta-agonists as needed.
- Severe, persistent asthma (frequent symptoms and exacerbations, peak flow <60%): Treat with high-dose corticosteroid (oral steroids may be necessary) and long-acting beta-agonist, along with albuterol inhaler as needed
  - Consider anti-IgE monoclonal antibody
- Acute exacerbations should be treated aggressively with beta-agonists, corticosteroids, and supplemental oxygen to maintain adequate oxygenation

PROGNOSIS & COMPLICATIONS

- Follows an episodic course with acute exacerbations separated by symptom-free periods
- The majority of patients will respond to therapy, which is aimed at reducing airway inflammation to preserve lung function
- Assure proper technique and regular administration of controller medications if the patient is not responding to conventional therapy
- The goal of therapy is to minimize disruption of everyday life
- Poorly controlled asthma can lead to airway remodeling with progressive loss of lung function and possible death
- Routine office spirometry should be followed yearly in asymptomatic patients and more frequently, if indicated

Pneumonia

INTRODUCTION

- A lower respiratory tract infection of the lung parenchyma, which results in inflammation, alveolar exudates, and lung consolidation
  - Community-acquired pneumonia (CAP): Occurs in nonhospitalized patients
  - Hospital-acquired pneumonia (HAP): Onset occurs 2–3 days after admission
  - Ventilator-associated pneumonia: Develops >48 hours after intubation
- Often distinguished by "typical" or "atypical" presentation, but the clinical picture alone is not sufficient for diagnosis of the microorganism or treatment
- Pneumonia is the 6th most common cause of death in the United States and the most common cause of infection-related mortality

ETIOLOGY, EPIDEMIOLOGY, & RISK FACTORS

- Microorganisms causing CAP include *Streptococcus pneumoniae*, *Haemophilus influenzae*, *Mycoplasma pneumoniae*, *Moraxella catarrhalis*, *Chlamydia pneumoniae*, *Legionella*, adenovirus, respiratory syncytial virus, influenza, and parainfluenza
- HAP is commonly caused by gram-negative enteric bacilli and *S. aureus*
  - Ventilator-associated pneumonia is also caused by these, particularly pseudomonas
- Patients treated with high-dose steroids for prolonged periods are susceptible to fungi (particularly aspergillosis) and *Pneumocystis carinii*
- Risk factors include smoking, alcoholism, immunodeficiencies (e.g., HIV, neutropenia), granulomatous disorders, structural lung diseases, and predisposing conditions (e.g., stroke)
- 3–4 million cases occur yearly in the United States, resulting in 500,000 hospitalizations and 45,000 deaths
- There is increased incidence during the winter months
- Mortality of CAP patients who need to be hospitalized is 14% (<1% mortality in those not hospitalized)
- HAP is the leading cause of nosocomial death (20–50% mortality)

PATIENT PRESENTATION

- "Typical" pneumonia is characterized by acute or subacute onset of fever, dyspnea, and productive cough
  - Constitutional signs include rigors, sweats, chills, chest discomfort, fatigue, myalgia, anorexia, headache, abdominal pain, and nausea and vomiting
  - Physical exam may reveal tachypnea, tachycardia, egophony, dullness to percussion, rhonchi, and hypoxia
- "Atypical" pneumonia is generally of more gradual onset and presents with a dry cough, headache, malaise, and minimal lung signs
  - Occurs primarily due to infection with *Mycoplasma*, *Legionella*, or chlamydia
- Patients with imparied neurologic status or severe reflux may aspirate

DIFFERENTIAL DX

- Upper respiratory infection
- Asthma or chronic obstructive pulmonary disease (COPD) exacerbation
- Pulmonary embolism
- Myocardial infarction
- Congestive heart failure
- Lung cancer
- Vasculitis
- Sarcoidosis
- Occupational exposure
- Goodpasture's disease
- Hypersensitivity pneumonitis
- Atelectasis

DIAGNOSTIC EVALUATION

- History and physical examination
- Pulse oximetry
- Chest X-ray ranges from diffuse patchy infiltrates to lobar consolidation
  - May reveal bilateral or unilateral changes
  - May show pleural effusion or cavitation
- Sputum gram stain and culture is generally indicated but has poor sensitivity and specificity
- Blood cultures are positive in 10% of cases
- Serologies for *Legionella*, *Mycoplasma*, and chlamydia may be tested
  - Testing for *Legionella* urinary antigen has better sensitivity and specificity than serology
- Consider HIV testing in young patients with repeated pneumonia
- Hospital-acquired pneumonia may require bronchoscopy with lavage to identify organism and guide management (blood and sputum cultures are often nondiagnostic)

TREATMENT & MANAGEMENT

- The Pneumonia Severity Index can be used to determine if hospitalization is necessary; factors favoring hospitalization include: Splenectomy or immune deficiency, age >65 years, underlying chronic diseases (e.g., AIDS, COPD, CHF, renal failure, diabetes), abnormal vital signs (e.g., high fever, tachypnea, tachycardia, hypotension), altered mental status, hematologic abnormality (anemia, neutropenia, or extreme neutrophilia), hypoxemia, multiple lobes involved, pleural effusion present, or rapid radiographic progression
- Outpatients with CAP are treated with a macrolide (e.g., azithromycin, clarithromycin), doxycycline, or a respiratory fluoroquinolone (e.g., moxifloxacin, levofloxacin, gatifloxacin)
- Hospitalized CAP patients are treated with a third-generation cephalosporin (e.g., IV ceftriaxone) plus a macrolide (e.g., azithromycin)
  - A respiratory fluoroquinolone (e.g., moxifloxacin, levofloxacin) alone can also be used
- If penicillin-resistant pneumococcus is possible, the regimen should include a respiratory fluoroquinolone or vancomycin
- HAP patients can generally be started on IV monotherapy with second- or third-generation cephalosporin or a quinolone
  - Severely ill patients requiring care in the ICU should be started on dual antibiotic therapy until an organism is identified and/or clinical improvement occurs
- Therapy should be tailored to specific organisms once identified

PROGNOSIS & COMPLICATIONS

- Complications include empyema, metastatic suppurative illness, meningitis, chronic bronchopleural fistula formation, and bronchiectasis
- The mortality of CAP ranges from 1% among outpatients to as high as 25% among hospitalized patients (factors that predict mortality include advanced age, associated comorbid illnesses [particularly diabetes], bacteremia, leukopenia, hypothermia, and renal failure
- HAP due to *Pseudomonas* or *Acinetobacter* carries the highest mortality
- In general, duration of therapy should be 10–14 days
- Chest X-ray clears in young healthy adults in 3–6 weeks, but may take up to 3 months in the elderly

Pulmonary Embolism

INTRODUCTION

- A thrombus from the deep venous system (legs, pelvis, and less commonly, the upper extremities) that embolizes to the lungs
- Infarction of the lung parenchyma occurs in about 10% of cases, resulting in a ventilation/perfusion (V/Q) mismatch
- It is estimated that 600,000 episodes occur each year in the United States, resulting in nearly 200,000 deaths yearly
- The clinical presentation overlaps significantly with numerous other cardiac and pulmonary diseases, making it one of the most commonly missed clinical entities; indeed, the majority of deaths are due to a missed diagnosis rather than a failure of existing therapies

ETIOLOGY, EPIDEMIOLOGY, & RISK FACTORS

- The majority of pulmonary emboli originate in the deep veins of the legs, most commonly the iliofemoral veins; saddle emboli often originate from upper extremity thromboses
- 50% of patients presenting with a deep venous thrombosis (DVT) have a concomitant pulmonary embolism (PE)
- Virchow's triad categorizes the risk factors for DVT and PE
  - Venous stasis: Immobility (especially after orthopedic surgery involving the pelvis or femur), chronic venous stasis (e.g., congestive heart failure)
  - Hypercoagulable states: Malignancy, inherited thrombophilias (e.g., factor V Leiden deficiency, protein C and S deficiency, antithrombin III deficiency), pregnancy (especially postpartum), oral contraceptives, estrogen therapy
  - Endothelial damage: Recent surgery or trauma, burns, indwelling catheters, drug abuse
- At least 1 risk factor for DVT is found in more than 80% of patients with PE
- Cancer is an important risk factor: About 10% of patients with no known source of DVT will eventually be diagnosed with a malignant neoplasm
- Nonthrombotic PE may occur due to fat, air, or amniotic fluid emboli
- More than 50% of PEs are undiagnosed
- 4–5% of all cardiac arrests occur secondary to a massive PE

PATIENT PRESENTATION

- The most common symptoms are dyspnea (90% of cases), chest pain (not necessarily pleuritic), anxiety, cough, and hemoptysis
  - Although dyspnea is the most common presenting symptom, its sensitivity and specificity have been reported as only 74% and 38%, respectively; however, a sudden onset of dyspnea or dyspnea on exertion is more useful
  - Other symptoms include palpitations, diaphoresis, wheezing, leg pain, and leg swelling are tachypnea (70–80%) and tachycardia
- Most common signs on physical examination are tachypnea (70–80%) and tachycardia
- Less common exam findings include wheezing, rales, presence of S4, prominent S2, fever, jugular venous distension, and right ventricular heave
- Syncope may occur; in fact, pulmonary embolism is estimated to be the underlying cause of 10–20% of syncopal episodes

DIFFERENTIAL DX

- Acute myocardial infarct
- Congestive heart failure
- Aortic dissection
- Pericarditis or cardiac tamponade
- Pneumonia
- Asthma
- Pleurisy
- COPD exacerbation
- Pneumothorax
- Anxiety attack
- Musculoskeletal pain (e.g., rib fracture, muscle strain, costochondritis)
- Gastroesophageal reflux disease or esophagitis
- Esophageal rupture
- Mitral valve prolapse
- Esophageal spasm

DIAGNOSTIC EVALUATION

- Laboratory tests include CBC, chemistries (note renal function because IV dye may be used for CT scan of lungs), coagulation studies, D-dimer, cardiac enzymes, and chest X-ray
- ABG may be normal and is no longer considered an essential workup component
- D-dimer less than 500 may help rule out PE but is nonspecific if above 500
- Electrocardiogram (EKG) most often reveals sinus tachycardia; other findings may include S1Q3T3 (rare, but pathognomonic for PE), right ventricular strain, left atrial deviation, or nonspecific ST-T wave changes (may mimic ischemic patterns, especially T-wave inversions in V1-V3 leads)
- Spiral CT scan has 95% sensitivity for segmental or large PE but only 75% sensitivity for subsegmental PE; newer, high-resolution CT-angiography scans have improved sensitivity
- V/Q scan is being used less frequently; however, it may be necessary as an adjunctive study for patients with nondiagnostic CT scans or contraindication to IV dye
  - A high-probability scan is virtually diagnostic for PE, and a normal scan rules out PE
  - However, most patients require further testing because 60% of scans are indeterminate
- Lower extremity venous duplex is used as an adjunct if CT and V/Q scans leave the diagnosis in doubt; a positive study with symptoms consistent for PE is considered diagnostic
- In unstable, high-risk patients (i.e., patients who are in shock) who cannot tolerate CT or V/Q scans, a bedside echocardiogram that shows right ventricular dysfunction or other evidence of high pulmonary arterial pressure suggests the diagnosis and should prompt consideration for immediate thrombolysis

TREATMENT & MANAGEMENT

- Initial treatment of includes supplemental oxygen, IV fluids, vasopressors (if IV fluids are inadequate to maintain blood pressure), and anticoagulation
- Anticoagulation should be initiated prior to imaging if there is a high likelihood of PE
  - Low molecular weight heparin (LMWH) has been shown to be as effective as unfractionated heparin in the initial management of PE and DVT and has a lower risk of heparin-induced thrombocytopenia and major bleeding events; furthermore, LMWH also has the benefit of not requiring frequent monitoring of coagulation studies
  - In unstable patients who may require thrombolytics or thromboembolectomy, unfractionated heparin is preferable to LMWH because it can be immediately discontinued
  - It is essential to use weight-based dosing for any form of heparin
  - LMWH should be used cautiously in patients with creatinine greater than 1.5
- Thrombolysis is generally reserved for patients who present in shock, those with evidence of right ventricular dysfunction on echocardiogram, or those with a large, proximal PE
  - May be considered up to 14 days after a diagnosis of PE
- In patients with contraindications to anticoagulation or who have failed therapeutic trials of anticoagulation, surgical placement of an inferior vena cava (IVC) filter should be considered; but, IVC filters increase the risk of DVT recurrence and may cause lower extremity edema
- Long-term treatment of PE and DVT generally includes compression stockings and/or anticoagulation (warfarin or low molecular weight heparin) for 3–6 months or longer

PROGNOSIS & COMPLICATIONS

- Clinical symptoms depend on the size of the embolus, which may range from insignificant to a large saddle embolus that obstructs the main pulmonary arteries; an embolus causing more than 50% occlusion of the pulmonary vascular bed can cause right ventricular failure
- Patients' initial cardiopulmonary status is an important predictor of outcome; further clinical course and likelihood of recurrence depend on the etiology of the clot
- Chronic, recurrent emboli may result in pulmonary hypertension with eventual respiratory failure and cor pulmonale
- Hypercoagulable states increase the risk of recurrence
- Mortality is 2–10% in treated patients and 20–30% in untreated patients
- Patients who present with hemodynamic compromise have a mortality rate of 20–30%

Lung Cancer

INTRODUCTION

- In the United States, lung cancer is the second most commonly diagnosed cancer in both men and women, but it is the leading cause of cancer-related death
- There are more deaths caused by lung cancer than caused by the next four most lethal cancers combined (colon, breast, prostate, non-Hodgkin's lymphoma)
- Lung cancer incidence rates are declining in men but increasing in women; mortality is decreasing in both men and women
- Lung cancer patients typically present late in the course of their disease, and the majority are inoperable at diagnosis; overall 5-year survival rate remains less than 15%

ETIOLOGY, EPIDEMIOLOGY, & RISK FACTORS

- Squamous cell, adenocarcinoma, and large cell cancers are collectively referred to as non-small-cell cancer (NSCLC)
  - NSCLCs are less aggressive and generally have a favorable response to surgical treatment
  - Small-cell lung cancer (SCLC) has rapid growth and early metastases (70% of cases have metastasized by the time of diagnosis); SCLC is treated by chemotherapy with or without radiation
- Risk factors include tobacco use, environmental (secondhand) tobacco smoke, marijuana smoking, occupational exposures (e.g., asbestos, arsenic, chromium, nickel), radon exposure, radiation exposure, polycyclic aromatic hydrocarbon exposure, and history of prior aerodigestive cancer
  - Risk increases with increasing age
- 90% of cases are due to smoking; the number of pack years is the major determinant of risk
- Mutations have been found in the *ras* and *myc* oncogenes and the *p53* suppressor genes

PATIENT PRESENTATION

- Pulmonary symptoms include cough, hemoptysis, dyspnea, chest pain, postobstructive pneumonia, and pleural effusion
- Superior vena cava (SVC) syndrome: Face and neck edema due to obstruction of the SVC
- Pancoast syndrome: An apical tumor may lead to Horner's syndrome or shoulder/arm pain due to involvement of the brachial plexus or chest wall
- Horner's syndrome: Miosis, ptosis, and anhidrosis
- Hoarseness may occur due to compression of the recurrent laryngeal nerve
- Extrathoracic symptoms may include anorexia, cachexia, fever, adenopathy, night sweats, or symptoms related to areas of metastases
- Paraneoplastic syndromes include syndrome of inappropriate antidiuretic hormone (SIADH), Eaton-Lambert syndrome, Trousseau's syndrome, and hypercalcemia

DIFFERENTIAL DX

- Tuberculosis
- Fungal infection
- Pneumonia
- Lymphoma
- Metastatic cancer
- AVM
- Sarcoid
- Bronchogenic cyst
- Pneumoconiosis
- Intrapulmonary lymph node
- Pulmonary-renal syndromes (Wegener's)
- Connective tissue disease
- Benign tumors: Lipoma, hamartoma, fibroma, leiomyoma, hemangioma

DIAGNOSTIC EVALUATION

- Appropriate diagnosis and management requires a tissue sample, evaluation of the extent of disease, and assessment of overall health status
- Chest X-ray may reveal a mass $+/-$ hilar adenopathy
  - 70–80% sensitive
  - Squamous cell, large cell, and small cell have a central mass
  - Adenocarcinoma has a peripheral mass
  - Pleural effusion, atelectasis, and mediastinal adenopathy may also be apparent
- Chest CT scan better visualizes the mass
  - May reveal lymphatic, mediastinal, or pleural spread
- Tissue diagnosis can be attained by sputum cytology or biopsy (via bronchoscopy, thoracoscopy, or CT-guided fine-needle aspiration)
- Staging workup to determine the extent of disease includes complete blood count, chemistries, electrolytes, liver function tests, amylase, lipase, chest X-ray, CT of the thorax/abdomen/pelvis, pulmonary function tests, and mediastinoscopy

TREATMENT & MANAGEMENT

- NSCLC: Stages I, II, and IIIA are resectable; adjuvant chemotherapy increases survival
  - Stage IIIB: Resection with preoperative chemotherapy is investigational
  - Stage IV: No curative options; survival of 6 months
  - Radiation to symptomatic sites for palliation
- SCLC responds very well to chemotherapy
  - Limited disease can be treated with radiation plus 4 cycles of chemotherapy; complete response is achieved in 50% of cases; median survival is 18 months, 5-year survival of 20%
  - Extensive disease is treated with chemotherapy; radiation does not improve survival; complete response is achieved in 25% of cases; median survival is 9 months; no 5-year survivors
- Smoking cessation decreases the risk of recurrence

PROGNOSIS & COMPLICATIONS

- NSCLC: Resection is effective in stage I or II disease, but few cases present this early
- SCLC: Most patients respond to chemotherapy (80–90%), but more than 90% relapse; thus, the 5-year survival is just 5%

Upper Respiratory Infection

INTRODUCTION

- Upper respiratory tract infections (URIs) constitute a broad range of infections involving the nose, sinuses, pharynx, larynx, trachea, and bronchi
- URI has been described as an acute rhinopharyngitis, although sometimes the term has been used interchangeably with "the common cold"
- The majority of cases are caused by viruses

ETIOLOGY, EPIDEMIOLOGY, & RISK FACTORS

- Usually of viral origin, but superimposed bacterial infection can occur
- Results in inflammation of the upper respiratory tract
- Most uncomplicated cases resolve spontaneously, although a small proportion become complicated by bacterial rhinosinusitis or bacterial pneumonia (particularly in high-risk patients with influenza, such as infants, elderly persons, and chronically ill patients)
- Symptoms caused by upper respiratory tract infection typically last 1–2 weeks, and most patients will feel much better within the first week
- Most URIs occur in the winter months, with the common cold accounting for the majority of these cases
- In 1995, URI was the most frequent reason for seeking ambulatory care in the United States, resulting in more than 37 million visits to physicians and emergency departments
- There are no clearly defined risk factors, although the very young, the immunocompromised, and the elderly are at higher risk for complications

PATIENT PRESENTATION

- Significant overlap in symptoms occurs between various URIs, which sometimes makes a specific diagnosis difficult
- In general, nasal congestion, sneezing, and sore throat suggest the common cold.
- Facial pain, maxillary toothache, headache, and purulent nasal discharge suggest sinusitis
- Sore throat with pain upon swallowing, fever, and absence of cough support a diagnosis of streptococcal pharyngitis, especially if there are sick contacts
- Additional symptoms of lethargy and muscle aches may suggest influenza

DIFFERENTIAL DX

- Pneumonia
- Influenza
- Bronchitis
- Otitis media
- Otitis externa
- Sinusitis
- Tonsillitis
- Laryngitis
- Pharyngitis
- Epiglottitis
- Rhinitis

DIAGNOSTIC EVALUATION

- As with all illnesses, a thorough history and physical exam is important
  - General questions include onset, duration of symptoms, and sick contacts
  - Head and neck examination should be done carefully: Observe the nasopharynx; look for boggy nasal turbinates, suppurative pharynx, and tender anterior cervical lymphadenopathy; and palpate the frontal and maxillary sinuses
  - Auscultate the lung fields to evaluate for consolidations, which may suggest pneumonia
- If the patient has exudates or an erythematous oropharynx, a rapid strep test may be warranted to evaluate for streptococcal pharyngitis
- Lungs: Always auscultate lung fields because signs of consolidation require more serious workup and treatment

TREATMENT & MANAGEMENT

- Symptomatic treatment and reassurance are generally sufficient; this includes fluids, rest, humidified air, and over-the-counter medications
- Symptoms generally improve spontaneously over a 3- to 10-day course, but cough could persist for 1–2 months
- If bacterial infection or superinfection is considered, antibiotic therapy aimed at *Streptococcus pneumoniae*, *Haemophilus influenza*, and *Moraxella catarrhalis* may be warranted; however, antibiotic treatment of upper respiratory tract infection has not been shown to alter the rates of bacterial superinfection or other rare complications

PROGNOSIS & COMPLICATIONS

- Symptoms are self-limited and usually resolve over a 1- to 2-week period
- Complications include otitis media, sinusitis (may develop after a URI because of obstruction of the sinus ostia), or, rarely, meningitis

Pleural Effusion

INTRODUCTION

- There is always a small amount of fluid in the pleural space; this fluid enters via the parietal pleura and exits via the parietal lymphatics
- Pleural effusions occur when the normal rate of entry and exit of fluid is disturbed
- The type of pleural fluid, exudate versus transudate, helps to determine the etiology of the excess fluid
- The most common cause is congestive heart failure

ETIOLOGY, EPIDEMIOLOGY, & RISK FACTORS

- There are several mechanisms of excess fluid accumulation within the pleural space
  - Increased fluid entry into the pleural space occurs when there is increased permeability, microvascular or hydrostatic pressure, decreased pleural pressure, or decreased oncotic pressure
  - Decreased fluid exit occurs when there is interference of lymphatic function, as seen in infiltration or obstruction by cancer or extrinsic compression by fibrosis or granuloma
  - Leaks across holes or tears in the pleura across the mediastinal or diaphragmatic surfaces
  - Other contributors include inflammation, injury caused by drugs or radiation, inherited anatomic abnormalities, decreased intrapleural pressure, or limitation of chest wall motion
- Transudate: The pleural surface is normal; rather, systemic factors influence the accumulation of pleural fluid
- Exudate: Arises from pleural inflammation, which causes increased capillary permeability, or from obstruction of the lymphatic drainage
- Empyema: A grossly purulent pleural effusion
- Hemothorax: Blood in the pleural space
- Chylothorax: Leakage of lymphatic fluid from the thoracic duct
- Pleuritic pain occurs with inflammation of the parietal pleura, where pain fibers are located

PATIENT PRESENTATION

- Many cases are asymptomatic
- Dyspnea
- Nonproductive cough
- Pleuritic chest pain
- Hypoxemia
- Fever
- Decreased breath sounds
- Egophony
- Dullness to percussion
- Decreased tactile fremitus
- Pleural rub
- Signs or symptoms of the primary disease process

DIFFERENTIAL DX

- Transudative effusion: CHF, cirrhosis, pulmonary embolism, nephrosis, hypoalbuminemia, trauma, hypothyroidism, superior vena cava (SVC) syndrome, sarcoidosis, peritoneal dialysis
- Exudative effusions: Pneumonia, tuberculosis, malignancy, asbestos, pulmonary embolism, pericarditis, coronary artery bypass graft (CABG), collagen vascular disease, uremia, drugs (e.g., amiodarone)
- Pleural thickening due to primary pleural tumors, asbestosis, collagen vascular disease, or metastatic disease
- Pancreatitis

DIAGNOSTIC EVALUATION

- The etiology can often be inferred from comorbid illnesses
  - Perform a thoracentesis if there is a symptomatic effusion, no clear etiology, or the patient does not improve as expected
- If the patient has CHF but does not have evidence of infection, and the effusions are bilateral and similar in size, treat the CHF first
  - Chest X-ray shows a blunted costophrenic angle (requires >175 cc of pleural fluid)
- Chest CT scan is more sensitive for effusion; also rules out other processes
- Thoracentesis with pleural fluid analysis should evaluate LDH, albumin, protein, cell count, gram stain and culture, glucose, cytology, amylase, pH, and markers of tuberculosis
  - First, determine transudate versus exudate: The effusion is considered an exudate if pleural fluid to serum protein ratio is greater than 0.5 OR pleural fluid to serum LDH ratio is greater than 0.6 OR pleural fluid LDH is greater than two-thirds of the serum normal limit
  - Elevated WBC suggests parapneumonic, rheumatologic, pancreatitis, or malignancy
  - Decreased glucose suggests malignancy, infection, or rheumatologic
  - Elevated amylase suggests esophageal rupture, pancreatitis, or malignancy
  - Elevated triglycerides (>110) suggests chylothorax
  - A pleural biopsy may be indicated if the cause of an exudate is in doubt

TREATMENT & MANAGEMENT

- Transudative effusion: Treat underlying cause; if symptomatic, consider draining the effusion via thoracentesis
- Exudative effusions often require further treatment
  - Malignant effusion: Repeated thoracentesis for symptomatic relief; perform pleurodesis (obliterate the pleural space with talc or doxycycline) or insert an indwelling catheter for frequent recurrences
  - Parapneumonic effusion: Treat with systemic antibiotics; perform thoracentesis (may need ultrasound- or CT-guided drainage) for large effusions (>10 mm); insertion of chest tube may be necessary to prevent the development of a loculated, more complex effusion that may require surgical intervention
  - Hemothorax: Insert chest tube; may require thoracotomy
- Video-assisted thoracic surgery (VATS) may be helpful for diagnosis of exudative effusions of unknown cause, staging of malignant mesothelioma, evaluation and staging of lung cancer when pleural involvement is suspected, and the treatment of recurrent malignant effusions with talc pleurodesis

PROGNOSIS & COMPLICATIONS

- All unexplained effusions and those that do not respond as expected to treatment require thoracentesis for analysis of the pleural fluid
- Symptoms depend on the size of the effusion and comorbid conditions
- The course of the effusion depends on the cause:
  - Malignant effusions rapidly recur and often require a sclerosing agent
  - Infectious effusions resolve with treatment of the infection
  - Transudative effusions resolve as the primary disease is corrected
  - Complicated parapneumonic effusions require urgent chest tube drainage; delay may allow formation of loculations, which require intrapleural streptokinase or surgery

Sleep Apnea

INTRODUCTION

- A syndrome of repetitive periods of apnea (at least 10 seconds without air flow) or hypopnea (decreased airflow) during sleep
- Results in frequent arterial oxygen desaturations and frequent awakenings from sleep
- Snoring is a major feature of obstructive sleep apnea
- Associated physiologic abnormalities may include hypoxemia, hypercapnia, elevation in systemic and pulmonary arterial pressures, sympathetic nervous system hyperactivity, and cardiac arrhythmias; appropriate treatment generally improves symptoms

ETIOLOGY, EPIDEMIOLOGY, & RISK FACTORS

- May be obstructive, central, or mixed (symptoms are similar regardless):
  - Obstructive sleep apnea: Upper airway soft tissue impedes airflow
  - Central sleep apnea: Absent signal to breathe from the CNS respiratory center (apnea without respiratory effort)
  - Mixed: An initial central component followed by an obstructive component
- Risk factors for obstructive sleep apnea include narrowed airways (obesity, macroglossia), alcohol, sedatives, upper respiratory infections, hypothyroidism, smoking, vocal cord dysfunction, or bulbar disease
- Obstructive sleep apnea has been linked to hypertension, myocardial infection, stroke, and premature cardiovascular death, as well as motor vehicle crashes caused by daytime sleepiness
- Occurs in 2% of women and 4% of men
- Most common in obese, middle-aged men
- Obstructive apnea is far more common than central apnea
- Central apnea is more common at the extremes of age
- There is often snoring for many years prior to the onset of actual obstruction; thus, snoring alone is not a reason for full workup

PATIENT PRESENTATION

- Loud snoring
- Excessive daytime sleepiness
- Witnessed periods of apnea by bed partner
- Restlessness or thrashing movements during sleep
- Nocturnal diaphoresis
- Nocturia and enuresis
- Nocturnal choking and gasping spells
- Mood and personality change
- Morning headaches
- Obesity
- Systemic hypertension
- Reduced libido
- Nonrestorative sleep
- Patients with central apnea tend to have insomnia, shortness of breath, and a witnessed crescendo-decrescendo respiratory pattern; they snore less often and may have features of CHF or neurologic dysfunction

DIFFERENTIAL DX

- Nocturnal oxyhemoglobin desaturation syndromes (e.g., chronic obstructive pulmonary disease, bronchial and nocturnal asthma, restrictive lung disease)
- Narcolepsy
- Periodic limb movement disorder
- Idiopathic hypersomnia
- Insomnia
- Hypothyroidism
- Circadian rhythm disorders
- Psychiatric disorders
- Dementia
- Primary alveolar hypoventilation ("Ondine's curse")
- Obesity-hypoventilation (Pickwickian) syndrome

DIAGNOSTIC EVALUATION

- Detailed history and physical examination
  - Inquire about snoring, breathing pauses, excessive daytime sleepiness or fatigue, choking or gasping spells, weight gain or obesity, environmental allergies, and ethanol or sedative use
  - Exam should include blood pressure, pulse, weight, and assessment for pharyngeal narrowing, nasal obstruction, small jaw, and receding lower jaw
  - Workup is appropriate when nocturnal problems are contributing to daytime sleepiness or behavioral/physiologic problems
- Testing may include complete blood count, thyroid function tests, and pulmonary function tests
- Screening nocturnal pulse oximetry may rule out sleep apnea if negative
  - A "saw-tooth" pattern of desaturations suggests sleep apnea or hypopnea and warrants confirmation by polysomnography
- Diagnostic polysomnography ("sleep study") is the gold standard for diagnosing sleep apnea; it should be performed during the patient's usual sleep episodes (usually at night)
  - Monitors EEG, EMG, electrocardiogram (EKG), pulse oximetry, airflow, respiratory effort, and body position
  - Sleep apnea or hypopnea is diagnosed if there are 5–10 or more events per hour
- Upper airway imaging studies are sometimes performed if surgery is anticipated

TREATMENT & MANAGEMENT

- Patients with increased upper airway muscle tone should avoid alcohol and sedatives
- Nighttime nasal continuous positive airway pressure (CPAP) is the treatment of choice; it is very effective but may be uncomfortable
- Patients with decreased upper airway lumen size may benefit from weight loss, an oral dental prosthesis, nasal septoplasty (if a deviated septum is present), or uvulopalatopharyngoplasty in selected patients
- Bypass occlusion: Consider tracheostomy in patients with life-threatening complications and failure of other therapies
- Prescribe supplemental oxygen carefully, as it may worsen apnea
- Tricyclic antidepressants may decrease episodes and improve daytime symptoms

PROGNOSIS & COMPLICATIONS

- Repetitive hypoxia may ultimately result in cardiac arrhythmias, pulmonary hypertension, and cor pulmonale
- Other sequelae include CHF (especially in patients with pre-existing left ventricular dysfunction), systemic hypertension, and erythrocytosis
- The disease usually follows a chronic, progressive course due to continued weight gain
- There is a good response to therapy, especially nasal CPAP
- Sleep apnea *does* cause increased mortality
- Sleep apnea syndrome is one of the leading causes of daytime sleepiness

Tuberculosis

INTRODUCTION

- Tuberculosis (TB) is a disease of major public health importance worldwide
- Caused by inhalation of *Mycobacterium tuberculosis* or ingestion of *Mycobacterium bovis* in milk (now rare due to pasteurization)
- After inhalation of *Mycobacterium tuberculosis*, the infection may cause symptomatic disease or be contained by the immune system and remain latent and asymptomatic
- Persons with latent infection are at risk for reactivation of the infection and development of active disease; risk of reactivation is highest within 2 years of the initial infection and in patients with medical or social risk factors for reactivation
- Resistance is primarily due to failure to complete the required long courses of therapy

ETIOLOGY, EPIDEMIOLOGY, & RISK FACTORS

- Persons with pulmonary or laryngeal tuberculosis may exhale mycobacteria droplets, which can travel large distances
- Inhaled mycobacteria cause a peripheral pneumonitis and drain to the hilar lymph nodes (called the primary complex); if the immune system contains the infection, the primary complex becomes calcified (sometimes visible on chest X-ray as the Ghon complex)
- Children and immunosuppressed patients are less likely to contain the infection at this stage and may develop miliary disease due to hematogenous dissemination (visible on chest X-ray as millet seed-sized nodules); infection may then spread to any organ
- A normal host infected with tuberculosis has a 5% risk within the first 2 years and 10% lifetime risk of developing active disease; an infected HIV patient has a 40% risk of disease in the first year, and then an 8% risk per year thereafter
- One-third of the world's population is infected
- 15 million persons are infected in the United States, with 5,000 cases of active disease reported yearly; more than 50% of cases occur in the foreign-born persons
- Most cases of active disease are due to reactivation of previous infection

PATIENT PRESENTATION

- Active tuberculosis of any organ system may present with fever, weight loss, and drenching night sweats
- Pulmonary involvement occurs in 85% of patients and may present with a productive cough, hemoptysis, and dyspnea
- Tuberculous lymphadenopathy occurs more commonly in children and foreign-born persons
- CNS involvement may be indolent and present with headaches, vomiting, and confusion
- Bone involvement is most common in the thoracic spine and large, weight-bearing joints
  - Spinal tuberculosis is known as Pott's disease
- Peritoneal TB causes abdominal swelling due to ascites and thickening of the abdominal wall
- Urogenital TB may present as hematuria, infertility, menorrhagia, or testicular swelling
- Laryngeal TB presents with cough and hoarseness and is highly contagious

DIFFERENTIAL DX

- Bacterial pneumonia
- Fungal pneumonia (histoplasmosis, cryptococcosis, blastomycosis, coccidiomycosis, aspergillosis)
- Primary or secondary lung malignancy
- Lung abscess
- Lymphoma
- Vasculitis
- Sarcoidosis
- CHF
- HIV

DIAGNOSTIC EVALUATION

- History and physical examination should include a thorough evaluation of recent contacts, previous treatment for tuberculosis, history of Bacille Calmette-Guérin (BCG) immunization (may cause positive PPD), and risk factors for tuberculosis
- A chest X-ray should be performed in patients with symptoms or a positive PPD
  - Primary tuberculosis: Lower lung infiltrates and adenopathy
  - Latent tuberculosis: Nodules and fibrosis in the upper lung
  - Reactivation tuberculosis: Upper lung infiltrates and cavitation
  - Miliary tuberculosis: Disseminated small nodules
  - Ghon complex: Granuloma with bacilli in center plus a calcified lymph node
- If cough or abnormal chest X-ray is present, send 3 sputum specimens or a bronchoscopy specimen for acid-fast bacilli smear and culture
- Tuberculin skin testing (PPD) is the most common screening test for latent TB
  - A negative PPD does not exclude active disease
  - 15 mm of induration is considered positive in patients without risk factors; 10 mm of induration is positive for patients at risk; 5 mm is positive in patients with HIV, recent exposure, or a suggestive chest X-ray
- HIV testing should be done in all patients with tuberculosis
- Biopsy (lymph node, liver, or bone marrow) to confirm diagnosis of extrapulmonary TB

TREATMENT & MANAGEMENT

- Tuberculosis cases should be reported to public health authorities
- Patients whose sputum or bronchoscopy specimens are "smear positive" and those with laryngeal tuberculosis are considered infectious and require respiratory isolation
  - Infection control precautions (including a negative-pressure room and N95 masks or personal respirators for health care workers) are essential until 3 sputum smears or a bronchoscopy specimen are confirmed as smear negative
- Active tuberculosis is treated with rifampin and isoniazid for 6 months plus pyrazinamide for the initial 2 months
  - Add ethambutol in areas of isoniazid resistance (most of United States), pending culture and sensitivity results
  - Add pyridoxine for patients with poor nutrition
  - Longer duration of treatment is indicated in patients with CNS disease or cavitary pulmonary disease with persistent positive sputum culture at 2 months
  - Steroids should also be given if there is CNS or pericardial disease
- If active disease is excluded, treatment for latent tuberculosis may be necessary due to the risk for active transformation (especially in high-risk groups): Treat with isoniazid for 9 months or rifampin for 4 months
- Directly observed therapy (DOT) should be considered for all patients

PROGNOSIS & COMPLICATIONS

- Monitor patients regularly for adherence, side effects, and response to treatment
- Patients with a fully sensitive *M. tuberculosis* organism who adhere to recommended treatment have a 2% risk of relapse
- Poor adherence is a risk factor for drug-resistant tuberculosis, which carries a higher mortality and requires treatment with more toxic drugs for a longer duration
- Rifampin, isoniazid, and pyrazinamide are hepatotoxic; liver function tests should be checked monthly if the patient has abnormal baseline liver function or known liver disease; patients should be asked to report nausea, impaired appetite, and abdominal pain
- Isoniazid may cause a peripheral neuropathy due to pyridoxine deficiency
- Ethambutol may cause optic neuritis; note baseline visual acuity and color vision

Pulmonary Function Testing

INTRODUCTION

- Pulmonary function tests (PFTs) are used to evaluate patients with dyspnea, particularly in patients with asthma and chronic obstructive pulmonary disease (COPD)
- The purposes of PFTs are to 1) determine the pattern of a pulmonary abnormality (restrictive ventilatory defect vs. obstructive ventilatory defect) in order to aid in the diagnosis of cardiac or pulmonary disease; 2) determine the severity of the abnormality; and 3) follow disease progression
- PFTs are usually performed in a specialized laboratory, although spirometry can be performed in the office or emergency room, and peak flow measurements can be performed by the patient at home

ETIOLOGY, EPIDEMIOLOGY, & RISK FACTORS

- The most common PFTs are peak flow, spirometry, lung volumes, and diffusion capacity
  - Peak flow and spirometry are performed by having the patient exhale as hard and for as long as possible through a measuring device
  - Lung volumes and diffusion capacity require various gases, body boxes, and measuring devices, which must be performed in a formal pulmonary function testing laboratory
- Obstruction (e.g., mucosal hyperplasia; edema; smooth muscle constriction or hypertrophy, as in asthma or chronic bronchitis; parenchymal destruction and airway collapse, as in emphysema) is typically defined by an FEV_1/forced vital capacity (FVC) ratio<70% of predicted
- Restriction (e.g., parenchymal pathology, such as interstitial edema, inflammation or fibrosis, or alveolar filling with fluid, blood, pus, or cells; pleural scarring; neuromuscular weakness; decreased extrathoracic compliance secondary to thoracic disease, such as kyphoscoliosis; abdominal factors, such as abdominal pain, ascites, or obesity) is typically defined by total lung capacity <80% of predicted
- Pulmonary function is normally determined by an individual's age, gender, and height
- 15–20% of cigarette smokers will develop airflow obstruction, typically after 20 pack years
- Asthma is increasing in prevalence and severity

PATIENT PRESENTATION

- Establish baseline PFT values
- Basic patterns:
  - Variable intrathoracic airflow obstruction
  - Variable extrathoracic airflow obstruction
  - Fixed airflow obstruction
- Isolated air trapping: Elevated residual volume (RV)/total lung capacity (TLC) ratio or RV >120% of predicted can suggest compensated asthma or COPD

DIFFERENTIAL DX

- Obstructive ventilatory deficit: Asthma; COPD; pharyngeal and laryngeal tumor, edema, or infection; foreign body aspiration; tumor, collapse, or stenosis of the trachea; obliterative bronchiolitis; hypersensitivity pneumonitis
- Restrictive ventilatory deficit: Interstitial disease (interstitial pneumonitis, pneumoconiosis, fibrosis, granulomatosis, edema), space-occupying diseases (cyst, tumor, BOOP), pleural disease (pneumothorax, pleural effusion, empyema, hemothorax), chest wall disease (neuromuscular disease, scoliosis, spondylitis), obesity, peritonitis

DIAGNOSTIC EVALUATION

- Peak flow measurements are most useful to evaluate patients with asthma and COPD
  - Patients perform the peak flow measurement twice per day and record results
  - A decrease of 25% from the maximum or baseline value on 2 consecutive measurements should prompt intervention (i.e., go to emergency room or call pulmonologist)
- Spirometry is most useful to follow patients after a diagnosis is established
  - Monitor the FVC in patients with restrictive diseases
  - Monitor the FEV_1 in patients with obstructive diseases
- Once the pattern of disease is established, the next step is to determine the severity
  - For obstructive disease, severity is based solely on the FEV_1: 80% or more is normal, 65–80% is mild, 50–65% is moderate, and 49% or less is severe
  - Restrictive disease is followed by the TLC (using the same percentages as above)
- Diffusion capacity (DLCO) is the transfer rate of carbon monoxide into the blood; it measures pulmonary capillary surface area, hemoglobin content, and alveolar microarchitecture and depends on total surface area of the alveoli, thickness of the alveolar wall, and the amount of hemoglobin in the lungs
  - DLCO is decreased in emphysema (by destroying alveoli), interstitial lung diseases (by causing thickening of the alveolar membranes), anemia (by decreasing the uptake of gas by the blood), and pulmonary hypertension
  - DLCO is increased in asthma and disorders with elevated left-sided cardiac filling pressures (by increasing the blood volume in the lungs)

TREATMENT & MANAGEMENT

- Refer to individual disease entries
- Medicare criteria for the use of supplemental oxygen:
  - Oxygen required while at rest if: Room air partial pressure of oxygen (pO_2) <55 mmHg or oxygen saturation <88%; pO_2 56–59 mmHg or saturation 89% with concurrent dependent edema or congestive heart failure, pulmonary hypertension, cor pulmonale, or hematocrit >56%
  - Oxygen required during sleep if: Meets criteria above OR pO_2 <55 mmHg or saturation <88% for at least 5 minutes
  - Oxygen required during exercise if: Normal oxygen saturation at rest (on room air) and hypoxemic (oxygen saturation <88%) during exercise (on room air), but normal oxygen saturation during exercise when given supplemental oxygen

PROGNOSIS & COMPLICATIONS

- Pulmonary function testing is underused in the evaluation of chest symptoms and management of respiratory tract disorders
- FEV_1 is an independent predictor of survival
- Asthma severity predicts risk of complications
- Patient complications during pulmonary function testing include headache, syncope, chest pain (typically musculoskeletal), and bronchospasm (uncommon)

Section 5

Ear/Nose/Throat

Acute Otitis Media

INTRODUCTION

- Acute otitis media is an infection of the middle ear
- It is more common in infants and young children than in older children, adolescents, or adults
- The diagnosis requires not only the presence of infected fluid behind the tympanic membrane, but also signs and symptoms of inflammation (e.g., erythema, pain)
- Adults and older children can suffer from complications of recurrent or severe middle ear infections during childhood; these sequelae include chronic perforations of the tympanic membrane, development of cholesteatoma, and hearing loss

ETIOLOGY, EPIDEMIOLOGY, & RISK FACTORS

- Infections (e.g., URI, sinusitis) or inflammation (e.g., allergic rhinitis) of the respiratory tract affect the mucociliary lining of the Eustachian tube and may impair its ability to drain secretions of the middle ear; this creates a favorable area for bacterial growth
- The bacteria that cause otitis media in healthy adolescents and adults are the same as those that cause infection in children: *Streptococcus pneumoniae*, nontypable *Haemophilus influenzae*, and *Moraxella catarrhalis*
- Children and adults with immunodeficiency may also have infections with gram-negative organisms, including pseudomonas species
- There is an inverse relationship between age and risk for development of otitis media
- Otitis media is more common during cold weather seasons
- Increased susceptibility in families with a history of recurrent otitis media
- Congenital anatomic anomalies that interfere with normal eustachian tube function, such as cleft lip and palate, can predispose patients to recurrent otitis media; a submucosal cleft palate may be occult and go undetected until adulthood
- Other risk factors include smoking or environmental exposure to cigarette smoke, nasal polyps or tumors of the nasopharynx, adenoidal hypertrophy, changes in barometric pressure (barotitis), and prolonged placement of nasogastric or nasotracheal tubes

PATIENT PRESENTATION

- Note the presence of signs and symptoms of systemic illness, including fever, lethargy, or irritability
- Patients may complain of ear pain, difficulty hearing or hearing loss, and/or drainage from the ear
- Patients may also complain of tinnitus or vertigo and may have nystagmus
- Fluid in the middle ear may cause bulging or abnormal motility of the tympanic membrane, an air-fluid level behind the tympanic membrane, or drainage of fluid into the ear canal (if the tympanic membrane is perforated)
- Inflammation of the middle ear may result in erythema of the tympanic membrane pain

DIFFERENTIAL DX

- Serous otitis media/otitis media with effusion
- Otitis media due to unusual organisms (e.g., *Corynebacterium diphtheria*, *Mycobacterium tuberculosis*, other mycobacteria, *Ascaris lumbricoides*)
- Otitis externa
- Chronic suppurative otitis media
- Pharyngitis
- Temporomandibular joint dysfunction
- Trauma
- Wegener's granulomatosis
- Relapsing polychondritis
- Tumor
- Cholesteatoma
- Mastoiditis
- Down syndrome

DIAGNOSTIC EVALUATION

- Focused history and physical examination of the head and neck, including pneumatic oto-scopy
  - Note the appearance of the tympanic membrane, looking for the bony landmarks of the middle ear and the light reflex
  - With pneumatic otoscopy, a normal tympanic membrane will move inward when the rubber bulb is squeezed and outward upon release of squeezing
  - Any fluid or negative pressure behind the tympanic membrane will affect mobility; the fluid must be visualized and be opaque or have the appearance of pus to be consistent with a diagnosis of otitis media (erythema or redness of the tympanic membrane is not sufficient)
- Tympanometry can be used to evaluate the compliance of the tympanic membrane
  - Compliance is reduced when there is fluid behind the tympanic membrane
- Acoustic reflectometry can also be used to determine the presence of fluid
  - Fluid behind the tympanic membrane will dampen the reflectivity of sound
  - However, this test does not distinguish infected from noninfected fluid
- Tympanocentesis (aspiration of the middle ear fluid) can be performed to determine the bacterial etiology of the infection
  - Recommended in patients who are severely ill, who do not respond to therapy, or who have a complication of infection
  - Should be considered in immunosuppressed patients in order to choose the appropriate antibiotic therapy

TREATMENT & MANAGEMENT

- Patients with severe infections, complications of infection, or immunosuppression should receive immediate antibiotic therapy
- For other patients, initial therapy should be directed at control of pain (e.g., acetaminophen, ibuprofen, topical analgesic drops); if symptoms do not resolve within 48–72 hours, an oral antibiotic directed at the most common bacterial etiologies is recommended
- Initial therapy should be with amoxicillin 875 mg twice daily for 5–7 days
  - Penicillin-allergic patients can be treated with an oral second- or third-generation cephalosporin or an oral macrolide
  - If there is no improvement in symptoms after 48 hours, the antibiotic regimen should be changed to cover beta-lactamase producing organisms; amoxicillin-clavulanate is recommended
  - A patient who fails these regimens should receive parenteral ceftriaxone or clindamycin to treat penicillin-resistant pneumococcal infections
- There is no proven role for decongestants, antihistamines, or steroids in the treatment of acute otitis media
- Surgical drainage of middle ear fluid is recommended only if there is concurrent mastoiditis

PROGNOSIS & COMPLICATIONS

- Symptoms may resolve without antibiotic therapy
- A patient treated with antibiotics will usually have significant or complete improvement in symptoms within 48 hours
- Fluid may persist for months after an acute episode of otitis media
- Fluid behind the tympanic membrane affects hearing acuity; a loss of about 25 dB is common when an effusion is present
- Complications include perforation of the tympanic membrane, chronic perforation, cholesteatoma formation, paralysis of the facial nerve, labyrinthitis, hearing loss, and infectious complications (e.g., mastoiditis, meningitis, osteomyelitis of the facial bones or bones of the calvarium, intracranial abscess, cerebral sinus thrombosis or thrombophlebitis)

Otitis Externa

INTRODUCTION

- Otitis externa is an infection of the external auditory canal
- Infection may be acute or chronic
- Acute infection may be localized or diffuse
- Invasive (malignant) otitis externa is a life-threatening infection

ETIOLOGY, EPIDEMIOLOGY, & RISK FACTORS

- Fluid and foreign material can become trapped within the narrow external canal of the ear, which can cause irritation and desquamation of the epithelium lining the canal
- Bacteria of the ear canal proliferate in this warm, moist environment, invade irritated skin in the canal, and cause inflammation of these tissues
  - The most common bacteria are *S. aureus*, *S. epidermidis*, corynebacteria, and anaerobes
  - *Pseudomonas aeruginosa* and other gram-negative bacteria can also cause infection
  - Fungal species can also cause infection but occur most commonly in patients who have systemic fungal infections or who are immunosuppressed
- "Swimmer's ear," or diffuse otitis externa, is an acute infection that occurs more commonly in warm weather months and areas of high humidity
  - Swimming increases the risk, but infection does not require water exposure
- Chronic otitis externa results from chronic suppurative drainage through a perforated tympanic membrane or irritation by foreign objects (Q-tip, hearing aid, earplug, earphone)
- Elderly, diabetic, and immunosuppressed patients are at risk for invasive otitis externa, which can be life threatening; it is caused by invasion and necrosis of the soft tissues and bone surrounding the ear canal
  - *Pseudomonas aeruginosa* is the most common cause of invasive otitis externa

PATIENT PRESENTATION

- Patients may complain of itchiness of the ear canal followed by pain
- Patients may complain of pain with movement or pressure on the pinna or tragus of the external ear or upon examination with an otoscope
- There may be drainage from the ear
- Patients may complain of difficulty hearing or hearing loss
- Acute, localized otitis externa is a localized infection of a hair follicle within the canal; it has the appearance of a pustule or furuncle
- Patients with invasive otitis externa have severe pain that is "deep" in origin and often does not respond to oral analgesics

DIFFERENTIAL DX

- Acute otitis media with perforation
- Infections (e.g., syphilis, tuberculosis, leprosy)
  - Scaling skin conditions (e.g., atopic dermatitis, seborrheic dermatitis, psoriasis, fungal infections)
- Neoplasm of the external auditory canal
- Trauma
- Polychondritis
- Mastoiditis

DIAGNOSTIC EVALUATION

- Perform a focused history to identify risk factors for infection
- Perform a complete examination of the head and neck
  - Note the appearance of the skin of the external canal: In acute, diffuse otitis externa, the skin is often red and swollen, and the canal is filled with white colored debris; in chronic otitis externa, the epithelium of the canal is reddened and scaling
  - Views of the involved skin may be obscured by discharge and debris in the canal
- Bacterial cultures of the discharge/debris in the canal are not routinely recommended
- In invasive otitis externa, granulation tissue occurs in the posteroinferior wall of the canal, at the junction of the bony and cartilaginous portions of the canal; biopsy of this tissue should be done to identify the etiology of the infection

TREATMENT & MANAGEMENT

- Debris can be removed with gentle irrigation using 3% saline or mixtures of isopropyl alcohol or acetic acid and water
- Rinsing with 50% Burrow's solution can reduce inflammation
- Treatment with a topical antibiotic or antibiotic-corticosteroid preparation reduces inflammation and treats infection
  - Regimens include topical quinolones (e.g., ofloxacin, ciprofloxacin-dexamethasone) or other antibiotics (e.g., neomycin, polymyxin-hydrocortisone combinations)
  - 10 days of therapy is recommended
- For localized infection, an oral antistaphylococcal antibiotic should be used
  - Furuncles may require incision and drainage
- Topical antibiotic preparations are recommended for the treatment of chronic otitis externa; treatment of concurrent middle ear disease may require oral antibiotics as well
  - Patients should discontinue use of any materials that may be causing irritation of the canal
- Early invasive otitis externa may respond to oral and topical antipseudomonal antibiotics, but most patients require parenteral therapy

PROGNOSIS & COMPLICATIONS

- Most patients with either acute diffuse or chronic otitis externa respond to topical therapy alone
- Patients with invasive (malignant) otitis externa can suffer intracranial infections including: osteomyelitis of the temporal bone, thrombophlebitis of the cranial sinuses, meningitis, and intracranial abscesses; permanent facial nerve paralysis often complicates this disease; other cranial nerves may be involved as well

Sinusitis

- Inflammation of 1 or more of the paranasal sinuses (maxillary, ethmoid, frontal, sphenoid)
- The term îrhinosinusitisî is often used since rhinitis almost always accompanies sinusitis
- May be classified on the basis of the length of time the process has been present (acute, subacute recurrent, chronic) or by the causative agent(s) (e.g., viral, bacterial, fungal, allergic)
- Multiple factors contribute to the development and perpetuation of rhinosinusitis, including intrinsic sinonasal mucosal factors, systemic disease, external agents, and obstructive phenomena
- Most cases are viral; acute bacterial rhinosinusitis should be considered if symptoms last longer than 7–10 days or worsen after 5 days

ETIOLOGY, EPIDEMIOLOGY, & RISK FACTORS

- There is no strict accepted definition that delineates acute sinusitis from chronic sinusitis
  - Acute sinusitis is present for less than 2 weeks and has typical symptoms of acute infections
  - Chronic sinusitis has persistent symptoms despite therapy or symptoms lasting >3 months
  - Acute exacerbations of sinusitis may occur in patients with chronic sinusitis
- Viruses are the most common cause of infectious sinusitis
- The normal bacteria of the nasopharynx are common causes of acute bacterial sinusitis (e.g., *Streptococcus pneumoniae*, *Haemophilus influenzae*, *Moraxella catarrhalis*, *S. aureus*)
- Common causes of chronic bacterial sinusitis include anaerobes, *Streptococcus* species, *H. influenzae*, and *Pseudomonas aeruginosa*
- Immunocompromised hosts may develop invasive fungal sinusitis
- Predisposing factors include allergy, exposure to irritants (e.g., smoke, chemicals, dust), immunodeficiency, anatomic obstruction (e.g., polyps, concha, bullosa, severe septal deviation), barotraumas (e.g., airplane trips, deep sea diving), dental infection, and nasal instrumentation (e.g., nasogastric tube)

PATIENT PRESENTATION

- Purulent anterior or posterior nasal discharge
- Nasal discharge
- Nasal congestion
- Facial pain or pressure
- Fever
- Cough
- Earache
- Headache
- Halitosis
- Some authorities suggest that the presence of purulent nasal secretions, maxillary dental or facial pain, unilateral sinus tenderness, and worsening symptoms after initial improvement are predictive for acute bacterial sinusitis

DIFFERENTIAL DX

- Allergic rhinitis
- Nonallergic rhinitis
- Allergic fungal sinusitis
- Vasomotor rhinitis
- Nasal foreign body
- Migraine
- Cluster headache
- Tension headache
- Periorbital cellulitis
- Sinus tumor
- Adenoiditis (children)
- Wegener's granulomatosis
- Sarcoidosis
- Cystic fibrosis

DIAGNOSTIC EVALUATION

- Most cases of acute sinusitis are diagnosed clinically
- CT scan is the best diagnostic test for chronic sinusitis
  - Coronal CT scans visualize the sinuses well but (due to cost) should only be considered if symptoms persist despite therapy
  - Positive findings on CT scan include opacification, mucosal swelling, and air-fluid levels
  - CT scans are less helpful in young children due to lack of specificity
- Plain X-rays and ultrasound have poor sensitivity and are usually more expensive than CT scans
- Transillumination of the sinuses may show opacification but is unreliable compared to imaging
- Culture of a direct sinus aspirate is considered the gold standard for microbiologic diagnosis, but this is not routinely performed in the initial management
  - Culture of nasal secretions is not helpful and may be misleading

TREATMENT & MANAGEMENT

- Initial therapy may include decongestants, antihistamines, and analgesics
- Antibiotic therapy for acute bacterial sinusitis is controversial
  - Antibiotics are indicated for severe symptoms or if moderate symptoms persist for 7 days
  - Treat with oral amoxicillin or a second- or third-generation cephalosporin if no antibiotics have been given in the proceeding month or if low rates of penicillin-resistant *Streptococcus pneumoniae* exist in the community
  - Treat with amoxicillin-clavulanate and fluoroquinolones if drug resistance is suspected
  - Treat for at least 10 days
  - Antibiotics are not usually effective for chronic sinusitis
- If treatment is indicated, use amoxicillin-clavulanate or a combination of antibiotics that includes anaerobic coverage, and continue antibiotics for 28 days
  - Surgical intervention may be considered in cases refractory to multiple courses of antimicrobials

PROGNOSIS & COMPLICATIONS

- Although most bacterial sinus infections self-resolve within 2 weeks, serious morbidity can result from persistent infection
- Antibiotics lead to resolution in 90% of cases of acute bacterial sinusitis
- Most complications result from direct spread (as opposed to hematogenous spread), including orbital cellulitis (often occurs with ethmoid involvement), frontal bone osteomyelitis, brain and subdural abscess, and meningitis
- Sinusitis associated with periorbital edema, mental status changes, or visual changes warrants immediate attention by a specialist

Rhinitis

INTRODUCTION

- Rhinitis is a heterogeneous disease that is often underdiagnosed and mistakenly considered as ˆnormalˆ
- Rhinitis consists of a variety of symptoms, such as sneezing, nasal itching, congestion, postnasal drip, and rhinorrhea
- The socioeconomic impact of rhinitis is high; rhinitis is linked to sleep disorders, emotional problems, and impaired functioning and learning in both children and adults
- Rhinitis can be divided into allergic and nonallergic etiologies

ETIOLOGY, EPIDEMIOLOGY, & RISK FACTORS

- The causes of rhinitis are multifactorial and are listed in the *Differential Dx* section
- Triggers for allergic rhinitis include pollens, molds, dust mites, and animal dander
- When IgE is cross-linked by allergen, mast cells release histamine that results in pruritis, rhinorrhea, and sneezing; other cytokines attract inflammatory cells, which lead to delayed congestion
- Allergic rhinitis is found in 10–25% of the population (up to 40% in some countries) and is increasing in frequency
- There is a genetic predisposition to allergic rhinitis
- Those with other allergic diseases (e.g., asthma, atopic dermatitis) are at higher risk for allergic rhinitis, as are those in higher socioeconomic groups

PATIENT PRESENTATION

- The most common symptoms are sneezing, itching, nasal congestion, postnasal drip, and rhinorrhea
- Patients may also have loss of smell, inability to taste, snoring, frequent throat clearing, functional decline, and daytime fatigue
- Allergic "shiners" (dark circles under the eyes) may occur due to venous congestion
- Many children develop a nasal crease, caused by chronic rubbing of the nose with the palm of the hand
- Turbinate edema and nasal passage occlusion can be visualized on exam; patients with nonallergic rhinitis may have erythema of the mucosa; allergic rhinitis causes a pale or blue nose
- Shiny polyps may be visualized
  - Cystic fibrosis should be considered in children with polyps

DIFFERENTIAL DX

- Allergic rhinitis
- Infectious rhinitis
- Structural rhinitis (e.g., deviated septum, tumor, adenoid hypertrophy, foreign body, polyps)
- Inflammatory rhinitis (e.g., Wegener's granulomatosis, sarcoidosis)
- Hormonal
- Medication-induced (rhinitis medicamentosa)
- Irritants
- Environmental (e.g., smoke, odors, temperature)
- Functional (e.g., ciliary dyskinesia, postural)
- NARES (nonallergic rhinitic eosinophilic syndrome)
- Cerebrospinal fluid leak

DIAGNOSTIC EVALUATION

- Complete history and physical examination, including occupational history, exposures (e.g., home environment, presence of mold, triggers, resolution of symptoms during vacation), and seasonal variability of symptoms
- Allergic rhinitis can be evaluated with IgE antibody testing, either via in vivo skin prick testing or in vitro serum analysis
  - In vivo testing is preferred, but serum analysis should be used if the patient has dermatographia (a condition in which gentle scratching of the skin causes raised, red lines), a history of anaphylaxis, is pregnant, or using beta-blockers
  - Antihistamines should be stopped several days prior to in vivo testing
- Other tests, such as blood eosinophil counts and total IgE levels, are less sensitive and specific and are not routinely recommended

TREATMENT & MANAGEMENT

- Avoidance allergens (e.g., bed and pillow casings for dust mite allergy)
- Intranasal corticosteroids are the preferred treatment for nasal congestion and other symptoms; these are safe and effective and have been shown to improve quality of life measurements, such as daytime somnolence
- Systemic antihistamines are useful in allergic rhinitis
  - Newer, second-generation medications, such as cetirizine, fexofenadine, loratadine, and desloratadine, have more favorable side effect profiles than older agents
- Topical nasal antihistamines (e.g., azelastine) can aide in the treatment of patients with allergic and nonallergic rhinitis
- Montelukast, a leukotriene receptor antagonist, has been approved for treatment of allergic rhinitis
- Nasal ipratropium bromide is effective for rhinorrhea
- Nasal cromolyn may be helpful as a prophylactic agent prior to allergen exposure
- Nasal saline lavage can reduce symptoms by 30%
- Immunotherapy for persistent symptoms in patients with allergic rhinitis can reduce medication needs and significantly improve quality of life

PROGNOSIS & COMPLICATIONS

- Allergic rhinitis is a chronic disease with significant morbidity and cost but can usually be managed effectively
- Complications of untreated rhinitis include poor school and work performance, otitis media and sinusitis, and exacerbations of asthma
- Mouth breathing due to nasal congestion can also lead to dental malocclusion, halitosis, and an increase in dental caries
- Uncontrolled nasal congestion can induce sleep disturbance

Hematology/Oncology

Bruising and Bleeding

INTRODUCTION

- There are 3 types of bruising: Subcutaneous (bleeding underneath the skin), intramuscular (bleeding within muscle), and periosteal (bleeding under the periosteum, which is the most severe and painful)
- As we age, the capillary walls become fragile and the skin thins, affording the capillaries less protection; this allows easier capillary rupture into the surrounding tissue, resulting in the familiar "black and blue" mark of a bruise
- After about 18 hours, a bruise may start to change colors to yellow, red, and/or green as the body resorbs the extravasated blood

ETIOLOGY, EPIDEMIOLOGY, & RISK FACTORS

- Bleeding may arise from direct injury, coagulation pathway defects, inhibitors of coagulation factors, platelet dysfunction, platelet consumption, or deficiencies in platelet production
- Bleeding disorders may be congenital or acquired
- During bruising, blood is extravasated from the bloodstream; significant bruising can lead to anemia, hypovolemia, hypotension, shock, or death
- Women are at higher risk for bruising as they age
- Disorders with balance impairment increase the risk for bruising, including Parkinson's disease, stroke, functional decline, and seizures
- Family history of bleeding disorders, nutritional deficiencies, alcoholism, liver disease, and hepatitis B or C increase the risk

PATIENT PRESENTATION

- Ecchymoses with minimal trauma
- Petechiae
- Excessive or repeated epistaxis
- Melena, bright red blood per rectum, hematemesis, hematuria, or gingival bleeding may also occur
- Fatigue, decreased exercise tolerance, lack of energy
- Pallor
- Tachycardia
- Angina
- Hypoxia

DIFFERENTIAL DX

- Trauma (accidental or abuse)
- Aging
- Medications (NSAIDs, aspirin, warfarin, clopidogrel, steroids, chemotherapy)
- Dietary supplements (fish oil, ginkgo biloba, ginger, garlic)
- Thrombocytopenia, ITP, TTP/HUS, HSP, platelet disorders
- Aplastic anemia
- Von Willebrand's disease
- Hemophilia
- Leukemia or lymphoma
- Cirrhosis, other liver disease
- Sepsis, DIC
- Nutritional deficiencies (vitamins C, K, B_{12}, folic acid)
- Surgery
- SLE
- HIV
- Uremia
- Cystic fibrosis

DIAGNOSTIC EVALUATION

- Complete history and physical examination, including medications, over-the-counter drugs, and alternative medicines, and family history of bleeding disorders
  - Evaluate for splenomegaly
- Initial labs may include complete blood count and peripheral smear, coagulation tests (prothrombin time, International Normalized Ratio, activated partial thromboplastin time), and bleeding time
- Consider mixing studies if concerned about coagulation factor deficiency or inhibitor
- Assess levels of fibrinogen, thrombin time, or D-dimer if suspect DIC
- Consider bone marrow biopsy/aspirate if suspect malignancy or abnormal platelets or other cell lines
- Other useful tests may include erythrocyte sedimentation rate (ESR), ANA, basic metabolic panel, liver function tests, and HIV testing
- Direct visualization of the gastrointestinal tract may be necessary for intractable bleeding (e.g., bleeding ulcers, bleeding varices, arteriovenous malformation, polyps)
- Hematology referral may be indicated

TREATMENT & MANAGEMENT

- Stabilize bleeding: Consider platelet transfusion (if <80,000 and actively bleeding, particularly in the presence of gastrointestinal bleeding or use of NSAIDs or other anticoagulants) and/or blood transfusion
- Fresh frozen plasma (FFP) may be indicated for warfarin overdose; deficiencies of coagulation factors (factors II, V, VII, VIII, IX, X, XI, XIII), antithrombin III, protein C, or protein S; severe liver disease; and vitamin K depletion
- Administer vitamin K (1 mg IV) for vitamin K deficiency or gastrointestinal bleeding due to warfarin use
- Treat the underlying cause as necessary
- Cease offending medications; consider NSAID avoidance
- Replace nutritional and/or factor deficiencies as necessary
- Heparin may be indicated for severe DIC
- Desmopressin (DDAVP) can be used for severe bleeding secondary to uremia or Von Willebrand's disease
- RhoGAM injection or splenectomy may be needed for recurrent ITP (steroids may also be an option)

PROGNOSIS & COMPLICATIONS

- Severe bleeding may be life threatening via exsanguination, MI, or stroke
- Prognosis is based on underlying condition
- Coagulation factor replacement or platelet transfusion may be necessary prior to surgery or procedures
- For chronic bleeding, periodic blood transfusions or iron replacement may be indicated depending on the degree of anemia
- At-risk patients should be cautious of trauma (e.g., refrain from contact sports or activities where head trauma is possible, such as sky diving or ice skating)

Hematology/Oncology

Lymphadenopathy

INTRODUCTION

- The lymphatic system is comprised of lymph vessels, nodes, and lymphoid tissues distributed throughout the body; it functions to drain interstitial fluids, ultimately returning fluid via the thoracic duct and right lymphatic duct to the thoracic venous system
- It also serves as an organ of the immune system; pathogens are brought through the lymphatics to regional nodes where cell-mediated immune functions respond to infections
- Lymphadenopathy refers to enlargement of the lymph nodes; localized lymphadenopathy involves 1 lymph region, while generalized lymphadenopathy involves more than 1 region
- The majority of cases are due to nonspecific causes or upper respiratory illnesses
- Less than 1% of cases are due to an underlying malignancy

ETIOLOGY, EPIDEMIOLOGY, & RISK FACTORS

- The most common cause of generalized lymphadenopathy is an immune response to an infection
    - Infections include viruses (e.g., EBV, CMV), bacteria (e.g., *Staphylococcus, Streptococcus,* tuberculosis), parasites (e.g., toxoplasmosis), and fungi
- Malignancies that tend to cause lymphadenopathy include lymphoma and leukemia (due to localized neoplastic proliferation) and metastases (due to infiltration by neoplastic cells)
- 10% of patients with unexplained lymphadenopathy are sent to specialists for further workup; 3.2% require biopsy; 1.1% are ultimately shown to have malignancy
- Risk increases with age: patients older than 40 with unexplained lymphadenopathy have a 4% risk of malignancy; patients younger than 40 have 0.4% risk
- Risk factors include exposures (cats, ticks, high-risk sex), travel, medications (e.g., allopurinol, penicillin, phenytoin, atenolol, captopril, cephalosporins, hydralazine, sulfonamides, quinidine)

PATIENT PRESENTATION

- Lymph node enlargement can be regional or localized, unilateral or bilateral, and may be further characterized as acute, subacute, or chronic
- Pain occurs due to expansion of the node capsule; this is *not* a predictor of malignancy
- Typically, enlargement >1 cm is considered abnormal
    - For the epitrochlear nodes, >0.5 cm is abnormal
    - For the inguinal nodes, >1.5 cm is abnormal
- The presentation of the enlarged node may help identify the underlying cause:
    - Hard nodes may suggest malignancy
    - Rubbery nodes may suggest lymphoma
    - Fluctuant nodes suggest a suppurative etiology
    - Fixed nodes (vs. mobile) may suggest malignancy or other inflammatory process

DIFFERENTIAL DX

- Lymphatic or hematologic malignancy (e.g., Hodgkin's and non-Hodgkin's lymphomas)
- Lymphoproliferative disorders
- Serum sickness
- Drug reactions (e.g., phenytoin)
- Addison's disease
- Hypothyroidism
- Sarcoidosis
- Chronic granulomatous disease
- Amyloid
- Systemic lupus erythematosus
- Rheumatoid arthritis
- Churg-Strauss vasculitis

DIAGNOSTIC EVALUATION

- History and physical examination should characterize the affected lymphatics (regional vs. generalized, number, size, tenderness, and associated systemic symptoms)
  - A history of arthropod (flea, tick) exposure may be present
  - There may be an associated rash, as in the case of Lyme disease
  - A travel history is important because many parasitic diseases are third-world (e.g., trypanosomiasis) or tropical (e.g., filariasis) diseases
  - Immune status is also important because of the prevalence of toxoplasmosis as an AIDS-associated disease
- Labs include complete blood count, erythrocyte sedimentation rate (ESR), liver function tests, and blood cultures
- Biopsy of affected lymph nodes may aid the diagnosis
  - Strongly consider biopsy if node is >2.0 cm, associated with abnormal chest X-ray, and/or age is >40 years
  - Biopsy should be performed on the largest, most abnormal node, if possible (in descending order of preference of location: supraclavicular, cervical, axillary, inguinal)
- HIV testing, skin testing for tuberculosis, or immune globulin titers to EBV or CMV may be indicated
- Ultrasound of regional lymphatics, chest X-ray, and chest CT scan may be indicated

TREATMENT & MANAGEMENT

- Management is focused on treating underlying condition
- If suspect bacterial infection, empiric antibiotics should cover staphylococci and streptococci (e.g., dicloxacillin, clindamycin)
  - Trimethoprim-sulfamethoxazole or doxycycline if suspect methicillin-resistant *S. aureus* (MRSA)
- If the node itself is infected, incision and drainage may be indicated
- If suspect viral infection, supportive care, including analgesia and cold compresses, is sufficient
- If suspect malignancy, refer to a specialist
- If medication-induced, discontinue the offending agent

PROGNOSIS & COMPLICATIONS

- Prognosis is based on underlying condition
- Malignancy is present in only 1% of unexplained causes of lymphadenopathy

Iron Deficiency Anemia

INTRODUCTION

- Anemia is a state of circulating erythrocyte deficiency
  - Assessed by measuring hemoglobin concentration or hematocrit level (the percentage of whole blood volume that is occupied by red blood cells)
- The World Health Organization criteria defines anemia as a hemoglobin or hematocrit level that is more than 2 standard deviations below the mean
  - Hemoglobin <13.0 g/dL in men or <12.0 g/dL in women
  - Hematocrit <41% in men or <36% in women
- Anemia may be the underlying cause of a presenting complaint or may be an incidental finding on physical or laboratory examination

ETIOLOGY, EPIDEMIOLOGY, & RISK FACTORS

- Iron deficiency is the most common nutritional deficiency worldwide and particularly affects women (especially pregnant women); however, in countries in which meat is a large part of the diet, iron deficiency due to nutritional inadequacy is uncommon
- In the body, iron exists as part of hemoglobin in red blood cells, as part of certain proteins (e.g., myoglobin), bound to transferrin in the blood, or stored as ferritin
- Iron homeostasis is a balance between absorption of dietary iron, iron loss in the feces and urine, and iron storage
  - Absorption (duodenum and jejunum) is regulated by the amount of iron in the diet
  - Diminished iron stores or increased erythropoiesis causes increased absorption
  - Iron is stored as ferritin, mostly in the bone marrow, liver, and reticuloendothelial system
- When increased hemoglobin is needed, iron stores are mobilized, resulting in iron deficiency without anemia; continued need for iron results in anemia
- In the U.S., iron deficiency anemia is present in 1–2% of adults
- Iron deficiency, with or without anemia, is most often associated with blood loss, either obvious or occult
- Teenage girls, menstruating women, and pregnant women are at highest risk for iron deficiency

PATIENT PRESENTATION

- Determine whether anemia is acute or chronic, whether the patient is actively bleeding or has recently bled, whether the patient is symptomatic, whether there is any underlying medical condition that may be causing the anemia, and whether the patient is taking medicines or drugs that may lead to anemia via hemolysis, marrow suppression, or bleeding
- Evaluate for signs of bleeding (stools for occult blood, ecchymosis or bleeding from sites of recent procedures), volume depletion, systemic illness
- Symptoms of anemia may include decreased exercise tolerance, dyspnea on exertion, dyspnea at rest, weakness, and lightheadedness
- Signs include pallor (conjunctival, nail bed, or palmar), bounding pulses, tachycardia, confusion
- Pica (an appetite for substances not fit for food, such as paper or dirt) and pagophagia (pica for ice) may occur

DIFFERENTIAL DX

- Dietary insufficiency
- Acute blood loss
  - Overt or obvious
  - Gastrointestinal source (active bleed, carcinoma)
  - Abnormal menstruation
- Decreased iron absorption
  - Malabsorption
  - Celiac sprue
  - Following gastric bypass
- Other forms of anemia
  - Microcytic (e.g., anemia of chronic disease, thalassemia)
  - Macrocytic (e.g., vitamin B_{12} or folate deficiency, hemolysis, liver disease, medications)
  - Normocytic (e.g., renal failure, thyroid disease, bone marrow suppression)

DIAGNOSTIC EVALUATION

- Laboratory evaluation in the emergent setting should include complete blood count, stool guaiac testing, basic metabolic panel, and blood type testing (type and screen or type and cross)
  - Complete blood count is indicated, with careful attention to the red blood cell distribution width (RDW) and mean corpuscular volume (MCV) for evaluation of possible etiologies
  - Peripheral smear will reveal microcytosis prior to a decrease in MCV
- The definitive test for iron deficiency anemia is a low serum ferritin level (10-15 ng/mL), which is diagnostic for iron deficiency
  - Other markers of iron deficiency include low serum iron, increased total iron-binding capacity, low transferrin saturation, and increased red blood cell distribution width
- Once iron deficiency is confirmed, further evaluate to determine the etiology (e.g., fecal occult blood testing, gynecology evaluation)
- Further evaluation for other types of anemia may be indicated (e.g., evaluate for hemolysis with peripheral smear, lactate dehydrogenase, haptoglobin, liver function tests, and appropriate autoimmune workup; vitamin B_{12} and folate levels)
  - Rarely, hemoglobin electrophoresis and bone marrow examination may be warranted
- If ongoing bleeding is suspected, immediate evaluation of the gastrointestinal tract with esophagogastroduodenoscopy (EGD) or colonoscopy may be indicated

TREATMENT & MANAGEMENT

- Oral iron is a cheap, safe, and effective means of restoring iron balance
  - In adults, a 300-mg ferrous sulfate tablet 3 times a day between meals provides 180 mg of elemental iron per day and should cause a 2 g/dL rise in hemoglobin within 3 weeks
  - Oral iron is absorbed best in the duodenum and proximal jejunum, so enteric-coated iron is not recommended
  - To improve iron absorption, ingest on an empty stomach; vitamin C or ascorbic acid also acidifies the stomach, thus increasing iron absorption
  - Length of therapy must be individualized; iron should be continued until stores are replenished and hemoglobin is normal
- Intramuscular or intravenous iron preparations (such as iron dextran or ferric gluconate) may be necessary in patients refractory to oral iron
  - In such cases, the iron deficit can be calculated to determine the correct dose
- Prophylactic iron therapy is warranted in high-risk groups, including pregnant women, women with menorrhagia, vegetarians, and adolescent girls
- In patients with symptomatic anemia, blood transfusions are often necessary

PROGNOSIS & COMPLICATIONS

- Look carefully for underlying causes, and have a high index of suspicion for occult gastrointestinal blood loss
- Iron deficiency, with or without anemia, is an easily treatable disease if the underlying cause of the deficiency is corrected
- Failure to respond to oral therapy can be a consequence of incorrect diagnosis, the presence of a coexisting disease, continued blood loss, noncompliance, or malabsorption
- Iron deficiency anemia is an uncommon cause of death; however, moderate to severe iron deficiency can worsen underlying pulmonary and cardiovascular disorders
- Chronic iron deficiency can produce defects of epithelial tissue (koilonychia, atrophic tongue, stomatitis, dysphagia), cold intolerance, or impaired immune tolerance

Outpatient Anticoagulation Therapy

INTRODUCTION

- Anticoagulation therapy with warfarin is commonly used to decrease the risk of arterial thromboembolism (i.e., stroke) in patients with atrial fibrillation/flutter or patients with prosthetic cardiac valves
- It is also used to prevent recurrent venous thromboembolism in patients with deep vein thrombosis or pulmonary embolism
- Less commonly, it is used for secondary prevention after myocardial infarction and in patients with hypercoagulable states
- The goal of anticoagulant therapy is to administer the lowest possible dose of anticoagulant that successfully prevents clot formation or expansion

ETIOLOGY, EPIDEMIOLOGY, & RISK FACTORS

- Warfarin is a Coumadin derivative that inhibits clotting by limiting the hepatic production of vitamin K-dependent clotting factors (activated factors II, VII, IX, and X)
- Reduction of the amount and activity of these factors inhibits the extrinsic and the common coagulation pathways, thus producing an anticoagulant response
- Warfarin is metabolized in the liver and kidneys
- The mean plasma half-life is approximately 40 hours, and the duration of its effect is 2–5 days; thus, the maximum effect occurs up to 48 hours after administration, and the effect persists for approximately 5 days
- The half-lives of the affected clotting factors differ (e.g., clotting factor II = 60 hours, VII = 6 hours, IX = 24 hours, X = 40 hours), so there is a delay before the full effect of warfarin is achieved; thus, patients should receive heparin as a "bridge" until warfarin achieves its antithrombotic effect
- The level of anticoagulation achieved is measured in terms of prothrombin time and the International Normalized Ratio (INR)
  - The INR was developed by the World Health Organization in response to variations in prothrombin time from lab to lab and across the world

PATIENT PRESENTATION

- Current recommendations for the initiation of warfarin therapy differ based on the urgency for achieving an anticoagulant effect
- While warfarin is being initiated, patients who require rapid anticoagulation should also be given unfractionated heparin or low molecular weight heparin
  - Patients who require nonurgent anticoagulation, such as those with stable chronic atrial fibrillation, may not need heparin

DIFFERENTIAL DX

Possible drug interactions
- Medications that increase INR or bleeding risk include amiodarone, imidazoles, statins, acetaminophen, cephalosporins, anabolic steroids, binding resins, thyroid hormone, and metronidazole
- Drugs that decrease INR or increase clotting risk include oral contraceptives, rifampin, penicillin, and carbamazepine

DIAGNOSTIC EVALUATION

- Upon initiating warfarin therapy, the INR should be checked daily or every other day until it is in the therapeutic range for 2 consecutive days, then every 3–5 days; once the INR and warfarin dose is stable for 1 week, the INR can be checked weekly for 2–3 weeks
  - Once a patient makes the transition from the initial dosing phase to a maintenance phase, INR should be monitored once every 4 weeks
  - Before adjusting the dosage, patients should be questioned regarding adherence, changes in any medications, current vitamin K consumption (including foods and supplements), and concomitant illnesses (e.g., heart failure, thyroid dysfunction)
- Recommended INR goals:
  - Deep venous thrombosis prophylaxis for high-risk surgery: INR of 2–3 after surgery
  - Venous thrombosis or pulmonary embolism, first episode: INR of 2–3 for 3–6 months
  - Venous thrombosis or pulmonary embolism, recurrent: INR of 2–3 indefinitely
  - Thrombosis associated with antiphospholipid antibodies: INR of 3–4 indefinitely
  - Chronic or intermittent atrial fibrillation: INR of 2–3 indefinitely (or for 3 weeks before and 4 weeks after cardioversion)
  - Cardiac valve replacement (tissue): INR of 2–3 for 3 months
  - Cardiac valve replacement (mechanical): INR of 2.5–3.5 for life
  - Cardiac valve replacement (bioprosthetic): INR of 2–3 for variable duration
  - Following MI: INR of 2–3, based on clinical judgment
  - Dilated cardiomyopathy with ejection fraction <30%: INR of 2–3 for life

TREATMENT & MANAGEMENT

- Avoid contact sports, skydiving, ice skating, and walking on icy areas
  - Risk of falling in the elderly may be an important consideration for use of anticoagulation
- Warfarin should be started at a dose of 5 mg/d
  - A lower starting dose is recommended in elderly patients, those with low body weight or low albumin levels, patients with congestive heart failure or liver disease, and patients who are taking certain medications (e.g., amiodarone, trimethoprim-sulfamethoxazole, metronidazole)
- The most common side effect of warfarin use is bleeding due to excessive anticoagulation
  - Characteristics associated with major risk for hemorrhage include age >65, history of gastrointestinal bleeding, and comorbid disease (e.g., hypertension, cerebrovascular disease, renal insufficiency)
- Management of warfarin-related hemorrhage is based on the severity of bleeding and intensity of anticoagulation at the time of the bleeding episode
  - Life-threatening hemorrhage is treated with IV vitamin K, fresh frozen plasma (FFP), and prothrombin complex concentrate (PCC)
  - Less severe hemorrhage may be treated by withholding warfarin for several days and/or administration of subcutaneous vitamin K

PROGNOSIS & COMPLICATIONS

- The duration of therapy with warfarin varies based on the indication for treatment and the need for anticoagulation
- In patients on anticoagulation therapy who are undergoing invasive procedures that carry moderate to high risks of bleeding, warfarin should be stopped 4 days prior to the procedure; heparin can be used perioperatively for thromboembolism prophylaxis
- For less invasive procedures with low risks of bleeding, warfarin may be stopped 3–4 days prior to surgery and restarted immediately following the procedure
- Among newer antithrombotic agents being developed for chronic anticoagulation, ximelagatran (Exanta) has shown promising results as a direct thrombin inhibitor

Cancer Screening

INTRODUCTION

- Breast cancer is the most common nonskin cancer in women and the 2nd most common cause of cancer death in women
- Cervical cancer is the 3rd most common gynecologic malignancy and 8th most common nonskin malignancy in women; mean age of diagnosis is 50
- Colon cancer is the 2nd leading cause of cancer death in the United States; most cases occur in individuals older than 50
- Prostate cancer is the most common nonskin malignancy in men older than 50 and the 2nd leading cause of cancer death in men; mean age of diagnosis is 72

ETIOLOGY, EPIDEMIOLOGY, & RISK FACTORS

- Breast cancer: Growth is likely estrogen dependent
  - Risk factors include increasing age, family history in a first-degree relative, previous history of breast cancer, prolonged unopposed estrogen exposure (e.g., early menarche, late menopause, late first pregnancy, use of hormone replacement therapy), and obesity
  - BRCA1 and BRCA2 genes confer a lifetime risk of 65–80%
- Cervical cancer: Infection with human papillomavirus (HPV) is a strong risk factor
  - HPV types 16, 18, 31, 33, 35, and 39 are strongly associated with increased risk
  - Other risk factors include smoking, early onset of sexual activity, multiple sexual partners, HIV infection or other immunosuppressive conditions, history of a sexually transmitted disease, and radiation exposure
- Colon cancer: Arises over long periods of time (6–10 years) from adenomatous polyps; thus, regular surveillance via colonoscopy provides an excellent means for prevention
  - Increased risk in hereditary syndromes, family history, inflammatory bowel disease, *Streptococcus bovis* bacteremia, ureterosigmoidostomy, tobacco use, age >40, obesity
- Prostate cancer: Hormonal influence plays a major role in the etiology of adenocarcinomas but not in other subtypes
  - Increasing age, African-American race, and family history increase the risk

PATIENT PRESENTATION

- Breast cancer: Most commonly discovered as a breast lump, breast pain, breast enlargement, nondescript thickening of the breast, or by screening mammogram.
- Cervical cancer: May present with irregular menstrual bleeding, abnormal vaginal discharge, pelvic pain, obstructive uropathy, back pain, or leg swelling
- Colon cancer: Weight loss, anorexia, or malaise
  - Proximal tumors (cecum, ascending colon): Anemia, heme-positive stools
  - Transverse colon tumors: Pain, cramps, obstruction, perforation
  - Sigmoid and rectal tumors: Tenesmus, small-caliber stool, hematochezia
- Prostate cancer: Asymptomatic, unless late stage
  - Local growth can cause dysuria, difficulty voiding, and urinary frequency or retention

DIFFERENTIAL DX

- Breast cancer: Cysts, fibrocystic changes, benign tumors (fibroadenoma, hamartoma, papilloma, lipoma, adenoma), infection (mastitis, tuberculosis, abscess), trauma, benign lymphadenopathy
- Cervical cancer: Necrosis, inflammation, and hemorrhage may produce false-positive results on Pap smear
- Colon cancer: Intestinal obstruction from nonmalignant causes, inflammatory bowel disease, malabsorption syndrome
- Prostate cancer: Benign prostatic hypertrophy, prostatitis, trauma with hematoma formation

DIAGNOSTIC EVALUATION

- Breast cancer: Annual mammogram beginning at 40 and regular breast examinations
  - Women with a positive family history may initiate screening earlier and be referred for genetic testing
- Cervical cancer: Annual Pap smear tests beginning with onset of vaginal intercourse but no later than age 21
  - Pap smears can be done every 3 years for low-risk women with 3 consecutive normal tests
  - More frequent screening is recommended for women at increased risk
  - Screening may not be necessary for women ≥70 years with at least 3 consecutive normal tests within the last 10 years or women with total hysterectomy (with the removal of cervix)
- Colon cancer: In patients with average risk, one of the following should be done beginning at age 50:
  - Fecal occult blood testing or fecal immunochemical testing annually *or*
  - Flexible sigmoidoscopy plus fecal occult blood testing every 5 years *or*
  - Double-contrast barium enema every 5 years *or*
  - Colonoscopy every 10 years
- Prostate cancer: Annual prostate-specific antigen (PSA) and digital rectal examinations beginning at age 50 or beginning at age 45 for men at increased risk
  - However, annual PSA testing is controversial
- Biopsy is necessary for definitive diagnosis following screening procedures

TREATMENT & MANAGEMENT

- Breast cancer: Preferred treatment is breast conservation surgery (lumpectomy followed by radiation therapy) or mastectomy
  - Chemotherapy is given to most patients
  - Hormone therapy (e.g., tamoxifen, aromatase inhibitors) in estrogen or progesterone hormone-positive tumors
- Cervical cancer: Treated by surgical excision, laser ablation, hysterectomy, chemotherapy, and/or radiation, depending on staging
  - A vaccine is now available to prevent initial infection with two HPV strains (16 and 18) that are associated with cervical cancer
- Colon cancer: Surgical resection is curative for early cancers; surgical resection plus adjuvant chemotherapy for advanced cancers
- Prostate cancer: Localized disease may be treated with prostatectomy, external-beam radiation, internal radiation (brachytherapy), or cryosurgery
  - Depending on patient age, health, and tumor status, "watchful waiting" (observation alone with no active treatment) may be acceptable
  - Gonadotropin-releasing hormone (GnRH) agonists (e.g., leuprolide) are also used
  - Chemotherapy is still under investigation

PROGNOSIS & COMPLICATIONS

- Breast cancer: 5-year survival rate of all patients with breast cancer is 85%, but prognosis varies widely based on stage, size, nodal status, hormone receptor status, and histology
  - Complications of screening include false-positives that lead to unnecessary procedures
- Cervical cancer: Prognosis primarily depends on stage and lymph node status
  - Early-stage tumors have up to 90% 5-year survival; advanced tumors have <15% survival
- Colon cancer: Survival time is directly related to the stage of the carcinoma at diagnosis
  - Potential complications of screening include bowel perforation, infection, bleeding, and splenic rupture
- Prostate cancer: Prognosis is excellent with early diagnosis (85% 10-year survival, even without treatment)

Neurology

Headache

INTRODUCTION

- Headache is one of the most common primary care complaints
- It may be an isolated or recurrent event
- It may be idiopathic (>90%) or secondary to an underlying cause (<10%)
- It may simply require an analgesic for pain relief or a complete and detailed workup to identify the source

ETIOLOGY, EPIDEMIOLOGY, & RISK FACTORS

- Although the pathophysiology of headaches is poorly understood, the proposed mechanisms include vascular, neuronal, and serotoninergic pathologies
  - Vascular spasms, dilation, and constriction, neuronal release of inflammatory cytokines, and serotonin imbalance have all been suggested as causes of headaches
  - Increased intracranial pressure can cause headaches
  - Compression of cranial or spinal nerves, muscle spasms, trauma, or inflammation of cranial or cervical musculature can also cause headaches
- Tension headache is the most common overall type
- Migraine headache is the most common diagnosis in patients who present to a physician
  - Affects 12% of the U.S. population
  - Migraines result in 150 million lost workdays and 329,000 lost school days each year
  - Migraines are three times more common in women
  - Migraine patients usually have positive family history of migraines
- Temporal arteritis should be strongly considered in headache patients older than 50
- At least 50% of patients with brain tumors develop a headache

PATIENT PRESENTATION

- Note location, duration, frequency, and character of the headache
- Assess for aura (occurs in 15% of migraine patients), which may include visual or sensory changes
- Nausea, vomiting, and photosensitivity may occur with migraine
- Sudden onset of severe headache may suggest intracranial bleeding
- Vision changes suggest temporal arteritis, optic neuritis, or glaucoma
- Fever, stiff neck, rash, or confusion suggest infection (e.g., meningitis)
- Assess blood pressure
- Jaw claudication suggests temporal arteritis
- Review medications, dosages, and durations of use
- Note signs of increased intracranial pressure (e.g., papilledema) and focal neurologic symptoms

DIFFERENTIAL DX

- Sinus pressure
- Increased intracranial pressure (e.g., hydrocephalus, tumor, pseudotumor cerebri)
- Tension headache
- Cluster headache
- Migraine headache
- Temporal arteritis
- Glaucoma
- Meningitis, encephalitis
- Stroke
- Optic neuritis
- Trigeminal neuralgia
- Temporomandibular joint
- Thyroid dysfunction
- Medication or substance withdrawal or overdose
- Posttraumatic (e.g., LP)
- Hypertension

DIAGNOSTIC EVALUATION

- History and physical exam often make the diagnosis
  - History should focus on onset, duration, frequency, possible triggers, severity, quality (e.g., throbbing, band-like), accompanying symptoms (e.g., aura, photophobia, visual changes, nausea/vomiting, lacrimation, nasal congestion), constitutional symptoms (e.g., weight loss, fever), medications, and dietary history
  - Is this the first and/or worst headache of life?
  - Physical examination should include complete neurologic exam, visual/retinal exam, head and neck exam, and gait exam
- Presence of red flags suggests possible serious etiologies and need for further workup: Constitutional symptoms, new headache in a patient older than 50, sudden onset, awakening from sleep, mental status changes, focal neurologic signs, visual/motor/balance disturbance, or papilledema
- CT scan may be indicated to assess for hemorrhage, mass lesions, or increased intracranial pressure
- MRI will identify posterior fossa tumors
- Lumbar puncture may be indicated if CT scan is normal but still suspect hemorrhage, infection, or tumor
- Serologies for bacterial, viral, and other causes of meningitis or encephalitis
- Elevated ESR suggests temporal arteritis or infection
- Carboxyhemoglobin measurement if history suggests carbon monoxide poisoning

TREATMENT & MANAGEMENT

- Assess for serious underlying conditions and treat accordingly
- Eliminate any potentially causative medications, including over-the-counter and alternative/complementary medications
- Educate patients about underlying headache physiology and have them try to identify triggers; if necessary, have patients keep a log of headache frequency and timing
- Tension-type headache: Regular exercise, stress management, tricyclic antidepressants, analgesics
- Migraine headache: Avoid triggers; serotonin agonists (e.g., sumatriptan), NSAIDs, ergotamines
- Temporal arteritis: High-dose corticosteroids
- Meningitis: Search for and treat the primary source (e.g., pneumonia, sinusitis, neoplasm) and administer immediate antimicrobial therapy for infections
- Subarachnoid hemorrhage requires attention to airway, breathing, and circulation and management of increased intracranial pressure (maintain blood pressure in the normal range as hypertension may cause the aneurysm to rebleed and hypotension may cause cerebral ischemia), administer nimodipine to prevent cerebral vasospasm, seizure prophylaxis with IV phenytoin, surgery
- Cluster headache: Oxygen inhalation for 5–10 minutes, serotonin agonists, ergotamines, and/or methysergide

PROGNOSIS & COMPLICATIONS

- Prognosis of secondary headaches depends on underlying illness
- The majority of patients with primary headaches will respond to treatment
- Severe migraines tend to be more difficult to control and may require multiple hospitalizations for IV therapy
- Some patients may require referral to a specialist
- Rarely, severe migraine can lead to a stroke, possibly because of prolonged constriction of blood vessels
- Conventional migraine treatments (triptans and ergotamines) are contraindicated for basilar and hemiplegic migraines (hemiparesis during aura period)

Dizziness and Lightheadedness

INTRODUCTION

- Lightheadedness is an extremely common symptom in clinical practice; however, the term is imprecise and may include symptoms of dizziness, vertigo, presyncope, or disequilibrium
  - Dizziness is more properly termed vertigo, which is a false sensation of movement (spinning, rotating, or swaying) of the patient or the environment
  - Presyncope is a syndrome of lightheadedness associated with a graying of vision, tinnitus, and expectation of syncope
  - Disequilibrium is a sense of imbalance that typically occurs when walking
  - In addition, postural hypotension, cardiogenic factors, and defective vasopressor mechanisms are common in the elderly

ETIOLOGY, EPIDEMIOLOGY, & RISK FACTORS

- Etiologies are numerous; most commonly caused by conditions that result in a relative decrease in cerebral perfusion
  - Vertigo is most commonly caused by peripheral vestibular dysfunction or CNS disease
  - Presyncope occurs secondary to cerebral hypoperfusion due to decreased cardiac output or decreased peripheral vascular resistance
  - Disequilibrium may occur due to problems with sensory proprioception or cerebellar system dysfunction
- The three most common peripheral disorders causing vertigo are benign paroxysmal positional vertigo (BPPV), vestibular neuronitis, and Ménière's disease
  - BPPV is usually caused by particles that float freely in the posterior semicircular canal of the inner ear
  - Ménière's disease is characterized by swelling of endolymphatic labyrinthine spaces and degeneration of the organ of Corti
  - Vestibular neuronitis involves inflammation of vestibular nerves and is usually preceded by viral infections

PATIENT PRESENTATION

- Acute vertigo presents with severe rotational dizziness, nausea/vomiting, diaphoresis, and tachycardia; examination reveals prominent nystagmus
  - Nystagmus of peripheral vestibular origin is typically horizontal and unidirectional; it is often suppressed with visual fixation and can be produced by head rotation
  - Nystagmus of central origin may be horizontal or vertical and may be associated with skew deviation of the eyes; not suppressed by fixation; may or may not be provoked by head rotation
- Dizziness secondary to central lesions is often associated with other central symptoms, such as diplopia, dysarthria, dysphagia, weakness, numbness, or palpitations

DIFFERENTIAL DX

- Otologic etiologies (e.g., positional vertigo, Ménière's disease)
- CNS etiologies (e.g., vertebrobasilar ischemia, cerebellar or brainstem infarct, cerebellar hemorrhage, basilar migraine, cerebellar pontine angle tumor, autonomic dysfunction)
- Other systemic etiologies include arrhythmia, orthostatic hypotension, acute or chronic alcohol intoxication, salicylate toxicity, antiepileptic drug toxicity, uremia, diabetes, hypoglycemia, thyroid disease, and hyperventilation
- Multiple medication use
- Anxiety/panic disorder

DIAGNOSTIC EVALUATION

- A complete history and physical exam should include signs of dehydration, questions about excessive pressure on the neck, headaches, palpitations, history of heart disease, hearing loss, cardiac auscultation, orthostatic blood pressures, and complete head and neck (including Weber/Rinne tests) and neurologic examinations
- Laboratory evaluation may include complete blood counts, electrolytes, calcium, glucose, BUN/creatinine, brain natriuretic peptide (BNP) level, ESR, carbon monoxide level, pulse oximetry and/or arterial blood gas, eosinophil count, and stool occult blood testing
- Further testing may include electrocardiogram (EKG), 24-hour EKG monitoring, echocardiography, electronystagmography, hearing evaluation, head CT, EEG, MRI (head and/or labyrinth) and/or magnetic resonance angiography (head or vertebrobasilar circulation)
- Vertigo may be evaluated via several specific maneuvers
  - Dix-Hallpike maneuver: With patient sitting, rapidly move the patient to the supine position with head over the back of the table, and observe for nystagmus (type and duration); repeat with head facing to the left and right (nystagmus that does not fatigue or is vertical is unlikely to be benign positional vertigo)
  - Barany (Nylan-Barany) maneuver is similar to Dix-Hallpike but is less sensitive

TREATMENT & MANAGEMENT

- Symptomatic management often involves vestibular suppressant drugs, such as prochlorperazine, cinnarizine, or meclizine
- Treat the underlying disorder as necessary
  - Rehydration
  - Treatment of cardiac disorders (e.g., medical therapy of heart failure, surgical intervention for valve disease)
  - Treat prodromal stroke (transient ischemic attack) with aspirin or warfarin
  - Carotid endarterectomy for significant carotid stenosis
  - Treat migraines with NSAIDs or triptans; valproate or tricyclic antidepressants for prophylaxis against future attacks
- Treatment of vertigo may include particle repositioning maneuvers (modified Epley maneuver), habituating exercises, vestibular rehabilitation, or surgical intervention for persistent disease
- If a specific etiology cannot be diagnosed, attempt to ameliorate contributing factors and symptoms by addressing anxiety, depressive symptoms, hearing impairment, balance impairment, and postural hypotension
- Consider reduction in causative medications

PROGNOSIS & COMPLICATIONS

- Most causes of dizziness can be identified and treated after detailed history and physical examination
- The physician should conscientiously investigate the possibility of an underlying organic pathology, which is often best accomplished by conducting a careful, thorough history and physical examination; if no organic disease is identified after a thorough investigation, a psychiatric or neurologic consultation may be warranted
- BPPV is usually self-limited
  - Up to 75% of cases improve within several months, even without treatment
  - Average duration of symptoms is 10 weeks
  - 25% of patients continue to have symptoms for years if not treated

Tremor

INTRODUCTION

- Tremor is the most common movement disorder; it is an involuntary, rhythmic oscillation of the hands, palate, or head
- Classified as resting tremor or intention tremor
  - Resting tremor occurs at rest or in a static position
  - Intention tremor occurs or increases with purposeful activity, such as reaching for an object; associated with a cerebellar deficit (e.g., multiple sclerosis, midbrain injury, stroke), which would otherwise inhibit the tremor
- May be worsened by caffeine or anxiety and relieved by alcohol ingestion

ETIOLOGY, EPIDEMIOLOGY, & RISK FACTORS

- Essential tremor is a visible postural tremor of the hands and forearms that may include a kinetic component
  - The specific pathophysiology of essential tremor remains unknown
  - May occurs sporadically or may be inherited
  - While the genetic defect has not been identified, familial transmission seems to be autosomal dominant with variable penetrance
- Physiologic tremor is a benign, visible, high-frequency, low-amplitude, postural tremor that occurs in the absence of neurologic disease
  - Caused by medical conditions (e.g., thyrotoxicosis, hypoglycemia, certain medications, withdrawal from alcohol or benzodiazepines) and is usually reversible once the cause is corrected
  - May be increased by emotions (e.g., anxiety, stress, or fear), exercise, fatigue, hypoglycemia, hypothermia, hyperthyroidism, and alcohol withdrawal
- Cerebellar tremors are kinetic (goal-directed) tremors that occur due to lesions of the lateral cerebellar nuclei (red nucleus), superior cerebellar peduncle, or their connections

PATIENT PRESENTATION

- Essential tremor initially presents as a postural distal arm tremor
  - Usually bilateral
  - May also involve head, voice, tongue, and legs
  - May slowly progress to a resting tremor
- Parkinsonian tremor occurs 4–8 cycles/second
  - May be the first sign of disease
  - Usually occurs at rest
  - 50% of patients have a postural component
  - Classically referred to as "pill rolling" tremor of hands, but may affect the head, trunk, jaw, or lips
- Cerebellar tremor is a medium-frequency intention tremor that has terminal accentuation (i.e., worse at end of movement)
  - Occurs primarily at the limbs, trunk, and head
  - The tremor is absent at rest
- Psychogenic tremor is abrupt in onset and may decrease or disappear when not watched

DIFFERENTIAL DX

- Essential tremor
- Parkinson's disease
- Drug- or toxin-induced (e.g., MPTP, alcohol)
- Medications (e.g., beta-agonists, lithium, amiodarone, valproic acid, metoclopramide, theophylline, methylphenidate)
- Postural tremor
- Stroke
- Cerebellar disease
- Wilson's disease
- Thyrotoxicosis
- Hypoglycemia
- Dystonia
- Choreoathetosis
- Psychogenic
- Anxiety
- Action myoclonus

DIAGNOSTIC EVALUATION

- History and physical examination is generally diagnostic
  - Assess onset, exacerbating and relieving factors, medications, family history, and associated symptoms
  - The physical examination should give attention to the body parts involved and the frequency and amplitude of the tremor; test the involved body parts at rest, with changes in posture, and during intended movement
- Diagnostic testing should be ordered based on the suspected etiology
  - Blood chemistry, hematology, thyroid function tests, and liver function tests may be ordered routinely
  - In patients with suspected Wilson's disease, 24-hour urine copper and serum ceruloplasmin determinations are helpful
  - Cerebrospinal fluid examination for oligoclonal IgG bands is appropriate in patients suspected of having multiple sclerosis
  - MRI may be useful when cerebellar tremor, stroke, or multiple sclerosis is suspected
  - PET scanning or single photon emission CT (SPECT) scanning may be useful in evaluating for parkinsonism
- Other evaluation tools used in research settings include surface electromyography, accelerometers, potentiometers, handwriting tremor analysis, and long-term tremor records

TREATMENT & MANAGEMENT

- Mild cases do not require treatment, and most forms of tremors do not have effective medical treatments
- Eliminate predisposing factors as necessary
- Medical therapy can be used as needed (e.g., during social events) for essential tremors
  - Primidone and propranolol are the most commonly used agents to decrease the tremor
  - Other agents may include topiramate, mirtazapine, and methazolamide
  - Alcohol use may also be effective, but abuse potential may limit its clinical utility
- There is no established treatment for cerebellar tremor; some patients may respond to isoniazid plus pyridoxine
- Parkinsonian tremor may be treated with anticholinergic medications (e.g., benztropine, trihexyphenidyl) and/or dopamine replacement therapy (e.g., levodopa plus carbidopa)
- Propranolol is very effective to reduce the tremor of alcohol withdrawal
- Orthostatic tremor often responds to clonazepam
- Surgical therapy (e.g., stereotactic thalamotomy, thalamic deep brain stimulation) may be considered in severe cases but is rarely necessary

PROGNOSIS & COMPLICATIONS

- Usually not disabling but may be socially embarrassing; severe tremors can interfere with daily activities, especially fine motor skills (e.g., writing) and speech, which may lead to social withdrawal and isolation
- May worsen with time, but patients should be assured that they do not have a life-threatening disorder

Weakness

INTRODUCTION

- The term "weakness" is used to mean different things by different patients, including decreased muscle strength, fatigue, fatigability, limitation of movement secondary to pain, and so forth
- Many different conditions, both general medical issues and specific neurologic etiologies, may lead to weakness
- Among primary neurologic etiologies, weakness can arise from damage to or dysfunction of nearly any level of the nervous system, from the motor cortex to the muscle

ETIOLOGY, EPIDEMIOLOGY, & RISK FACTORS

- Dysfunction at any level of the pathway from brain to muscle can result in weakness
- The upper motor neurons arise from layer V of the cerebral cortex (primary motor cortex, premotor cortex, supplementary motor cortex, and even the primary sensory cortex), arranged somatotopically, as represented by the familiar "homunculus"
  - The axons of these neurons descend through the corona radiata and internal capsule to form the corticospinal tract
  - 90% of these fibers decussate in the lower medulla and continue to descend through the corticospinal tracts of the spinal cord
- The axons synapse in the anterior horn of the spinal cord, with neurons that project out of the cord via the ventral nerve roots; these "anterior horn cells" represent the lower motor neurons
  - After passing through the peripheral nerves, the axons of the lower motor neurons transmit their signals directly to muscle via the neuromuscular junction
- The output of motor neurons is modulated by contributions from the basal ganglia, cerebellum, and other areas of the CNS
- Stroke is a common cause of weakness and the leading cause of disability in the U.S.

PATIENT PRESENTATION

- Muscle strength is graded using the Medical Research Council scale:
  - 0 = no movement
    1 = flicker of movement
    2 = movement possible with gravity removed
    3 = movement against gravity but not resistance
    4 = some movement against resistance
    5 = full movement against resistance
- Determine the pattern of weakness:
  - Time course: Acute versus chronic
  - Fatigable versus constant weakness
  - Distribution: Proximal versus distal; one-sided weakness (often brain pathology) versus bilateral (often spinal cord pathology); upper motor neuron (spasticity, increased reflexes) versus lower motor neuron (atrophy, fasciculations, decreased or absent reflexes)
- Associated features may include pain, sensory changes, cranial nerve or bladder dysfunction

DIFFERENTIAL DX

- Brain: Stroke, neoplasm, trauma, multiple sclerosis (MS)
- Spinal cord: Trauma, MS, neoplasm, myelopathy, infarct
- Anterior horn cell: ALS, spinal muscular atrophy, polio
- Ventral root: Degenerative disc disease, Guillain-Barré
- Plexus: Infiltrating mass or hemorrhage, radiation plexopathy, diabetic amyotrophy, inflammatory
- Peripheral nerve: Guillain-Barré, CIDP, Charcot-Marie-Tooth, trauma, HIV, porphyria
- Neuromuscular junction: MG, botulism, Lambert-Eaton
- Muscle: Myositis, myopathy, MD, thyroid disease

DIAGNOSTIC EVALUATION

- Thorough history and physical examination is essential
- Creatine phosphokinase is often elevated in muscle disease but normal in other conditions
- Consider CNS imaging if upper motor neuron signs or other associated features are present
- Consider lumbar puncture if suspect Guillain-Barré syndrome, CIDP, MS, or Lyme disease
- Consider electromyography and nerve conduction studies if suspect spinal root, plexus, peripheral nerve, neuromuscular junction, or muscle disease
- Muscle or nerve biopsy may be indicated if suspect neuromuscular disease

TREATMENT & MANAGEMENT

- Treat the underlying etiology as appropriate
- Stroke: Treat per accepted protocols
- Neoplasm requires urgent neurosurgery consultation
  - Multiple sclerosis: IV steroids for acute exacerbation, interferon-beta 1 or glatiramer acetate for long-term management
  - Amyotrophic lateral sclerosis (ALS): Riluzole is the only treatment available
  - Guillain-Barré syndrome: Intravenous immunoglobulin or plasma exchange
  - CIDP: Steroids, immunosuppression.
  - Myasthenia gravis: Pyridostigmine, consider thymectomy

PROGNOSIS & COMPLICATIONS

- Prognosis and complications are generally related to the underlying diagnosis
- Physical and occupational therapy may improve strength and purposeful function
- Continued weakness can lead to muscle atrophy and possible contractures

Dementia

INTRODUCTION

- Dementia is a syndrome where focal brain regions undergo premature neuronal death, resulting in loss of function in multiple cognitive and emotional abilities
- More than 50 illnesses may cause dementia; Alzheimer's disease is the most common cause (50–60%), followed by vascular (multi-infarct) dementia (20%)
  - Potentially treatable causes (e.g., syphilis, vitamin B_{12} deficiency) account for 5–10%
- Affects 1% of the population by age 60; the prevalence then doubles every 5 years to affect 30–50% by age 85

ETIOLOGY, EPIDEMIOLOGY, & RISK FACTORS

- Cortical etiologies: Alzheimer's disease, amyotrophic lateral sclerosis dementia complex, Pick's disease
- Subcortical etiologies: Parkinson's disease, multisystem atrophy, progressive supranuclear palsy, Huntington's disease
- Mixed etiologies: Multi-infarct dementia, corticobasal degeneration, Lewy body dementia, chronic alcohol abuse, prion diseases
- Risk factors include increasing age, family history, tobacco use, stroke, female gender, head trauma, endocrine dysfunction, hypertension, diabetes mellitus, low education level, and alcohol or substance abuse

PATIENT PRESENTATION

- Cognitive decline (e.g., memory loss, inattentiveness, poor recall, progressive disorientation to time and place)
- Language disorders (e.g., decreased spontaneous speech, word finding difficulty)
  - Anomia: Difficulty finding words and naming objects
  - Aphasia: Disordered speech, comprehension, naming, reading, and writing
  - Apraxia: Inability to perform previously learned tasks, such as combing hair
  - Agnosia: Impaired recognition or comprehension of specific auditory, visual, or tactile stimuli
- Impairment performing activities of daily living
- Behavioral symptoms (e.g., depression, emotional lability, hallucinations, delirium [more common with Lewy body dementia], disinhibition, and personality changes)

DIFFERENTIAL DX

- Normal cognitive aging
- Pseudodementia of depression
- Metabolic and endocrine disorders (e.g., vitamin B_{12} deficiency, Wernicke's encephalopathy)
- Medication effects
- Infections (e.g., Creutzfeldt-Jakob disease, neurosyphilis, HIV, cryptococcal meningitis)
- Complex partial seizures
- Inflammatory diseases (e.g., sarcoidosis, CNS vasculitis, SLE, paraneoplastic syndromes)
- Normal pressure hydrocephalus
- Wilson's disease
- Tumors

DIAGNOSTIC EVALUATION

- A complete history and physical is essential to rule out underlying medical, neurologic, or psychiatric illnesses that may mimic symptoms of dementia
  - Distinguish dementia from delirium (an acute, metabolically induced state of fluctuating consciousness) and depression
  - Perform Mini-Mental Status Examination
  - Medication history should be elicited to identify drugs that may contribute to cognitive changes (e.g., analgesics, sedatives, anticholinergics, antihypertensives)
  - Diagnostic criteria require memory impairment and abnormalities in at least one of the following areas: language, judgment, abstract thinking, praxis, executive function, or visual recognition
- Labs testing may include CBC, electrolytes, renal and liver function tests, glucose, thyroid function tests, vitamin B_{12} and folate, screening for inflammatory and infectious causes, and toxicology screen; consider screening for syphilis, HIV, and Wilson's disease
- Head CT scan without contrast to rule out structural lesions (e.g., infarct, malignancy, hydrocephalus, extracerebral fluid collection)
- EEG is not routinely used; however, it may identify toxic and metabolic disorders or Creutzfeldt-Jakob disease
- Genetic testing may be indicated if family history suggests Alzheimer's disease (especially early-onset disease)
- Cerebrospinal fluid analysis may be indicated

TREATMENT & MANAGEMENT

- There is no cure for most cases of dementia; treatment is palliative
- Treat reversible causes as necessary (e.g., hypothyroidism, vitamin deficiency, cerebral vasculitis, neurosyphilis, HIV)
- Eliminate all unnecessary medications, especially those with known CNS and anticholinergic effects
- Anticholinesterase inhibitors (e.g., donepezil, galantamine, rivastigmine) may initially slow progression of Alzheimer's disease; N-methyl-D-aspartate (NMDA) receptor antagonists (e.g., memantine) are now being used as well
- In select cases, antidepressants (avoid tricyclic antidepressants) and neuroleptics (e.g., quetiapine, risperidone) may be tried
- Social support (e.g., structured environments; social services to assess safety of the home environment, nutrition, medication, and placement issues)
  - Counseling for caregivers may be necessary
- Optimize blood pressure and control diabetes
- Involve neurology or neuropsychiatry early in the course of disease

PROGNOSIS & COMPLICATIONS

- Most cases are relentlessly progressive
- Death occurs over 6–10 years
- Patients gradually lose independence, cannot drive, are unable to care for themselves, and require significant assistance, which may include nursing home placement
- Patients are at increased risk for falls, infections, malnutrition, skin breakdown, and abuse

Stroke

INTRODUCTION

- This chapter will concentrate on ischemic stroke, which constitutes >80% of cases
  - The remainder of cases are hemorrhagic strokes, which are classified as subarachnoid hemorrhage, intracerebral hemorrhage, and nontraumatic epidural/subdural hematoma
- Thrombotic stroke is the most common type of ischemic stroke; lacunar infarcts account for 30% of ischemic strokes; cardioembolic infarcts account for 25%; arterial dissection are the most common cause of ischemic stroke in younger patients (younger than 50)
- Many strokes are preventable with appropriate risk factor modification and medical or surgical interventions
- An acute stroke is a medical emergency requiring immediate management ("time is brain")

ETIOLOGY, EPIDEMIOLOGY, & RISK FACTORS

- Thrombotic strokes are most common and occur due to arteriosclerosis
  - May be intracranial or extracranial (e.g., carotid or vertebral stenosis or occlusion)
  - May be associated with hypercoagulable states (e.g., antiphospholipid antibody syndrome, factor V Leiden, pregnancy, oral contraceptive use)
- Lacunar infarcts are small-vessel occlusions that produce limited neurologic deficits
- Arterial dissections most commonly occur due to trauma
- The vascular territory involved determines associated neurologic deficits
  - Carotid ischemia results in anterior circulation stroke causing dysfunction of the cerebral hemispheres and eyes
  - Vertebrobasilar ischemia results in posterior circulation stroke, causing dysfunction of the structures of the posterior fossa (e.g., cerebellum, brainstem), portions of the temporal lobe, and the occipital lobe
- Advancing age is the number 1 risk factor; other risk factors include family history, smoking, hypertension, diabetes mellitus, dyslipidemia, cardiac disease, atrial fibrillation, carotid artery disease, alcohol use, and obesity
- Transient ischemic attack (TIA) is a strong risk factor for subsequent stroke (50% of strokes occur within 2 days following TIA)

PATIENT PRESENTATION

- Abrupt onset of negative symptoms, such as photopsias, visual loss, paresthesias, numbness
- Headache occurs in 25% of cases
  - Severe headache, particularly with decreased level of consciousness, seizure, or progressive deficits, may occur with hemorrhagic stroke
  - Severe headache in association with Horner's syndrome (with recent trauma history) strongly suggests arterial dissection
- Anterior circulation strokes result in focal weakness, sensory alterations, or aphasia
- Posterior circulation stroke syndromes often have a more complex presentation depending on the area involved (e.g., thalamus, midbrain tegmentum, midbrain peduncle, pons, occipital lobe, lateral medulla, medial medulla)
- Amaurosis fugax suggests carotid artery disease

DIFFERENTIAL DX

- Hemorrhagic stroke
- Complicated migraine
- Seizure, postictal state, or Todd's paralysis
- Hypertensive urgency or emergency
- Hypo- or hyperglycemia
- Syncope
- Positional vertigo
- Brain tumor
- Multiple sclerosis
- Meningitis/encephalitis
- Brain abscess
- Drug overdose
- Trauma
- Conversion hysteria
- Bell's palsy
- Mononeuropathy

DIAGNOSTIC EVALUATION

- Prompt diagnostic workup should be performed in all TIA/stroke patient; essentially, all patients should be admitted to the hospital
- History and neurologic examination
- Initial laboratory studies include complete blood count, glucose, lipid profile, homocysteine level, and C-reactive protein
  - Coagulation profile is indicated in younger patients
- Head CT scan without contrast to evaluate for hemorrhage, tumor, and infarct; however, acute infarcts will not show up on CT scan for at least 24 hours
- MRI with diffusion weighting will reveal acute infarct within minutes of occurrence
- Echocardiogram to evaluate for cardiac source
  - Transesophageal echocardiogram is much more accurate than transthoracic echocardiogram to detect cardiac emboli
- CT scan or MRI is used to evaluate for extra- and intracranial arterial stenosis or occlusion
- Carotid and vertebral Doppler studies are also used to evaluate for arterial stenosis or occlusion
- Catheter angiogram is now used less frequently but is still the gold standard to diagnose arterial stenosis

TREATMENT & MANAGEMENT

- Acute therapy includes stabilization of glucose and blood pressure
  - Treat elevated blood pressure only when >220/115 because hypertension may be necessary to maintain cerebral perfusion (do not lower systolic blood pressure below 180)
- Thrombolytic therapy (tissue plasminogen activator) may be indicated if within 3 hours of symptom onset
  - Note: Thrombolytic therapy carries a 6% risk of inducing hemorrhage
- Anticoagulation with heparin is often used, but there is no evidence that it improves outcomes
- Secondary prevention includes antiplatelet therapy (e.g., aspirin, clopidogrel [Plavix], dipyridamole plus aspirin), statin therapy for hyperlipidemia, and blood pressure control
- If a cardiogenic source is found (e.g., atrial fibrillation), chronic anticoagulation with warfarin is indicated
- Carotid endarterectomy (or percutaneous stenting) is indicated in cases of carotid stenosis with >70% stenosis in the symptomatic artery

PROGNOSIS & COMPLICATIONS

- 20% immediate mortality
- 70% have some degree of disability
- Recurrence of stroke occurs at a rate of about 10% per year in untreated patients
  - Antiplatelet agents reduce the rate of stroke recurrence by 20%
  - Statins and blood pressure control (especially ACE inhibitors) reduce recurrence by 30%
  - Further risk factor modification includes smoking cessation, weight loss and exercise, and appropriate management of diabetes
- 50–70% of patients regain independence; up to 80% regain the ability to walk
- Nearly 50% of stroke victims will eventually die of myocardial infarction
- Physical, occupational, and speech therapy are extremely helpful

Seizures

INTRODUCTION

- Seizures are either a symptom of some underlying cause or idiopathic
- Seizures are discrete events that occur due to transient, synchronous, abnormal neuronal output; they may or may not be associated with convulsive activity
- Seizures are classified into 2 major groups: Focal or partial seizures (onset in 1 cortical area) include simple partial, complex partial, or secondarily generalized; and primary generalized seizures (diffuse cortical onset) include absence, tonic-clonic, tonic, clonic, atonic, and myoclonic
- 10% of the population will have a single, unprovoked seizure during their lifetime; 1% of the population is diagnosed with epilepsy

ETIOLOGY, EPIDEMIOLOGY, & RISK FACTORS

- Seizures are classified as generalized (global onset) versus partial (focal onset)
- Partial seizures are further classified as complex (accompanied by a change in consciousness) or simple (no change in consciousness)
- Etiologies are varied and may include central nervous system (CNS) or systemic infections, trauma, metabolic (e.g., hypoglycemia, hyperglycemia, hyponatremia, hypomagnesemia, hypocalcemia, uremia, hyperammonemia, hypoxia), toxic (e.g., cocaine, amphetamines, tricyclic antidepressants, antibiotics, alcohol or benzodiazepine withdrawal), tumors, vascular (e.g., stroke, hemorrhage, vascular malformation, sinus thrombosis, hypertensive encephalopathy, eclampsia), and degenerative dementias
  - Seizures may also be idiopathic (e.g., cryptogenic, hereditary)
  - The most common cause of acquired epilepsy worldwide is neurocysticercosis
- Psychogenic seizures result from stressful psychological conflicts (e.g., major trauma) and almost always occur in patients with a significant underlying psychiatric history
- 6% of the population will have a seizure at some point in their lifetime; only 0.5–1% of the population has epilepsy
- Risk factors for epilepsy include prior seizure, history of head trauma or central nervous system infection, family history of seizures, and history of febrile seizures

PATIENT PRESENTATION

- Aura may precede the seizure (simple partial)
- Generalized tonic-clonic seizures begin with tonic posturing during which the patient is rigid, hypoxic, and produces a characteristic cry from tonic contraction of the respiratory muscles
  - The clonic phase follows, consisting of rhythmic contractions that begin with low-amplitude, high-frequency jerks and progress to high-amplitude, lower frequency jerks
  - A postictal period follows with confusion and lethargy, which can last for minutes to hours
- Focal seizures can begin with focal contractions involving one limb or a focal sensation; they can also present with staring spells lasting a few minutes with associated automatisms (e.g., lip smacking or picking at clothes)
- Focal seizures can secondarily generalize and resemble generalized seizures; these may be followed by a hemiparesis (Todd's paralysis)

DIFFERENTIAL DX

- Syncope
- Convulsive syncope
- Psychogenic seizures (e.g., anxiety attack, panic attack)
- Cardiac arrhythmia
- Conversion disorder ("pseudoseizure")
- Drug-induced seizure (e.g., tricyclic antidepressant, alcohol withdrawal, lidocaine, cocaine)
- Metabolic abnormalities (e.g., hypoglycemia, electrolyte abnormalities)
- Sleep disorders (especially if seizures are purely nocturnal)
- Movement disorders
- Meningitis
- Hypoxia
- Brain metastases

DIAGNOSTIC EVALUATION

- History and physical examination gives valuable information
  - An observer's account of the seizure can be useful (duration, time of onset, tongue biting, loss of bowel or bladder control); most importantly, a thorough description of the seizure activity (e.g., focal vs. generalized) is helpful
  - Note recent illness or change in medications
  - Note risk factors for epilepsy (see opposite page)
  - Neurologic examination should evaluate for focal findings (e.g., weakness, reflex asymmetry, Babinski's sign)
  - General examination should evaluate for fever, elevated blood pressure, meningismus, and dermatologic abnormalities (e.g., rash, birthmarks)
- Initial laboratory testing includes screening for metabolic abnormalities (e.g., sodium, calcium, magnesium, glucose) or evidence of infection (e.g., blood cultures, urine cultures)
- Lumbar puncture may be indicated if the patient has fever, meningismus, or HIV
- CT scan may be indicated to rule out an acute bleed
- Some patients will need an MRI to look for structural lesions and an EEG to characterize seizures; these can both be performed as an outpatient once the above workup has been completed
- If the diagnosis is in doubt (i.e., suspect pseudoseizures), inpatient monitoring can be performed to directly observe seizure activity with video and EEG
- Prolactin levels are rarely useful and may lead to misdiagnosis

TREATMENT & MANAGEMENT

- Most seizures are self-limiting, last only a few minutes, and do not require sedation
- Initial treatment includes protecting the patient: Place the patient on their side so they do not aspirate, protect them from injuring themselves on sharp objects or hard surfaces
  - Nothing should be placed in their mouths, and they should not be held down
- Administer supplemental oxygen
- Some neurologists do not recommend benzodiazepine administration immediately in a new-onset seizure patient because it will interfere with the neurologic exam; however, it is common practice to abort the seizure with intravenous benzodiazepines
- Treatment after the first seizure is determined by weighing the risks and benefits of medical treatment versus observation; consider withholding treatment in low-risk patients until the second seizure occurs since the majority of patients have only 1 lifetime seizure
  - If drug treatment is initiated, monotherapy is always preferred; do not add a second drug until monotherapy with two different drugs has failed
  - Older antiepileptic drugs (e.g., carbamazepine, phenobarbital, valproate) are as effective as newer drugs (e.g., gabapentin, lamotrigine, topiramate, oxcarbazepine); however, newer drugs may have less side effects and easier dosing and may not require frequent monitoring
  - For most seizures, valproate, carbamazepine, and phenytoin are the initial choices
  - Change to a second drug or refer to a neurologist if increasing dose of the first drug fails
- Regular sleep patterns may be important because sleep deprivation can trigger seizures

PROGNOSIS & COMPLICATIONS

- Neurology consultation may not be necessary; consider neurologic consultation or outpatient neurologic follow-up if the workup, etiology, or management is in doubt
- Aspiration, hypoxia, and trauma are the most important complications
- The underlying etiology may carry its own morbidity and mortality risks
- Patients may have breakthrough seizures during periods of stress or drug noncompliance
- Patients with 1 seizure have a 20% chance of a recurrent seizure within 1 year in the absence of focal brain lesions; after 2 seizures, the risk increases to 85% chance of recurrence
- State laws for reporting of seizures are highly variable

Bell's Palsy

INTRODUCTION

- A sudden, unilateral facial paralysis or weakness involving the distribution of cranial nerve VII to the muscles of facial expression
- The most common cause of facial nerve paralysis; affects men and women equally
- Most patients recover completely; however, more than 8000 people per year in the United States are left with potentially disfiguring facial weakness
- The early use of corticosteroids and acyclovir may lead to improved facial function outcomes
- Differentiating whether the facial palsy is from a central or peripheral cause guides management
- Accounts for 60-75% of cases of unilateral facial paralysis

ETIOLOGY, EPIDEMIOLOGY, & RISK FACTORS

- Pathophysiology involves edema of the facial nerve, which likely becomes compressed in the facial canal or foramen spinosum
- Often follows exposure to cold or wind (for unclear reasons)
- There is some association with elevated herpes-1 titers
- Bell's palsy is a peripheral (lower motor neuron) palsy; differentiate supranuclear facial palsy from peripheral facial palsy
  - Supranuclear (central) palsy predominantly involves the lower part of the face; emotional responses may be intact (e.g., the patient may not be able to show you his teeth but will smile in response to a joke)
  - Peripheral palsy affects all ipsilateral muscles of facial expression, resulting in paralysis of the entire ipsilateral side; the angle of mouth is pulled to the normal side and may droop on the affected side, facial creases are effaced, and the affected eyelid may not close
- Incidence is 20-30 cases per 100,000 people per year, and higher during pregnancy

PATIENT PRESENTATION

- Paresis or paralysis of facial muscles, including eye closure, reaching maximum weakness within 48 hours
- Retroauricular pain often precedes the paralysis
- Occasional tingling sensation of face
- Ipsilateral loss of taste due to involvement of chordae tympani
- Bell's phenomenon (upward deviation of eye with attempted eye closure)
- Drooling of mouth at side of paresis
- Irritation of cornea may occur secondary to impaired eye closure
- May have hyperacusis, decreased tearing, and decreased sensation in the C2 dermatome

DIFFERENTIAL DX

- Stroke (Bell's palsy involves the entire face with inability to close eye completely, whereas strokes affect the lower part of the face primarily)
- Hemifacial spasm
- Lyme disease
- Guillain-Barré syndrome
- Acoustic neuroma
- Herpes zoster (Ramsay-Hunt syndrome)
- Ectatic basilar artery and compression of facial nerve
- Hysterical facial contractures, including blepharospasm
- Multiple sclerosis
- Acoustic neuroma
- Diabetes
- Trauma

DIAGNOSTIC EVALUATION

- History and physical examination
  - Attempt to distinguish central palsy from peripheral palsy: Sparing of the forehead muscles suggests a central palsy
- In central palsies, brain MRI is indicated to rule out ischemia, infection, or inflammatory diseases
- In general, peripheral palsies do not warrant immediate tests
- EMG and nerve conduction studies of the facial nerve may be useful for prognostic purposes in patients with complete loss of function
- Lumbar puncture is not necessary unless Lyme disease or Guillain-Barré syndrome is suspected
- Lyme antibody titer is only indicated if other clinical features of Lyme disease are present (e.g., arthralgias, characteristic rash)

TREATMENT & MANAGEMENT

- Early treatment with acyclovir in combination with prednisone may be effective in improving facial functional outcomes; it will relieve the retroauricular pain, but it is uncertain whether it helps to improve the facial palsy
- Eye protection is necessary, including lubricating drops during the day and eye ointment and patch at night
- Gentle massage of the face is recommended
- Electrical stimulation has not been shown to be of benefit
- Surgical decompression is not beneficial and not recommended

PROGNOSIS & COMPLICATIONS

- 80% of cases recover within 2–3 weeks
- 10% of cases may take up to a year to recover
- 10% of cases do not recover and develop synkinesis of face (contracture of muscles)
- Ability to close eye and recovery of taste are favorable prognostic signs
- Diabetics and hypertensive patients may have a worse prognosis for full recovery
- Poor prognostic factors include age over 60, hypertension, diabetes, pregnancy, impairment in taste, pain other than in the ear, complete facial weakness, and no recovery by 3 weeks

Multiple Sclerosis

INTRODUCTION

- A relatively common, acquired, demyelinating disease of young adults that tends to follow a relapsing-remitting course with variable degrees of disability
- Results from damage to myelin; the location of the lesion(s) is the major factor determining disability
- Causes demyelination and sclerosis of the brain, spinal cord, or both
- The most common autoimmune inflammatory disease of the CNS
- Patients may experience one of four clinical courses that can be mild, moderate, or severe: 1) Relapsing-remitting (most common and best prognosis); 2) primary progressive; 3) secondary progressive; and 4) progressive relapsing

ETIOLOGY, EPIDEMIOLOGY, & RISK FACTORS

- Presumed to be an autoimmune process; some evidence suggests that the disease is contracted in early life when a viral antigen stimulates the immune system, resulting in complex B- and T-cell dysregulation
- Affects the central nervous system and optic nerves
- Destruction of myelin sheaths results in demyelination and inflammation of CNS white matter; multiple plaques of demyelination of different ages and in different locations are seen ("separated by both time and space")
- Unknown etiology; probably an autoimmune process that occurs in genetically susceptible persons
  - Familial incidence of about 15%, suggesting an infectious etiology
  - There are certain histocompatibility antigens in patients with multiple sclerosis, suggesting a genetic predisposition
- Peak onset during ages 20–40; rarely occurs after 50
- Increasing incidence with increasing latitude: <1/100,000 at the equator; up to 80/100,000 in northern United States and Canada
  - Studies have suggested an association with smoking

PATIENT PRESENTATION

- Optic neuritis (visual loss)
- Myelitis (Lhermitte's sign: a sensation of electricity down the back upon passive flexion of the neck)
- Brainstem and cerebellar dysfunction: Diplopia, ataxia, dysarthria, dysmetria
- Weakness: Monoparesis, hemiparesis, or paraparesis
- Sensory symptoms may include a sensory level in spinal cord disease
- Bladder/bowel dysfunction
- Psychiatric features include depression and cognitive complaints
- Marcus-Gunn pupil
- Ophthalmoplegia
- Upper motor neuron signs (e.g., Babinski, hyperreflexia)
- Internuclear ophthalmoplegia

DIFFERENTIAL DX

- Acute disseminated encephalomyelitis
- Other demyelinating syndromes (e.g., central pontine myelinolysis, Devic's disease, Baló's disease)
- Autoimmune disorders (e.g., SLE, vasculitis, antiphospholipid antibody syndrome, sarcoidosis)
- Neoplastic and paraneoplastic syndromes (especially lymphoma)
- Gliomatosis cerebri
- Adrenoleukodystrophy
- Metachromatic leukodystrophy
- HIV encephalopathy
- Vitamin B_{12} deficiency
- Lyme disease

DIAGNOSTIC EVALUATION

- History, physical examination, and ancillary tests determine the likelihood of disease as "clinically definite," "lab-supported definite," "clinically probable," or "lab-supported probable"
- MRI is the most sensitive test; shows multiple white matter abnormalities in periventricular locations
  - For patients with classic demyelinating lesions on MRI scan, minimal additional workup is needed
  - Multifocal demyelinating lesions separated in "space and time" are classic
  - Essentially always shows lesions; if absent, the diagnosis should be reconsidered
  - In patients with optic neuritis, if the MRI reveals typical lesions of multiple sclerosis, the full disease will likely develop
- Cerebrospinal fluid analysis reveals oligoclonal bands and increased IgG; mild lymphocytic pleocytosis in acute attacks; protein may be mildly elevated
- Slowed evoked potentials (visual, auditory, and sensory)

TREATMENT & MANAGEMENT

- There is no cure, but existing therapies often give good results
- Steroids are indicated for acute attacks (high-dose IV steroids for moderate to severe attacks, low-dose oral steroids for mild attacks)
- Immunomodulators (e.g., interferons, glatiramer acetate) for prophylaxis of relapsing events
- Consider IVIG or plasmapheresis for unusually severe attacks
- Consider immunosuppressive agents and chemotherapy for unusually severe progressive cases
- Supportive care includes physical therapy, prostheses/orthotics, amantadine to reduce fatigue, antispasmodics (e.g., baclofen), antidepressants, bladder dysfunction agents (e.g., oxybutynin), and analgesia
  - Spasticity: Stretching exercises, medications (e.g., baclofen, tizanidine, gabapentin, diazepam)
  - Fatigue: Lifestyle adjustments, education, heat avoidance, exercise, medications (e.g., amantadine, modafinil, methylphenidate)
  - Depression: Counseling, antidepressants (e.g., amitriptyline, fluoxetine)
  - Cognitive dysfunction: Use of memory aids, trial of cholinesterase inhibitors (e.g., donepezil)

PROGNOSIS & COMPLICATIONS

- The clinical course is marked by exacerbations and remissions: Relapsing-remitting (episodes of acute worsening and recovery), secondary progressive (gradual deterioration with superimposed relapses), primary progressive (gradual deterioration from onset), progressive relapsing (gradual deterioration from onset with relapses superimposed)
- Predictive factors are weak but identifiable: Worse prognosis in males, later onset, progressive form from onset, motor symptoms from onset, or poor recovery from first attack
- MRI is weakly predictive (high lesion load suggests worse prognosis)
- Patients who do well in the first 5 years tend to do well for the next 5–10 years or longer; those who do well for the first 10 years have a 90% chance of doing well for another 10 years
- 50% of patients with optic neuritis will go on to develop multiple sclerosis

Myasthenia Gravis

INTRODUCTION

- An autoimmune disease caused by the development of antibodies to acetylcholine receptors at the neuromuscular junction, which inhibit muscle membrane depolarization
- Results in interference of neuromuscular transmission, leading to muscular weakness
- Occurs primarily in young women and older men, but may occur at any age

ETIOLOGY, EPIDEMIOLOGY, & RISK FACTORS

- Pathogenesis may begin in the thymic tissue, which provides an area for autoantibody production in susceptible patients
- There is a 20% concurrence with autoimmune hypothyroidism, suggesting a more generalized autoimmune disorder
- Associated with thymic hyperplasia in 80% of cases, thymoma in 15% of cases (30% of these are malignant), thyrotoxicosis, rheumatoid arthritis, and systemic lupus erythematosus
- Myasthenic crises are associated with infections and may result in respiratory muscle weakness necessitating intubation
- Congenital myasthenia is a rare disorder that is relatively refractory to treatment
- Neonatal myasthenia occurs in 12% of pregnancies in myasthenic women via placental transfer of antiacetylcholine receptor antibodies
- Can be triggered by illness, stress, thyroid dysfunction, pregnancy, and many drugs
- Familial occurrence is rare, but first-degree relatives do have a higher incidence of other autoimmune diseases

PATIENT PRESENTATION

- Fatigable weakness
  - Ocular and facial muscles are most frequently involved (e.g., diplopia, ptosis, dysphagia, drooling, difficulty chewing); indeed, 75% of cases are restricted to ocular involvement
  - Symmetrical limb weakness
  - Respiratory failure due to respiratory muscle weakness
  - Weakness often fluctuates
  - Especially prominent following persistent activity
- Head lolling (inability to hold up head)
- Symptoms may be subtle as to suggest hysteria
- Normal reflexes and cerebellar and sensory function

DIFFERENTIAL DX

- Guillain-Barré syndrome
- Botulism
- Lambert-Eaton syndrome
- Nondepolarizing muscle relaxants
- Brainstem stroke
- Ocular myopathy
- Thyroid disease
- Cranial neuropathy
- Tic paralysis
- Organophosphate poisoning
- Amyotrophic lateral sclerosis
- D-penicillamine (temporary reaction)
- Periodic paralysis
- Muscular dystrophy
- Myopathies

DIAGNOSTIC EVALUATION

- History and physical examination
  - Subacute onset of fluctuating diplopia and ptosis with normal pupillary responses strongly suggests myasthenia gravis
- Anticholinergic challenge with edrophonium will rapidly and temporarily reverse symptoms in most patients
  - Used for the initial diagnosis
  - Also used to distinguish myasthenic crisis (worsening of disease) versus cholinergic crisis (supratherapeutic drug levels secondary to medications): Edrophonium will reverse myasthenic crisis but exacerbate cholinergic crisis
- Acetylcholine receptor antibody assay is positive in more than 80% of cases
- Routine laboratory tests and cerebrospinal fluid analysis are normal
- TSH is often abnormal
- Imaging of mediastinum to rule out thymoma
- Repetitive nerve stimulation results in a decremental response in motor unit amplitude
- Single-fiber EMG is the most sensitive electrophysiologic test

TREATMENT & MANAGEMENT

- Symptomatic treatment with acetylcholinesterase inhibitors (e.g., neostigmine, pyridostigmine) allows more time for acetylcholine to compete for binding at active acetylcholine receptor sites, thereby allowing the patient to maintain strength
- Frequent measurement of vital capacity and negative inspiratory force is necessary to evaluate respiratory muscle function; intubation may be necessary
- Corticosteroids (must start slowly because high initial doses may worsen the disease), IVIG, and immunosuppressive agents (e.g., azathioprine, cyclosporine, methotrexate, mycophenolate)
- Plasmapheresis for severe cases and myasthenic crises
- Thymectomy may be curative but may take months to take effect
- Avoid immunoglycosides, sedative hypnotics, beta-blockers, and other medications that may decrease neuromuscular transmission

PROGNOSIS & COMPLICATIONS

- Mortality is low if the disease is diagnosed early and appropriate supportive measures are taken
- Characterized by remissions and exacerbations of fluctuating weakness, but does not follow a steadily progressive course
- If limited to ocular muscles for more than 2 years, the disease rarely extends to other muscles
- Patients with a forced vital capacity <1.5 L usually require prophylactic intubation or observation in an intensive care unit
- Patients should be admitted if they cannot walk or have signs of respiratory distress
- Starting steroids without the direction of a neurologic consultant is discouraged

Parkinson's Disease

INTRODUCTION

- A common, progressive, degenerative, CNS disorder that affects dopamine-containing neurons and is characterized by impoverished movements, rigidity, and tremor
- Second in frequency only to Alzheimer's disease as a neurodegenerative disorder in U.S.
- Affects 1% of Americans older than 50
- The most common variety, idiopathic Parkinson's disease (paralysis agitans), has an onset between 40 and 70 years
- May be associated with dementia, depression, daytime sleepiness, hallucinations, and psychosis
- Dementia occurs in up to 35% of cases

ETIOLOGY, EPIDEMIOLOGY, & RISK FACTORS

- Results from the loss of dopaminergic neurons in the substantia nigra and other CNS areas
- Dopamine plays a modulatory role in the basal ganglia, differentially regulating movement
- Most cases are idiopathic
- Parkinsonism can also be drug induced due to a postsynaptic blockade of dopamine receptors; usually caused by psychotropic or antidopaminergic agents
  - Exposure to 1,2,3,6-tetrahydropyridine (MPTP), which is a byproduct of synthetic heroin, rapidly causes parkinsonism
- Average age of onset is about 60 years
- Autopsy shows Lewy bodies in the brainstem and basal ganglia
- Risk factors include rural living, agrochemical exposure, well water consumption, living near wood pulp mills, exposure to herbicides, and proximity of residence to industrial plants, printing plants, or quarries

PATIENT PRESENTATION

- The classic triad consists of tremor (a resting, "pill-rolling" tremor that decreases with movement), "cogwheel" rigidity, and bradykinesia (slow initiation of movement)
- Positive symptoms include tremor, rigidity, and flexed posture
- Negative symptoms include loss of reflexes, bradykinesia, and freezing
- Masked facies
- Difficulties with activities of daily living (e.g., dressing, eating, writing)
- Subcortical dementia
- Seborrhea (oily skin), excess salivation
- Unstable posture with flexion of trunk and extremities and shuffling gait
- Festinating gait (propulsive tendencies)
- Postural hypotension late

DIFFERENTIAL DX

- Drug-induced parkinsonism (e.g., metochlopramide, phenothiazines, haloperidol)
- Diffuse Lewy body disease
- Progressive supranuclear palsy
- Shy-Drager syndrome
- Essential tremor
- Wilson's disease
- Gait apraxia
- Corticobasal ganglionic degeneration
- Normal pressure hydrocephalus
- Poisonings (e.g., carbon monoxide, methanol, manganese)

DIAGNOSTIC EVALUATION

- History and physical examination are generally diagnostic
  - At least 2 of the 4 cardinal symptoms (resting tremor, rigidity, akinesia, gait disturbance) should be present for diagnosis
- Clinical response to therapy with dopamine agonists strongly suggests Parkinson's disease
- No laboratory test or imaging is diagnostic
- Be sure to exclude Wilson's disease in young patients (low serum ceruloplasmin, high urine copper, Kayser-Flescher rings)
- MRI should be obtained if dementia occurs

TREATMENT & MANAGEMENT

- Discontinue all drugs with Parkinson's effects (e.g., metoclopramide, phenothiazines, haloperidol)
- Early cases can be observed for a period of time if no significant functional impairment is present
- Treatment is aimed at increasing the levels of dopamine in the CNS
  - Dopamine agonists are initially used, including ropinirole and pramipexole
  - Eventually, patients require levodopa plus carbidopa combinations
  - With time, patients develop wearing off of the effects of levodopa; entacapone may be tried
- Amantadine may be helpful for short periods of time; useful for dyskinesias
- Selegiline is of variable benefit
- Surgical intervention with subthalamic deep brain stimulation is beneficial in patients with intractable dyskinesia, tremor, or rarely, rigidity
- Emotional and social support, exercise, and good nutrition are important
- Supplemental use of coenzyme Q10 has been suggested to be neuroprotective but requires clinical trials for evidence of benefit

PROGNOSIS & COMPLICATIONS

- Disease advances in all cases, but the degree of progression varies from patient to patient
- Medications have prominent side effects, such as dyskinesia
- Severe side effects of medications and dementia generally occur within 5 years
- Hallucinations, often of animals or children, are commonly seen in late stages
- In terminal cases, aspiration pneumonia, sepsis, and pulmonary emboli occur
- Physical therapy is often beneficial

Genitourinary

Hematuria

INTRODUCTION

- Hematuria is the intermittent or persistent excretion of red or brown urine; it is relatively common, can arise from nearly any site in the urinary tract, and has a variety of etiologies ranging from the benign and self-limited to the malignant and lethal
- Approximately 2.5% of the general population has asymptomatic hematuria
- A single urinalysis showing hematuria may be due to exercise, fever, menstruation, mild trauma, sexual activity, or viral illness; persistent hematuria warrants further investigation
- It is important to evaluate the cause of hematuria carefully because gross painless hematuria is considered a urinary tract cancer until proven otherwise (even though a malignancy is found in only 10% of cases of hematuria in outpatient populations)

ETIOLOGY, EPIDEMIOLOGY, & RISK FACTORS

- The amount of blood can be grossly evident or microscopic (often found indirectly by urine dipstick and verified by microscopic visualization of the urine sediment)
- Gross hematuria occurs from disruption of the urinary tract epithelium
- The source of microscopic hematuria may be classified as follows:
  - Glomerular: Occurs due to disruption of the glomerular capillary walls and is often associated with proteinuria
  - Nonglomerular: Occurs due to disruption of the uroepithelium
- Nearly 50% of cases of microscopic hematuria are caused by infection or kidney stones
- The prevalence of hematuria ranges from 0.2–16%, depending on patient demographics
- The prevalence of uroepithelial malignancy associated with hematuria ranges from 0–25%, with higher rates found in men and the elderly
  - Risk factors for uroepithelial malignancy include age >40, irritative voiding symptoms, previous urologic disease, analgesic abuse, cyclophosphamide use, history of pelvic irradiation, tobacco abuse, and occupational exposure to benzenes and other aromatic amines (e.g., painters, machinists, chemical workers, and textile workers)

PATIENT PRESENTATION

- Note the timing of hematuria during urination:
  - Hematuria throughout urination suggests renal or ureteral disease
  - Hematuria at the onset of urination suggests urethral disease
  - Hematuria at the culmination of urination suggests bladder or prostate disease
- Note irritative voiding symptoms (e.g., dysuria, frequency, nocturia, urgency), which may suggest infection or uroepithelial malignancy
- Hematuria may occur alongside a variety of clinical symptoms; perform a complete review of systems, with attention to arthralgias, fatigue, fever, pain, pulmonary symptoms, rash, weakness, and weight loss

DIFFERENTIAL DX

- Transient hematuria (e.g., UTI, kidney stones, exercise, trauma, endometriosis)
- Glomerular bleeding (e.g., IgA nephropathy; thin basement membrane disease; Alport's syndrome; postinfectious glomerulonephritis, SLE, Wegener's granulomatosis, Churg-Strauss disease, cryoglobulinemia, endocarditis)
- Nonglomerular bleeding: Infection, kidney stones, uroepithelial malignancy, BPH, prostate cancer, renal cell cancer, stricture, polycystic kidney disease, AVM, renal infarction, renal trauma, sickle cell disease
- Menses

DIAGNOSTIC EVALUATION

- Complete history and physical examination
  - Review medications, doses, and duration of use; commonly implicated medications include analgesics, cyclophosphamide, and extended-spectrum penicillins
  - Physical examination should include evaluation for hypertension, abdominal and back examination for pain or masses, dermatologic examination for rash, musculoskeletal examination for arthritis, and prostatic, urethral, and vaginal examinations
- Nearly all patients require a urinalysis; consider catheterization to distinguish vaginal bleeding from other sources
  - Blood clots can occur with extraglomerular etiologies
  - Glomerular sources of bleeding result in RBC casts, large proteinuria, dysmorphic RBCs
  - Urinary tract infection results in pyuria, nitrates, and leukocyte esterase
- Laboratory tests include microscopic analysis of a freshly voided, midstream, clean-catch urine specimen; urine protein:creatinine ratio; coagulation studies; BUN/creatinine; uric acid
- Microscopic hematuria can be classified by associated findings in the urine sediment:
  - A glomerular origin is suggested by >20% dysmorphic RBCs with or without RBC casts and is often accompanied by proteinuria on dipstick
  - Pyuria suggests infection; verify by urine gram stain or culture
  - Bleeding from the lower urinary tract is indicated by (80% of normal RBCs
- Glomerular sources of bleeding should be further evaluated with ESR, ANA, C-ANCA, P-ANCA, complement levels (C3, C4), ASO titers, anti-DNAse B Abs, and anti-GBM Abs

TREATMENT & MANAGEMENT

- Hematuria is often a sign of an underlying disease; treatment is generally directed at the underlying disease process
- Patients with gross hematuria should undergo a full urologic evaluation
- Eliminate any potentially causative medications, including over-the-counter medicines and herbal agents
- Older patients with transient hematuria should always be evaluated fully due to increased risk of urinary tract cancers; consider referral to urologist for further evaluation and treatment
- Glomerular sources of hematuria: Follow BUN/creatinine levels, blood pressure, creatinine clearance, and 24-hour urine protein, and refer for a kidney biopsy if worsening
- Nonglomerular source: Refer to urologic specialist if imaging indicates a renal, bladder, or urethral lesion
- Urinary tract infection should be treated with the appropriate empiric antibiotic or based on results of urine culture
  - Urinalysis should be repeated to ensure resolution of hematuria

PROGNOSIS & COMPLICATIONS

- Persistent isolated microscopic hematuria that is undiagnosed after a complete evaluation requires further follow-up, which may include repeated urinalyses and voided urine cytology at 6, 12, 24, and 36 months
- Nephrology referral should be considered if hypertension, proteinuria, or evidence of glomerular bleeding develops
  - Renal failure or significant proteinuria (urine protein:creatinine >1) is an indication for renal biopsy
- Urology referral (which may require intravenous urography, CT scan, or ultrasound) should be considered if abnormal voided urine cytology, gross hematuria, nonglomerular microscopic hematuria, or irritative voiding symptoms develop

Proteinuria

INTRODUCTION

- Whereas a small amount of protein is normally present in the urine, proteinuria is defined as urinary protein excretion exceeding 150 mg/d; it is relatively common and most often benign, but it may signify underlying disease
- Proteinuria >3.5 g/d is consistent with nephrotic syndrome, which may occur secondary to primary renal disease, systemic diseases (e.g., amyloidosis, diabetes), or infection
- A single urinalysis with proteinuria may be an isolated, benign occurrence (e.g., due to decompensated heart failure, dehydration, uncontrolled diabetes, excessive exercise, fever, medications [e.g., NSAIDs, ACE inhibitors], stress, or urinary tract infection); however, persistent proteinuria warrants further investigation

ETIOLOGY, EPIDEMIOLOGY, & RISK FACTORS

- The pathophysiology of proteinuria involves increased permeability of the glomerulus and may be classified as glomerular, tubular, or overflow:
  - Glomerular: Often due to structural renal injury, which causes loss of size and charge selectivity of the glomerular capillary wall, resulting in increased filtration of protein
  - Tubular: Due to inability of the proximal tubules to reabsorb low molecular weight proteins
  - Overflow: Due to increased production of low molecular weight proteins that exceeds the reabsorptive capacity of the proximal tubules
- Proteinuria may be found in about 15% of patients on a single dipstick urinalysis; however, most of these patients do not have significant underlying disease and less than 2% of these patients have serious urinary tract disease
- Patients at increased risk of chronic kidney disease should be screened for proteinuria with an albumin-specific dipstick
  - Risk factors for chronic kidney disease include autoimmune diseases, diabetes mellitus, hypertension, malignancy, and vasculitides
- Nephrotic syndrome is characterized by urinary protein excretion >3.5 g/d, hypoalbuminemia, hyperlipidemia, and edema (which may manifest as hypertension)

PATIENT PRESENTATION

- Peripheral and/or periorbital edema (due to decreased oncotic pressure from protein loss) may occur in severe cases (e.g., nephrotic syndrome)
- Note evidence of underlying disease processes (e.g., diabetes mellitus, heart failure)
- Review all medications, dosages, and duration of use; commonly implicated drugs include NSAIDs, gold, ACE inhibitors, heroin, lithium, and penicillamine
- Note family history of renal disease
- Complete review of systems should include arthralgias, fatigue, fever, pain, pulmonary symptoms, rash, weakness, and weight loss
- Complete physical examination should include evaluation for hypertension and edema, abdominal and back examination for pain or mass, dermatologic examination for rash, and musculoskeletal examination for arthritis

DIFFERENTIAL DX

- Primary glomerular: IgA nephropathy, thin basement membrane disease, FSGS, idiopathic membranous glomerulonephritis, membranoproliferative glomerulonephritis
- Secondary glomerular: Diabetes, CHF, cirrhosis, amyloidosis, infection (e.g., HIV, viral hepatitis), SLE, drug-induced, Goodpasture syndrome, Wegener's granulomatosis, malignancy, endocarditis
- Tubular: Hypertensive nephrosclerosis, AIN
- Overflow: Amyloidosis, multiple myeloma, monoclonal gammopathy, leukemia

DIAGNOSTIC EVALUATION

- Initial laboratory tests include microscopic analysis of a freshly voided, midstream, clean-catch urine specimen; sulfosalicylic acid (SSA) test, urine protein:creatinine ratio, complete blood count, and creatinine clearance
  - SSA will detect the presence of low molecular weight proteins missed by urine dipstick
  - False-positive results may occur due to alkaline or concentrated urine, gross hematuria, presence of leukocytes, presence of semen or vaginal secretions, or recent iodinated contrast
- Assessment of the urine sediment can help classify the source of proteinuria:
  - A glomerular origin is suggested by >20% dysmorphic RBCs with or without RBC casts
  - Infection may result in pyuria and a positive urine gram stain or culture
  - Eosinophils suggest drug-induced acute interstitial nephritis (AIN)
- Postural proteinuria should be ruled out in any patient younger than 30 with <2 g of protein excretion per day and normal renal function
  - In postural proteinuria, nighttime urinary function is normal (<50 mg of proteinuria per 8 hours), but daytime function is impaired
- A glomerular source of bleeding should be further evaluated with ESR, ANA, complement levels (C3, C4), C-ANCA, P-ANCA, anti-GBM Abs, hepatitis and HIV serologies, VDRL, and serum levels of albumin, electrolytes, lipids, and urate
- Renal ultrasound may be indicated to evaluate renal size and to rule out obstruction
- Significant proteinuria (urinary protein >3.5 g/d or urine protein:creatinine ratio >1) with renal failure should prompt referral to nephrologist for renal biopsy

TREATMENT & MANAGEMENT

- Treat the underlying disease (e.g., infection, malignancy, diabetes) as necessary
  - Control of hypertension decreases proteinuria and delays the progression to renal failure
  - Urinary tract infection should be treated with the appropriate empiric antibiotic or tailored antibiotics based on urine culture results; urinalysis should be repeated to ensure that proteinuria resolves
- Eliminate potentially causative medications
- Ensure appropriate fluid and electrolyte balance
- Primary glomerulopathies may require immunosuppression with either systemic corticosteroids or cyclophosphamide
- ACE inhibitors and angiotensin receptor blocker (ARB) medications may reduce proteinuria and slow the progression of chronic renal disease by decreasing intraglomerular pressure

PROGNOSIS & COMPLICATIONS

- The prognosis depends on the underlying disease and the development of chronic renal failure
- Patients with isolated proteinuria have a 20% risk of progressing to chronic renal failure within 10 years; they should be monitored carefully for hypertension, worsening proteinuria, and renal failure every 6 months
- Protein excretion >1 g/d places patients at higher risk of progression to chronic renal failure
- Proteinuria is an independent risk factor for cardiovascular disease, cardiovascular mortality, and all-cause mortality

Penile Discharge

INTRODUCTION

- Penile discharge is a common primary care complaint that occurs as a result of an acute inflammatory process within the urethra
- Etiologies include infection, neoplasm, and foreign bodies
- Sexually transmitted diseases are a common cause
  - A thorough history, including a complete and accurate sexual history, as well as focused physical examination and penile cultures are generally indicated
  - Less commonly, non-sexually transmitted diseases are the cause of penile discharge

ETIOLOGY, EPIDEMIOLOGY, & RISK FACTORS

- Infection is the most common cause
  - *Neisseria gonorrhea*: Primary gonorrhea infection may progress to disseminated gonococcal infection (triad of tenosynovitis, dermatitis, and arthritis)
  - *Chlamydia trachomatis*: The most common cause of nongonococcal urethral discharge
  - *Trichomonas vaginalis*: Usually asymptomatic in men; female partner tends to be symptomatic with pelvic pain, itching, and vaginal discharge
- Nonspecific urethritis
- Reiter's syndrome is associated with chlamydia infection
  - Triad of urethritis, conjunctivitis, and arthritis ("can't see, can't pee, can't climb a tree")
  - Skin lesions involve the palms and soles, begin as vesicles, and become hyperkeratotic
- Lack of circumcision may increase the risk of HIV, gonorrhea, and syphilis

PATIENT PRESENTATION

- Patients with urethral discharge are often otherwise asymptomatic
  - Gonorrhea: Profuse, purulent, thick yellow or gray discharge, dysuria, and urinary urgency or frequency
  - Chlamydia: Thin, scant, and mucoid (watery) discharge
- *Trichomonas vaginalis*: Usually asymptomatic in men but may present with penile discharge and dysuria; female partner tends to be symptomatic with pelvic pain, itching, and vaginal discharge
- Carcinoma of the urethra: Bloody discharge
- Foreign body in the urethra: Pain and bloody discharge
- Reiter's syndrome: triad of urethritis, conjunctivitis, and arthritis ("can't see, can't pee, can't climb a tree")

DIFFERENTIAL DX

- Gonococcal urethritis
- Nongonococcal urethritis
- Indwelling Foley catheter or other foreign body
- Prostatitis
- Urethral carcinoma
- Reiter's syndrome

DIAGNOSTIC EVALUATION

- History and physical examination
  - Assess onset, duration, and character of discharge, voiding symptoms, and hematuria
  - Obtain a complete sexual history
  - Note prior instrumentation of genitals and urinary tract, and inquire about inserting foreign objects into the meatus (especially in children)
  - Physical exam should include complete examination of meatus, phallus, and testes and digital rectal exam
- Urethral cultures are the gold standard for diagnosis of gonorrhea and chlamydia
  - Obtain cultures by holding the penis up and carefully inserting the tip of the culture swab into the meatus about 1/2 inch, and twirl; remove and place in culture medium
- Urinalysis and urine culture
- Wet mount to evaluate for trichomonads
  - To express penile discharge, have the patient "milk" the penis from the base up to the tip
- Further workup for sexually transmitted diseases may include HIV testing, RPR, hepatitis B studies, and hepatitis C antibody
- Consider blood cultures, CBC, and joint fluid aspiration if suspect disseminated gonorrhea
- If suspect foreign body, obtain plain film X-rays of the penis and pelvis and consider urology referral

TREATMENT & MANAGEMENT

- Penile discharge without dysuria or frequency should be treated as a sexually transmitted disease until proven otherwise
- Begin empiric antibiotic therapy upon clinical suspicion
  - Gonorrhea: Single-dose IM ceftriaxone (give in office for 100% compliance) or oral cefixime, ciprofloxacin, levofloxacin, or ofloxacin (note that fluoroquinolone resistance exists in Asia, Hawaii, and California)
  - Chlamydia: Single-dose azithromycin, doxycycline (7 days), ofloxacin (7 days), or erythromycin (7 days)
  - *Trichomonas*: Metronidazole (single dose or 7-day course)
- If positive cultures, treat accordingly, and obtain test of cure 6–8 weeks after initiating antibiotic treatment
- Prostatitis is treated with 3 weeks of fluoroquinolones
- Encourage patients to inform sexual partners of disease so that they can be treated
  - Inform the health department, if required
- Use this visit with the patient to educate on safe sex and the use of barrier methods to decrease transmission of infections, and consider testing for other sexually transmitted diseases
- Emergent urology consult is required for foreign bodies or carcinoma of the penis

PROGNOSIS & COMPLICATIONS

- Chlamydial and gonococcal urethritis may result in pelvic inflammatory disease, leading to female infertility and/or Fitz-Hugh-Curtis perihepatitis; there is also a risk for disseminated gonococcal infection (3%), including arthritis, tenosynovitis, dermatitis, meningitis, and/or sepsis
- Gonorrhea has been associated with urethral stricture; the classic presentation involves a patient with multiple short strictures and a history of sexually transmitted diseases or penile discharge
- Gonorrhea may cause epididymitis
- Reiter's syndrome occurs in 1–3% of patients

Testicular Pain and Scrotal Masses

INTRODUCTION

- Orchalgia is chronic pain of the testicles or scrotum that typically lasts >3 months
- Acute or chronic scrotal or testicular pain may occur at any age and may or may not be associated with a scrotal or testicular mass
- Although most etiologies are not serious or emergent, testicular pain must be considered an emergency because of the possibility of testicular torsion or Fournier's gangrene
- Scrotal masses and swelling can involve the contents of the scrotum, the wall of the scrotum, and the scrotum itself
  - Swelling of the scrotum without a mass is usually associated with an underlying medical condition, such as heart failure or anasarca

ETIOLOGY, EPIDEMIOLOGY, & RISK FACTORS

Testicular pain
- Epididymitis: A bacterial (*Chlamydia*, *Enterobacter*) or viral infection (mumps, mononucleosis, adenovirus) of adolescent boys and young adults
- Testicular torsion: Twisting of the spermatic cord that results in testicular ischemia/infarct
- Hydrocele: A collection of fluid between the layers of the tunica vaginalis around the testicle
- Varicocele: A mass of dilated veins; the most common correctable cause of male infertility
- Fournier's gangrene: Necrotizing fasciitis of the perineum; seen primarily in older men

Scrotal mass or swelling
- Painful masses include torsion of the spermatic cord, epididymitis, orchitis, strangulated hernia, and trauma
- Nonpainful masses include hernia, varicocele, testicular cancer, spermatocele, hydrocele, epididymal cyst, and scrotal edema due to cardiac, hepatic, or renal failure
  - Testicular cancer is most common in men aged 20–50 and is 40 times more common in patients with cryptorchidism

PATIENT PRESENTATION

- A painless scrotal mass should be considered testicular cancer until proven otherwise
  - Masses that are easily separable from the testicle are much more likely to be benign
- Epididymitis: Gradual, insidious onset of scrotal pain and swelling; elevation of testicle may relieve pain
- Torsion: Sudden onset of severe testicular pain, often radiating to the lower abdomen
  - May result in a transverse lie of the testicle
- Hydrocele: Vague pain or asymptomatic
- Varicocele: "Heaviness" of the hemiscrotum; dilated veins may be seen on the affected side
- Postvasectomy syndrome: Dull achy pain arising after vasectomy

DIFFERENTIAL DX

In addition to the diagnoses described in the etiology section, additional etiologies include:
- Torsion of the appendix testes
- Renal or ureteral stones
- Postvasectomy syndrome
- Inguinal hernia
- Chord lipoma
- Chord adenoma
- Peritonitis
- Ruptured abdominal aortic aneurysm
- Referred pain due to constipation
- Henoch-Schönlein purpura

DIAGNOSTIC EVALUATION

- History and physical examination, including abdomen, back, genitalia, and rectal exam
  - Note character of onset (sudden vs. subacute), duration (minutes vs. hours vs. days), location (generalized vs. localized), quality (sharp vs. dull, moderate vs. severe, constant vs. intermittent), and previous episodes
  - Palpate testicle and spermatic cord to assess for tenderness, effusion, subcutaneous emphysema, size, and lie of testicle, and assess for hernias
  - Transilluminate for presence of fluid
  - "Blue dot sign": Bluish discoloration along upper pole seen in about 20% of cases of torsion of the testicular appendix and due to infarction and necrosis
  - "Prehn's sign": Relief of pain with elevation of the testis in testicular torsion
- If testicular torsion is suspected, emergent detorsion (usually) by a urologist is necessary
- Scrotal ultrasound is usually indicated
- Initial laboratory testing includes complete blood count, urinalysis, and urethral gram stain and culture
- CT scan and/or MRI may be warranted

TREATMENT & MANAGEMENT

- Testicular torsion is a surgical emergency
  - If surgery is not available, manual detorsion may be attempted
  - Detorsion maneuver: Infiltrate spermatic cord with 10–20 mL of 1% lidocaine, then twist the testes counterclockwise on left or clockwise on right; successful detorsion is indicated by immediate relief of pain
- Incarcerated inguinal hernias and testicular rupture require immediate surgical repair
- Epididymitis and orchitis are treated with antibiotics
  - Patients younger than 35 (presumed to be sexually acquired): Treat with ceftriaxone or a fluoroquinolone plus doxycycline or azithromycin or tetracycline
  - Patients older than 35: Treat with trimethoprim-sulfamethoxazole or a fluoroquinolone, unless history reveals that infection is sexually acquired
  - Analgesics and scrotal support may be used
- Testicular cancer found on exam or ultrasound should prompt immediate urologic consultation for emergent orchiectomy
  - Beta-human chorionic gonadotropin, alpha-fetoprotein, LDH, chest X-ray, and CT scan of the abdomen and pelvis should be ordered but should not delay referral to urologist

PROGNOSIS & COMPLICATIONS

- Testicular cancer classically spreads to the para-aortic and paracaval nodes
- Torsion results in permanent ischemic changes within 6 hours of the initial insult
- Epididymitis may result in a chronic pain state or testicular scarring and fibrosis that could cause infertility
- Varicocele and spermatocele may recur after surgical resection
- The majority of cases of postvasectomy pain resolve over 6 weeks with minimal intervention

Erectile Dysfunction

INTRODUCTION

- Erectile dysfunction (ED) has been defined by the NIH as "a consistent inability to obtain and maintain an erection satisfactory for sexual function"
- The risk of ED increases with age in a linear fashion, affecting 40% of 40-year-old men to 70% of 70-year-old men
- May be situational (specific times, places, or partner)
- Less than 10% of symptomatic men in the United States (20 million) are being treated
- ED is intimately related to cardiovascular disease and may precede symptomatic coronary artery disease
- Female sexual dysfunction is also prevalent, affecting 40% of women

ETIOLOGY, EPIDEMIOLOGY, & RISK FACTORS

- Organic etiologies are most common:
  - Vascular (70% of cases): Arterial atherosclerosis (e.g., diabetes), which leads to decreased blood flow to the penis; venous leak or occlusion, which leads to decreased blood remaining in the penis during erection; trauma; or surgical disruption
  - Neurologic: Postoperative, stroke, spinal cord injury, diabetic neuropathy
  - Endocrine: Andropause, hypogonadism, hyperprolactinemia, thyroid abnormalities
- Psychogenic (10% of cases): Stress, depression, anxiety
- Medication-related (10% of cases): Antidepressants, antihypertensives (especially beta-blockers, thiazides, and clonidine), cimetidine, spironolactone, and anticholinergics
- Common risk factors include hypertension (which predisposes to atherosclerosis and endothelial dysfunction); diabetes (which is directly toxic to nerves and arteries); pelvic surgery, trauma, or radiation (which can cause both nerve and vascular dysfunction); depression and stress; substance abuse, including tobacco and alcohol use; and Peyronie's disease (40% of patients suffer from some degree of ED)

PATIENT PRESENTATION

- Inability to obtain or maintain an adequate erection
- May be "sometimes" or "always"
- If the patient can achieve an adequate morning erection, consider nonorganic causes
- Most cases of ED are undiagnosed (most men consider it a normal part of aging)
- Men undergoing ED treatment for should be screened for predisposing conditions, particularly risk factors for cardiovascular disease (e.g., diabetes, hypertension, hyperlipidemia, thyroid disorders)
- Consider screening for ED in patients with established risk factors; sexual dysfunction is often a treatable component of their medical condition(s)
- Consider screening all patients over 40 years for declining sexual function and libido

DIFFERENTIAL DX

- Peyronie's disease
- Rapid ejaculation
- Penile fracture
- Hormonal abnormalities (e.g., thyroid dysfunction)
- Kidney or liver disease
- Medications, including herbal and over-the-counter drugs
- Neurologic (e.g., stroke, seizures, multiple sclerosis)
- Anxiety
- Depression

DIAGNOSTIC EVALUATION

- Focused history and physical examination
  - Attention to medications, substance abuse, cardiovascular risk factors, and psychosocial and relationship factors
  - Detailed sexual history, including onset and duration of ED, ability to sustain erection, morning erections, libido, ejaculatory difficulties, and penile curvature
  - Physical exam should assess testis size, penile sensation, bulbocavernosal reflex (absent in 30% of normal men), peripheral pulses, penile plaque, and gynecomastia
- Laboratory testing generally includes complete blood count, chemistry panel, random glucose, and early morning total testosterone
  - If early morning total testosterone is less than 300–400, further evaluate levels of free testosterone, luteinizing hormone, and prolactin
  - Consider thyroid function tests
- Validated questionnaires, such as the International Index of Erectile Function (IIEF) and Sexual Encounter Profile (SEP), may be useful
- Consider urology referral
- Nocturnal penile tumescence and rigidity scans may be used to distinguish psychogenic from organic etiologies

TREATMENT & MANAGEMENT

- Treat underlying disorders (e.g., stress, depression, cardiovascular disease, hypertension, diabetes, liver or kidney disease, thyroid disease) as necessary
- Eliminate or adjust causative medications
- Avoid tobacco use, alcohol, and drugs
- Lifestyle modifications, including behavioral therapy and support
- Oral agents (e.g., sildenafil, vardenafil, tadalafil) can be effective in appropriate cases
  - Contraindicated in patients taking nitrate medications (e.g., nitroglycerin)
  - Avoid vardenafil and tadalafil in patients taking alpha-blockers; separate use of sildenafil and alpha-blocker by at least 4 hours
  - Avoid in patients with recent myocardial infarction (within 2 weeks), unstable angina, or poor cardiac performance status
  - Medications that compete with the liver's P-450 pathway (e.g., erythromycin, ketoconazole, itraconazole, ritonavir, indinavir) may affect drug dosing
- Second-line therapies include intracavernous injections and intraurethral prostaglandin injections (e.g., alprostadil)
- Other treatments include surgical prostheses, vacuum erection devices, hormone therapy, and sex therapy

PROGNOSIS & COMPLICATIONS

- Oral agents are effective in up to 70% of patients and have limited side effects (10–15% headache, 7–9% flushing, 5–9% dyspepsia)
- Injection therapy is effective in 60–90% of patients with 5–10 minutes of onset
  - 3% risk for local complications, such as hematoma or scarring
  - May result in priapism
  - Contraindicated in patients taking MAO inhibitors
- Intraurethral alprostadil is effective in 30–40% of patients
  - Contraindicated for use with pregnant partners
- Penile implants have high patient satisfaction rates (over 85%)
  - 2–3% infection rate, 2% mechanical malfunction rate, 15% reoperation rate at 10 years

Dysuria

INTRODUCTION

- Dysuria is a painful or burning sensation during or immediately after urination
- A common symptom in primary care: Nearly 20% of women aged 20–55 will have one episode of dysuria per year, resulting in over 8 million physician office visits yearly
- Women are affected much more frequently than men
- The most common cause of dysuria in adult women is lower urinary tract infection

ETIOLOGY, EPIDEMIOLOGY, & RISK FACTORS

- Dysuria is usually caused by irritation of urothelium and its innervation.
- Pain with micturition may be primarily urethral in origin or referred from distal ureter, bladder, or prostate.
- Most commonly caused by infection or inflammation
- Commonly due to an anatomic abnormality such as a tumor or outflow obstruction, presence of calculus or foreign body, or recent instrumentation such as a catheter or urologic procedure, or a consequence of intravesical chemotherapy, systemic medications, or inflammation of adjacent organs
- Despite extensive investigation, dysuria may remain idiopathic, although this is a diagnosis of exclusion after more serious etiologies have been eliminated.
- Risk factors: Urinary tract infection, sexually transmitted disease, female sex, urethral instrumentation, renal calculi, urothelial carcinoma, benign prostatic hypertrophy, pelvic radiation, atrophic vaginitis

PATIENT PRESENTATION

- Subjective pain or burning with micturition
- Differentiate dysuria at initiation of, throughout, or at termination of micturition
  - Pain at the start of micturition usually indicates urethral involvement
  - Pain throughout micturition (strangury) suggests bladder and urethral spasm
  - Pain at the end of micturition (suggests a bladder etiology
- Dysuria is usually accompanied by other lower urinary tract symptoms, such as urinary frequency and urgency
- Vaginal discharge suggests sexually transmitted disease or bacterial vaginosis
- Tender, boggy, swollen prostate suggests prostatitis; enlarged prostate is associated with nocturia; and urinary frequency suggests BPH
- Tender epididymis suggests infection

DIFFERENTIAL DX

- Cystitis (e.g., infection, interstitial cystitis, radiation, instrumentation)
- Urethritis (e.g., infection, urethral diverticulum, caruncle, prolapse, radiation, instrumentation)
- Nephrolithiasis/urolithiasis
- Obstruction to outflow (e.g., stones, bladder neck contracture, posterior urethral valves, prostatic hypertrophy, urethral stricture, meatal stenosis)
- Cancer (e.g., uroepithelial, prostate, tumors adjacent to or invading the lower urinary tract)
- Foreign bodies (e.g., urethral catheter, recent instrumentation)

DIAGNOSTIC EVALUATION

- History, physical examination, and genital exam
  - Male genital exam may include DNA test, culture, and gram stain
  - Female genital exam may include KOH prep, wet mount, gram stain, and DNA tests/culture
- Urinalysis is indicated in all patients
  - Hematuria suggests urolithiasis, pyelonephritis, or cystitis; painless hematuria may suggest bladder cancer
  - Positive nitrites, leukocyte esterase (highly sensitive and specific for infection), or WBCs with suprapubic tenderness suggests uncomplicated cystitis
- Urine culture is indicated if there is a positive urinalysis and in pregnant women, diabetic or immunocompromised patients, and males with urethral discharge
- Urine cytology to evaluate for uroepithelial carcinoma is indicated if there is persistent microscopic hematuria, dysuria, urinary urgency, or frequency in the absence of infection
- Imaging of the genitourinary tract may be warranted in some cases: KUB films if suspect renal calculi or foreign body; CT scan is more definitive for calculi and urologic tumors and to assess the upper urinary tract

TREATMENT & MANAGEMENT

- Refer to a urologist for anatomic or functional abnormalities revealed in evaluation that cannot be adequately addressed in primary care setting
- Symptomatic therapy with phenazopyridine hydrochloride (Pyridium) can be given to alleviate dysuria
  - Contraindicated in renal insufficiency and hepatic dysfunction
  - Side effects include renal or hepatic toxicity, methemoglobinemia, and hemolytic anemia
  - Will turn urine and other body fluids orange (patients should be warned that contact lenses can be stained orange)
- Treat underlying disease as appropriate:
  - Cystitis/prostatitis: Appropriate antibiotics
  - Pyelonephritis: Outpatient antibiotic treatment in patients who tolerate liquids and have no significant comorbidities; otherwise, admission for IV hydration and antibiotics
  - Urolithiasis: Hydration, pain control while attempting to pass stones; urology referral if stones will not pass
  - Atrophic vaginitis: Consider estrogen creams or systemic replacement if other symptoms
  - BPH: Symptomatic relief with α-blockers, 5α-reductase inhibitors, or saw palmetto extract
  - Sexually transmitted diseases: Treat the specific disease and screen for other STDs (e.g., HIV, hepatitis B)

PROGNOSIS & COMPLICATIONS

- Prognosis depends on the underlying etiology
- Dysuria usually responds well to alleviation of the offending abnormality
- Rarely, subjective dysuria with no demonstrable etiology is recalcitrant to treatment
- Persistent dysuria should be periodically re-evaluated for underlying malignancy by upper urinary tract imaging, cystoscopy, and urine cytology by a urologist

Genitourinary

Incontinence

INTRODUCTION

- Urinary incontinence is an involuntary loss of urine
- It is one of the 10 most common medical problems in the Unites States, with prevalence estimated at 13–60 million Americans, particularly geriatric patients (affects 15–30% of women over 65); however, most patients do not seek treatment despite the significant effects on self-esteem and social interactions
- Classified as stress, urge, overflow, or mixed incontinence

ETIOLOGY, EPIDEMIOLOGY, & RISK FACTORS

- <u>Stress incontinence</u>: Loss of urine upon increases in intra-abdominal pressure (e.g., laughing, coughing, change in position, exercise)
  - Caused by weakness of the pelvic floor due to urethral hypermobility or sphincter dysfunction; these can occur due to urethral trauma (e.g., prostate surgery), vaginal childbirth, or deconditioning
- <u>Urge incontinence</u> ("overactive bladder"): Due to spontaneous bladder contractions caused by central neurologic disorders, local bladder disorders (e.g., cystitis, bladder cancer), or idiopathic
- <u>Detrusor hyperreflexia</u>: Involuntary bladder contractions due to a neurologic lesion above the sacral spinal cord (e.g., multiple sclerosis, Parkinson's disease, stroke, spinal cord injury, hydrocephalus)
- <u>Overflow incontinence</u>: Overdistention of the bladder due to an outlet obstruction (e.g., benign prostate hypertrophy, prostate cancer, prolapse) or contractility dysfunction (e.g., diabetic or alcoholic neuropathy, anticholinergic medications)
- <u>Mixed incontinence</u>: Combined elements of stress and urge incontinence are common in older females; combined elements of overflow and urge incontinence are most common in men and frail nursing home patients

PATIENT PRESENTATION

- <u>Stress incontinence</u>: Leakage of urine upon abdominal straining (e.g., cough, sneeze, laugh, exercise, going from sitting to standing position)
- <u>Urge incontinence</u>: Leakage of urine associated with a strong urge to urinate, having to run to the restroom, urinary frequency, urgency, and/or nocturia, or suprapubic discomfort due to bladder spasm
- <u>Overflow incontinence</u>: Leakage of urine upon abdominal straining, weak stream, urinary hesitancy/intermittency, nocturia, urinary dribbling, palpable bladder, no sensation of bladder filling (neurogenic) or suprapubic discomfort from full bladder (obstruction)
- Continuous leakage may indicate fistula or ectopic ureter
- Postvoid dribbling in women may indicate urethral diverticulum or vaginal pooling of urine

DIFFERENTIAL DX

Transient, acute incontinence
- Delirium
- Urinary tract infection
- Atrophic vagitis/urethritis
- Drugs (e.g., diuretics, sedatives, alcohol, beta-blockers, ACE inhibitors, antidepressants)
- Endocrine disorders (e.g., hypercalcemia, hyperglycemia)
- Urinary retention
- Fecal impaction

Persistent/chronic incontinence
- Stress incontinence
- Urge incontinence
- Overflow incontinence
- Functional incontinence (poor mobility, mental status decline)
- Mixed incontinence
- Diabetes insipidus

DIAGNOSTIC EVALUATION

- History and physical examination
  - Note whether the patient has problems holding urine versus emptying bladder; leakage of urine with cough, exercise, sneezing, laughing, lifting; frequency of urination; nocturnal urination; strong urge to urinate; lose of urine before reaching toilet; hesitancy, dribbling, slow stream, incomplete voiding, dysuria; bowel habits (e.g., constipation); medications; fluid intake; and medical and surgical history
  - Full neurologic and mental status examinations, assessment of physical frailness (e.g., use of walking aids, dysfunction secondary to stroke), abdominal exam (e.g., lower quadrant distention, pregnancy, fecal impaction), and genital and rectal exam (evaluate for cystocele, vaginal atrophy, and strength of pelvic muscles in women; rectal tone; penis and prostate exam)
  - Voiding diaries may be used to track urinary habits
- Urinalysis and urine culture; consider urine cytology
- Measurement of postvoid residual volume via catheterization and/or pelvic ultrasound (>100 cc of residual urine is abnormal)
- A "cough stress test" may be attempted: Immediate leakage suggests stress incontinence; delayed leakage suggests urge incontinence
- Specialized urodynamic tests (e.g., cystometrogram, cystourethrogram) are reserved for ambiguous results or treatment failure
- Cystoscopy may be indicated to evaluate for bladder and prostate pathology

TREATMENT & MANAGEMENT

- Goals of treatment are to preserve renal function, optimize quality of life, and treat and/or prevent infections and other reversible causes
- Stress incontinence: Increase bladder outlet resistance to prevent leakage
  - Behavioral therapy: Timed voiding, Kegel exercises, biofeedback
  - Occlusion devices: Urethral plug, pessaries
  - Pharmacologic therapy: Alpha-adrenergics, tricyclic antidepressants, estrogens, duloxetine
  - Surgical intervention: Urethral bulking (e.g., collagen, Deflux) procedures, sling procedures, Burch, artificial sphincter, urinary diversion
- Urge incontinence: Decrease bladder contractility to improve urine storage
  - Behavioral therapy: Timed voiding, pelvic floor physiotherapy and biofeedback
  - Pharmacologic therapy: Anticholinergics, muscle relaxants, magnesium supplementation, tricyclic antidepressants, estrogens
  - Surgical intervention: Hydrodistention, Botox injection, percutaneous nerve stimulation, implantable sacral nerve stimulator, and/or augmentation cystoplasty
- Overflow incontinence: Decrease outlet resistance to improve urine outflow
  - Pharmacologic therapy to open bladder neck and decrease prostate size (e.g., alpha-adrenergic blockers, 5-alpha-reductase inhibitors)
  - Emptying bladder with clean, intermittent catheterization
- Surgical intervention: Prostatectomy, bladder neck incision, urethral dilation, urethroplasty

PROGNOSIS & COMPLICATIONS

- With newer and more effective anticholinergic medicines coming to the market and the development of less invasive surgical procedures to correct incontinence, patients suffering with this problem have many options to choose from
- In a vast majority of these patients, a durable solution can be found

Benign Prostatic Hyperplasia

INTRODUCTION

- Benign prostatic hyperplasia (BPH) is a common cause of lower urinary tract symptoms in aging men
- Often incorrectly called benign prostatic *hypertrophy*; however, the disorder is truly hyperplastic and is associated with an increased number of prostate cells
- Androgens are necessary for development of BPH but are not necessarily causative
- Not all patients with enlarged prostates have symptoms, and not all patients with symptoms have enlarged prostates; about half of men with a histologic diagnosis have moderate to severe symptoms
- About 50% of men over 50 have BPH, about 60% of patients over 60 have BPH, and so on

ETIOLOGY, EPIDEMIOLOGY, & RISK FACTORS

- BPH is characterized by an increase in the number of epithelial and stromal cells in the periurethral transitional zone of the prostate, which transmits pressure to the urethra and results in increased resistance to urinary flow
- Urethral obstruction and obstruction-induced changes in detrusor function are compounded by age-related changes in both bladder and nervous system function
- Androgens, estrogens, stromal-epithelial interactions, growth factors, and neurotransmitters may play a role
- No established link has been made between socioeconomic status, smoking, religion, diet, sexual activity, or hypertension
- Abdominal obesity may increase the frequency and severity of lower urinary tract symptoms

PATIENT PRESENTATION

- Symptoms can be measured by the American Urological Association symptom score
  - Measures 7 symptoms: Straining to urinate, urgency, nocturia, weak urinary stream, incomplete emptying, frequency of urination, and intermittency of urine stream
  - Graded from 0 (not at all or none) to 5 (almost always)
  - The summed score stratifies symptoms into mild (0–7), moderate (8–19), or severe (20–35)
  - Quality or life (or bother) is measured as well from 0 (delighted) to 6 (terrible)
- May be asymptomatic
- Rectal examination reveals an enlarged prostate without nodules or tenderness
- The challenge is establishing that the urinary tract symptoms are due to BPH versus other disorders

DIFFERENTIAL DX

- Prostate cancer
- Urethral stricture
- Urinary tract infection
- Neurogenic bladder
- Prostatitis
- Bladder cancer
- Bladder neck contracture
- Stroke
- Parkinson's disease
- Polyuria
- Medication side effect (e.g., anticholinergics, alpha-agonists)

DIAGNOSTIC EVALUATION

- History and physical examination with digital rectal exam and neurologic exam
  - Note prior genitourinary surgery and family history of BPH or prostate cancer
  - Evaluate for medications that can exacerbate BPH and medical conditions or medications that can cause polyuria
- Calculate the American Urological Association symptom score (see *Patient Presentation*)
- Urinalysis to rule out infection
- Consider PSA testing if knowledge of the presence of cancer would change treatment
- Urine cytology to rule out bladder cancer may be indicated if the symptoms are primarily irritative (e.g., urgency, frequency) and if there is a history of smoking
- A voiding diary may be helpful to assess polyuria and voided volumes
- Cystourethroscopy can help rule out stricture or bladder cancer
- Urine flow rate may be suggestive of obstruction, but pressure-flow study is better
- Transrectal ultrasound or MRI may be helpful to establish prostate size for surgical planning

TREATMENT & MANAGEMENT

- Watchful waiting is an option if symptom score is 0–7 or if bother from symptoms is low
- If symptoms are moderate to severe and bothersome, options include watchful waiting, medical management, minimally invasive treatments, or surgical therapies
- Medical therapy includes alpha-blockers (e.g., alfuzosin, tamsulosin, terazosin, doxazosin), 5-alpha-reductase inhibitors (e.g., dutasteride, finasteride), and saw palmetto (not FDA approved but has been shown to be effective)
- Minimally invasive therapies include transurethral microwave thermotherapy (TUMT), which uses heat to destroy prostate tissue, and transurethral needle ablation (TUNA), which uses radiofrequency waves to ablate tissue
  - These are generally more effective than medical therapy but have higher retreatment rates and failure rates than surgical therapies
- Surgical therapies include transurethral resection of the prostate (TURP), transurethral electrovaporization, transurethral incision of the prostate, transurethral holmium laser resection/enucleation, visual laser ablation, transurethral laser vaporization, and open prostatectomy

PROGNOSIS & COMPLICATIONS

- Failure of watchful waiting and indications for surgery include urinary retention, urinary tract infection, bladder stone, recalcitrant hematuria, incontinence, azotemia, and kidney deterioration
- Alpha-blocker therapy has been shown to improve symptom score by 4–6 points; side effects include orthostasis, dizziness, tiredness, retrograde ejaculation, and nasal congestion
- 5-alpha-reductase inhibitors help prevent progression of symptoms and usually improve symptom score by about 3 points; side effects are uncommon, but some users may experience decreased libido, ejaculatory dysfunction, and erectile dysfunction
- TURP syndrome: Hyponatremia due to absorption of irrigant

Nephrolithiasis

INTRODUCTION

- Nephrolithiasis is a relatively common clinical problem; it is estimated that more than 10% of men and about 5% of women will have a symptomatic stone before the age of 70
- Incidence increases with age and is higher in men and Caucasians
- Most often occurs due to increased concentrations of stone-forming material in the urine, either from increased excretion or decreased urinary volume
- Common in patients with urinary stasis (e.g., bladder outlet obstruction) and/or chronic infection
- Prompt identification and treatment is important because untreated, chronic nephrolithiasis can lead to significant renal disease and infection

ETIOLOGY, EPIDEMIOLOGY, & RISK FACTORS

- The majority (>75%) of cases are due to calcium stones
  - Calcium oxalate is the most common type, followed by calcium phosphate
  - Can occur due to hypercalciuria (often secondary to excessive intestinal absorption of calcium), hyperparathyroidism, excess vitamin D, or bone metastases
  - Hyperoxaluria occurs due to oxalate-rich foods, short gut syndromes, metabolic disorders
  - Ironically, high dietary calcium intake may *decrease* the risk of stone formation because it forms ligands with oxalate and phosphate, preventing stone formation
- Uric acid stones are associated with low urine pH (e.g., chronic diarrhea) and hyperuricosuria (e.g., gout, myeloproliferative states)
  - May occur with severe dehydration despite normal uric acid levels
- Struvite stones (composed of magnesium ammonium phosphate) occur in patients with chronic urinary tract infections caused by urea-splitting bacteria (e.g., *Proteus*)
  - These stones often fill the entire renal collecting system, resulting in "staghorn" calculi
- The pathophysiology of stone formation is not completely understood
  - The initial step is thought to be development of crystals: When high levels of calcium, oxalate, or another normally soluble material appear in the urine, the urine becomes supersaturated and crystals develop; they then aggregate into a stone around the initial nidus

PATIENT PRESENTATION

- Pain is the most common symptom
  - Severe, acute, colicky pain
  - Often located in the flank region, but can radiate towards the pelvis
- Hematuria
  - May be microscopic or gross
  - As many as one-third of patients may not have hematuria.
- Nausea, vomiting
- Costovertebral angle tenderness
- Many patients complain of dysuria and urinary urgency

DIFFERENTIAL DX

- Pyelonephritis
- Ectopic pregnancy
- Pelvic inflammatory disease
- Renal cell carcinoma
- Abdominal aortic aneurysm
- Flank or abdominal trauma
- Small bowel obstruction
- Polycystic kidney disease
- Biliary colic
- Appendicitis
- Diverticulitis
- Epidural abscess
- Pancreatitis
- Hyperparathyroidism
- Tumor lysis syndrome
- Familial hypocalcemic hypercalciuria
- Gout

DIAGNOSTIC EVALUATION

- The clinical presentation is highly predictive, especially in patients with a past history of urolithiasis
- Urinalysis is an essential part of the workup
  - Will reveal hematuria, unless a complete urinary tract obstruction is present
  - The urine pH may differentiate stones caused by infection versus other causes: Those caused by infection often occur in an alkaline urine with pH >7.5
- Noncontrast abdominal CT scan is the test of choice to detect stones and urinary tract obstructions
  - Uric acid stones are the only radiolucent stone; thus, they will not show up on X-ray but are opaque on CT scan
  - Small stones may be missed by CT scan
- Intravenous pyelogram (IVP) and ultrasound are now used less frequently and are less sensitive than CT scan
- In the nonacute setting, a 24-hour urine collection may be sent for analysis of volume, pH, calcium, citrate, oxalate, uric acid, and creatinine
- Strain the urine to catch a passed stone for composition analysis

TREATMENT & MANAGEMENT

- Pain control is most often achieved with narcotics or NSAIDs
  - A recent meta-analysis found NSAIDs and narcotics to be equivalent in analgesia
  - The use of NSAIDs may have the benefit of less nausea and vomiting
  - However, NSAIDs are nephrotoxic, and their use can be associated with acute renal failure; they should be held for 3 days prior to use of extracorporeal shock wave lithotripsy (see below)
- Small (<5 mm) stones will often pass spontaneously; urology should be consulted for stones >5 mm and for patients who present with fever, renal failure, intractable pain, persistent nausea, or urinary tract infections
- Stones in the kidney are often treated with extracorporeal shock wave lithotripsy (ESWL)
  - Large stones and struvite stones are best treated by surgical removal
  - Uric acid stones can be dissolved by hydration and urinary alkalinization with potassium citrate
- Stones in the ureters are treated with ESWL, ureteroscopy, or intracorporeal laser lithotripsy
- Stones in the bladder are often treated by endoscopic stone crushing and extraction of fragments; very large or hard stones may require a small open cystostomy for removal

PROGNOSIS & COMPLICATIONS

- Recurrence is common; patients should be instructed in methods of stone prevention
  - General measures include increased fluid intake, restriction of animal foods and salt, avoidance of oxalate-containing foods (e.g., tea, dark greens, chocolate), and consumption of citrate (e.g., lemons)
  - Potassium citrate is a good supplement for most calcium stone formers and those with uric acid or cysteine stones
  - A complete metabolic analysis and specific medication regimen may be necessary in severe cases
- Stones that are unable to pass may serve as a nidus of infection and lead to acute or chronic pyelonephritis or renal failure

Prostatitis

INTRODUCTION

- The term prostatitis categorizes a large group of adult men with varied acute and chronic complaints referable to the lower urogenital tract and perineum
- Among otherwise healthy young men, prostatitis is the most common urologic diagnosis
- Accounts for nearly 2 million physician visits annually (represents 8% of visits to urologists and 1% of visits to primary care physicians in the U.S.)
- Bacterial prostatitis is a common clinical diagnosis, but well-documented bacterial infections of the prostate, whether acute or chronic, are uncommon; most patients have no history of bacteriuria and little objective evidence of bacterial infection; indeed, most men with this diagnosis do not have prostatitis, but rather noninflammatory prostatic symptoms

ETIOLOGY, EPIDEMIOLOGY, & RISK FACTORS

- Most patients with prostatitis syndromes are classified into 4 categories:
  - Acute bacterial prostatitis (type I): Acute bacterial infection of the prostate associated with bacteriuria
  - Chronic bacterial prostatitis (type II): Recurrent episodes of bacteriuria associated with a persistent focus of infection in the prostate gland
  - Chronic prostatitis/chronic pelvic pain syndrome (type III): Represents more than 90% of symptomatic patients; presents with chronic symptoms in the absence of bacteriuria
  - Asymptomatic inflammatory prostatitis (type IV): Documented prostatic inflammation in a patient who has no genitourinary tract symptoms
- When infectious, the most common etiologic organisms are *E. coli*, *Klebsiella*, *Enterococcus*, *Staphylococcus*, and *Candida*
- May be associated with sexually transmitted diseases, such as gonorrhea and chlamydia
- Structural genitourinary tract abnormalities associated with bacterial urinary tract infections are important risk factors for acute and chronic bacterial prostatitis

PATIENT PRESENTATION

- Most patients have perineal, penile, or lower abdominal pain, or ejaculatory pain
- Other symptoms may include sexual dysfunction, voiding dysfunction, and depression
- Acute bacterial prostatitis: Lower urinary tract symptoms (e.g., dysuria, frequency); may have urinary tract obstruction due to acute edema of the prostate; high fever; lower abdominal discomfort with an exquisitely tender prostate
- Chronic bacterial prostatitis: Recurrent bacterial urinary tract infections caused by the same organism; often asymptomatic between episodes; the prostate gland is usually normal on exam
- Chronic pelvic pain syndrome: No history of bacteriuria; pelvic pain or discomfort (may be perineal, suprapubic, lower abdominal, penile, or scrotal); pain may be exacerbated by ejaculation
- Asymptomatic inflammatory prostatitis: Patients have no genitourinary tract symptoms

DIFFERENTIAL DX

- Musculoskeletal low back pain
- Constipation
- Psychogenic
- External hemorrhoids
- Dysfunctional voiding
- Seminal vesiculitis
- Urolithiasis
- Inguinal hernia
- Bladder stones
- Bladder malignancy
- Urethritis
- Other causes of suprapubic pain (e.g., cystitis, appendicitis, diverticulitis, epididymitis)
- Trauma

DIAGNOSTIC EVALUATION

- History and physical examination with digital rectal exam
  - If acute bacterial prostatitis is suspected, avoid prostatic massage because this may cause bacteremia and exacerbate the situation
- All patients require urinalysis and urine culture
- The Meares-Stamey four-glass test may be used for urine culture
  - Sample #1 includes the first 10 mL of voided urine (a urethral specimen)
  - Sample #2 is a midstream urine collection
  - Sample #3 is of expressed prostatic excretions
  - Sample #4 is the first 10 mL of urine after prostatic massage
- Further evaluations may help direct therapy, including lower urinary tract localization cultures, symptom index (e.g., NIH Chronic Prostatitis Symptom Index), urine flow rate, and residual urine determination
  - Lower urinary tract localization cultures constitute the cornerstone for diagnosis for chronic bacterial prostatitis
- Selected patients merit additional evaluation including semen analysis and/or culture, evaluation of urethral leukocytes and pathogens, prostate-specific antigen, pressure-flow and urodynamic studies, or urinary cytology
- Some patients with chronic pelvic pain syndrome have leukocytes in their prostatic secretions or postprostate massage urine
- Prostate-specific antigen (PSA) levels may be falsely elevated during acute prostatitis

TREATMENT & MANAGEMENT

- Acute and chronic bacterial prostatitis: Treat with antimicrobial therapy based on culture results
  - Empiric therapy can be started prior to culture results with a systemic fluoroquinolone (e.g., levofloxacin, ciprofloxacin) or trimethoprim-sulfamethoxazole for 2–4 weeks
- Chronic pelvic pain syndrome: Optimal therapy remains unclear
  - Current first-line therapies include antibiotics (e.g., fluoroquinolone or trimethoprim-sulfamethoxazole), alpha-adrenergic blockers (e.g., terazosin or doxazosin), or anti-inflammatory agents (e.g., ibuprofen)
- Asymptomatic inflammatory prostatitis: There is active debate on whether these patients merit antibiotics, anti-inflammatory therapy, or no therapy at all
- Consider treatment for sexually transmitted infections in younger populations (e.g., tetracycline, fluoroquinolone)
- Penicillins and cephalosporins have poor prostatic penetration and should be avoided
- Chronic cases may benefit from prostatic massage, herbal therapies (e.g., saw palmetto), intraprostatic injections, or transurethral resection of the prostate (TURP)

PROGNOSIS & COMPLICATIONS

- Acute and chronic bacterial prostatitis have good prognoses with appropriate antimicrobial therapy
  - Complications include urosepsis, prostatic abscess, and granulomatous prostatitis
- Chronic pelvic pain syndrome: Patients may remain symptomatic for prolonged periods
- Asymptomatic inflammatory prostatitis: Prognosis is uncertain
- Epidemiologic studies suggest that patients with a history of prostatitis may be at increased risk for prostate cancer and benign prostatic hypertrophy

Sexually Transmitted Diseases

INTRODUCTION

- 15 million persons in the United States acquire a sexually transmitted disease (STD) each year, many of whom are asymptomatic
- Prompt diagnosis and treatment of symptomatic patients, screening of patients at risk, and partner notification and treatment are all necessary because STDs can cause long-term complications and increase the risk of HIV acquisition and transmission
- Screening should be offered to asymptomatic persons at higher risk of infections or complications, including men who have sex with men, sexually active women under 24, patients with new or multiple sexual partners, pregnant women, and commercial sex workers

ETIOLOGY, EPIDEMIOLOGY, & RISK FACTORS

- STDs are primarily transmitted by sexual (mucosal-to-mucosal) contact, although occasional reports suggest that fomite transmission of selected infections can occur
  - Infections with long incubation periods (e.g., HIV, hepatitis B) are maintained in the population even with low-level sexual activity or sequential partners (serial monogamy)
  - Infections with short incubation periods (e.g., gonorrhea) are maintained by high-level sexual activity and concurrent sexual partners
- Herpes simplex anogenital disease is most commonly caused by HSV-2; genital infection with HSV-1 is less likely to be recurrent
  - HSV-2 is the most common cause of genital ulcers in the United States; 22% of the population is seropositive
- Syphilis is caused by the spirochete *Treponema pallidum*, which may cause an initial painless chancre followed by dissemination (secondary and tertiary disease)
- 3 million cases of chlamydia are reported annually, most commonly in women 15–19
- Chancroid (*Haemophilus ducreyi*), donovanosis (also known as granuloma inguinale, caused by *Calymmatobacterium granulomatis*), and lymphogranuloma venereum (*Chlamydia trachomatis*) are rare causes of genital ulcer disease in the U.S. but should be considered following recent travel abroad or if initial investigations fail to confirm HSV or syphilis

PATIENT PRESENTATION

- Symptoms depend both on the infecting organism and sexual activity (e.g., receptive vs. insertive; oral vs. vaginal vs. anal sex)
- Cervical, vaginal, or urethral infections: Urethral or vaginal discharge, dysuria, pelvic pain
- Anal or rectal infections: Pain, diarrhea, or rectal discharge, or may be asymptomatic
- Chlamydia and gonorrhea: Cervicitis, urethritis, proctitis, and pelvic inflammatory disease
  - Gonococcus may cause pharyngitis after oral sex; it may also disseminate hematogenously and cause fever, arthralgia, tenosynovitis, and pustular skin rash on the extremities
- Syphilis may present with a painless ulcer of the anogenital or pharyngeal region and may then spread hematogenously to cause disseminated secondary or tertiary disease
- HSV may present as painful recurrent crops of ulcers

DIFFERENTIAL DX

- Genital ulcer disease: HSV, syphilis, chancroid, LGV, donovanosis, trauma, Behçet's syndrome, malignancy, SLE
- Vaginitis: Trichomoniasis, candidiasis, bacterial vaginosis, atrophic vaginitis
- Urethritis: Chlamydia, gonorrhea, trichomoniasis, *Mycoplasma hominis*, ureaplasma urealyticum
- Cervicitis: Gonorrhea, chlamydia, HSV, syphilitic ulcer, cervical cancer
- More than one infection may be present

DIAGNOSTIC EVALUATION

- History and physical examination
  - A history of symptoms, previous STDs, sexual activity, number and sex of partners, and condom and contraceptive use should be taken in a nonjudgmental manner
  - Pregnancy testing and cervical cancer screening should be considered in all females
  - All patients should be offered syphilis and HIV testing
- Vaginal discharge should be evaluated with an endocervical culture for gonorrhea and chlamydia or nucleic acid amplification testing (NAAT), vaginal swab for KOH and wet preparation, and pH testing
  - pH <4.5 and pseudohyphae suggests *Candida* ("yeast") infection; pH >6 with motile forms suggests trichomoniasis; pH >6 with clue cells suggests bacterial vaginosis
- Urethral discharge should be evaluated by urethral swab for gonorrhea and chlamydia culture or NAAT
  - More than 5 WBC/HPF is diagnostic of urethritis
- The presence of intracellular gram-negative diplococci suggests gonorrhea
- Receptive anal sex or symptoms of proctitis: Culture for gonorrhea and chlamydia
- Pharyngitis or history of oral sex: Pharyngeal culture for gonococcus
- Asymptomatic screening can be accomplished by first-void urine testing for gonorrhea and chlamydia or NAAT
- Anogenital or pharyngeal ulceration should be evaluated by dark-field microscopy, HSV culture, RPR (may be negative in primary syphilis)

TREATMENT & MANAGEMENT

- Patients may initially be treated empirically for the most likely disease based on clinical presentation and epidemiologic circumstances (e.g., cervicitis should be treated for chlamydia and gonorrhea, genital ulceration should be treated for syphilis and/or HSV); however, diagnosis based solely on history and physical examination is insensitive because "classic" findings are only seen in some cases
- To ensure compliance, directly observed, single-dose therapies are preferred, if possible
- Patients with confirmed gonorrhea (by microscopy and/or culture) should be treated for chlamydia also, unless a reliable test for chlamydia is negative
- Directed treatment for confirmed infections should follow CDC guidelines:
  - Uncomplicated gonorrhea: Single-dose cefixime, ceftriaxone, or ciprofloxacin
  - Chlamydia: Single-dose azithromycin or doxycycline for 7 days
  - Trichomoniasis: Single-dose metronidazole (avoid in pregnancy)
  - Genital herpes: Acyclovir 3 times daily or valacyclovir twice daily for 5–10 days
  - Primary syphilis: Single-dose benzathine penicillin
- All patients should be counseled for HIV testing, educated about condom use and reduction of sexual partners, and offered vaccination against hepatitis B
- Notify the State Health Department of STDs and all sexual partners for reportable diseases

PROGNOSIS & COMPLICATIONS

- Completed courses of treatments are generally highly effective; however, poor adherence to treatment and antibiotic resistance, especially gonorrhea, is increasingly common
- All STDs are associated with an increased risk of HIV transmission
- Chlamydia and gonorrhea are leading causes of pelvic inflammatory disease, female infertility, and ectopic pregnancies
- Urethritis in men may be complicated by the development of a urethral stricture
- Secondary or tertiary syphilis may occur if the initial infection is untreated
- Chlamydia and gonorrhea both cause neonatal conjunctivitis, and babies infected with chlamydia at birth may also present with pneumonia; disseminated herpes may develop in a neonate born to a mother with genital HSV infection at the time of delivery

Acute Renal Failure

INTRODUCTION

- Acute renal failure is a fairly common syndrome (1% of all hospitalized patients, 20% of intensive care patients) that results in an inability to excrete metabolic wastes and maintain proper fluid and electrolyte balance
- It is usually defined as a drop in glomerular filtration rate (GFR) by more than 25%, combined with an increase in serum creatinine by 50% over a period of hours to days
- Etiologies can be divided into prerenal, postrenal, and intrinsic causes
- 50–75% of patients who survive an episode of acute renal failure will regain renal function

ETIOLOGY, EPIDEMIOLOGY, & RISK FACTORS

- <u>Prerenal failure</u> (70% of outpatient cases, 30% of inpatient cases) is caused by conditions that reduce renal perfusion: Decreased circulating volume (e.g., acute hemorrhage, profuse vomiting, excessive diuresis, decreased oral intake), decreased cardiac output (e.g., congestive heart failure), or extracellular fluid accumulation (e.g., sepsis, cirrhosis, severe acute pancreatitis)
- <u>Intrinsic renal failure</u> (10% of outpatient cases, 50% of inpatient cases) is caused by diseases that affect the renal glomerulus or tubules: Acute tubular necrosis, renal artery obstruction, vasculitis, thrombotic thrombocytopenic purpura, postinfectious, systemic lupus erythematosus, interstitial nephritis (e.g., due to beta-lactam antibiotics, H2 receptor blockers, NSAIDs), drug toxicity (e.g., acyclovir, methotrexate), rhabdomyolysis, multiple myeloma, atheromatous emboli
- <u>Postrenal failure</u> (20% of outpatient cases, <5% of inpatient cases) is caused by processes that block urine outflow: Benign prostatic hypertrophy, urethral stricture, urolithiasis, pelvic mass, neurogenic bladder
- Intravenous contrast is an important risk factor for acute renal failure, particularly in patients with diabetes, severe congestive heart failure, hypotension, glomerular filtration rate less than 35 mL/min, or large boluses of contrast (e.g., during cardiac catheterization)

PATIENT PRESENTATION

- Alteration of urine output: Patients may be anuric, oliguric (urine output <30 mL/h), or nonoliguric
- Symptoms of renal failure include nausea, vomiting, metallic taste, nonspecific abdominal pain, lethargy, and morning headaches
- Patients may present with signs of volume overload (e.g., pulmonary edema, crackles, peripheral edema, elevated jugular venous pressure)
- Severe uremia may present with encephalopathy, change in mental status, asterixis, pericarditis, electrolyte disorders and arrhythmias, metabolic acidosis, hypertension, or heart failure
- Uremia also predisposes to bleeding due to platelet dysfunction

DIFFERENTIAL DX

- Chronic renal failure
- Acute prerenal, intrinsic renal, or postrenal failure (see etiologies, above)
- If anuric, consider bilateral ureteral obstruction and shock
- If unilateral flank pain occurs, consider nephrolithiasis, renal infarction, infection, obstruction
- If peripheral edema, hematuria, and hypertension are present, consider vasculitis and glomerulonephritis
- If dyspnea occurs, consider pulmonary embolus, MI, CHF
- If rash occurs, consider acute interstitial nephritis due to medications, vasculitis, or atheroemboli

DIAGNOSTIC EVALUATION

- History and physical examination should evaluate for possible etiologies and evaluate the time course of renal failure
- Assess urine output
  - Anuria (<100 mL/d) suggests postrenal obstruction, severe intrinsic renal injury, or renal artery occlusion
  - Oliguria (100–400 mL/d) suggests prerenal disease
  - Nonoliguria (>400 mL/d) is typical of intrinsic renal processes
- Evaluate for electrolytes abnormalities: Hyperkalemia, hyperphosphatemia, and metabolic acidosis are common in renal failure
- Obtain urine sodium (U_{Na}), urine creatinine (U_{Cr}), plasma sodium (P_{Na}), and plasma creatinine (P_{Cr}) levels, and calculate the fractional excretion of sodium (FeNa) to distinguish prerenal failure versus intrinsic renal failure
  - FeNa $= (U_{Na}/P_{Na}) * (P_{Cr}/U_{Cr}) * 100$ (note that FeNa is only useful in oliguric renal failure)
  - FeNa <1 indicates a prerenal etiology (a prerenal etiology is also suggested by BUN:Cr ratio greater than 20:1, elevated plasma CO_2 level, elevated uric acid, low urine sodium [<20 mEq/L], and normal urine microscopy)
  - FeNa >1 implies an intrinsic renal etiology (an intrinsic renal etiology is also suggested by proteinuria, microscopy with casts [granular, WBC, and RBC], and urine sodium >20 mEq/L)
- Renal ultrasound or CT scan may be indicated to evaluate for postrenal obstruction

TREATMENT & MANAGEMENT

- Place a Foley catheter to rule out urethral/bladder obstruction, and monitor urine output
- Correct hydration and electrolyte abnormalities, and optimize hemodynamics
  - Patients with volume depletion require IV fluids; however, administer conservative fluid loads (e.g., 500 mL) to patients with congestive heart failure or pulmonary edema
  - Patients with hyperkalemia require immediate treatment and cardiac monitoring
  - Bicarbonate administration may be necessary to counter severe acidosis (pH <7.2)
- Adjust drug doses (e.g., antibiotics, insulin, digoxin) according to glomerular filtration rate
- Discontinue nephrotoxic drugs (e.g., NSAIDs, aminoglycosides, ACE inhibitors); consider discontinuation of drugs associated with interstitial nephritis (e.g., penicillins, cephalosporins, NSAIDs, thiazide diuretics, allopurinol, furosemide, sulfonamides, ciprofloxacin)
- Dialysis or continuous hemofiltration is indicated for symptomatic uremia (e.g., encephalopathy), fluid overload (e.g., pulmonary edema), or severe electrolyte or acid-base abnormalities that are refractory to standard measures (e.g., severe hyperkalemia, acidosis)
  - Dialysis is also indicated for toxins that have no antidote and cannot be chelated by charcoal (e.g., lead, iron, lithium, alcohols, theophylline)
- Note that loop diuretics do not improve renal function but may decrease volume overload, thereby preventing the need for emergent hemodialysis
- In patients with poor cardiac output, afterload reducers (e.g., hydralazine) and positive inotropes (e.g., dobutamine) will increase cardiac output and may improve renal perfusion

PROGNOSIS & COMPLICATIONS

- 20% overall mortality rate (50% mortality rate for patients who develop acute renal failure while hospitalized and 70% mortality rate if develop acute renal failure while in ICU)
- Early nephrology consultation has been shown to improve outcomes
- Prognosis depends on the etiology, the presence of comorbid conditions, pre-existing renal disease, and the degree of oliguria
- 20–60% of hospitalized patients require hemodialysis at some point
- Prerenal failure is reversible if treated appropriately
- Acute tubular necrosis usually resolves within 3 weeks
- Contrast nephropathy often recovers within 3–7 days (patients at highest risk are those with diabetes, chronic renal insufficiency, or intravascular volume depletion)

Chronic Kidney Disease

INTRODUCTION

- Chronic kidney disease (CKD) (formerly known as chronic renal failure or chronic renal insufficiency) is defined by either a glomerular filtration rate (GFR) $<$60 mL/min/1.73 m^2 for at least 3 months *or* by functional or structural damage to the kidney for 3 or more months as seen on imaging or blood or urine testing
  - Stage 1 CKD: GFR $>$90 mL/min/1.73 m^2 with persistent proteinuria
  - Stage 2 CKD: GFR 60–89 with persistent proteinuria
  - Stage 3 CKD: GFR 30–59 (~4% of the population)
  - Stage 4 CKD: GFR 15–29 (~0.2% of the population)
  - Stage 5 CKD: GFR $<$15 (~0.2% of the population)

ETIOLOGY, EPIDEMIOLOGY, & RISK FACTORS

- Diabetic nephropathy accounts for nearly 50% of cases, hypertension accounts for 25%, and glomerulonephritis accounts for 10%; less common etiologies include renal cystic disease, other urologic pathology (e.g., congenital disease, urinary obstruction), multiple myeloma, amyloidosis, atheroemboli, Fabry's disease, hemolytic uremic syndrome (HUS), and analgesic abuse
- The pathophysiology varies based on the underlying etiology:
  - Immune deposition diseases (e.g., SLE) lead to CKD by immune complex deposition in the glomerulus with subsequent activation of the complement system
  - Obstructive diseases (e.g., urolithiasis) lead to CKD by increasing pressure proximal to the obstruction, which is reflected back to the glomerulus and may cause renal ischemia
  - Longstanding diabetes leads to glomerular sclerosis
  - Poorly controlled hypertension leads to glomerulosclerosis and nephron loss
- $>$8 million Americans have chronic kidney disease, and many more have proteinuria
- CKD is underdiagnosed and undertreated, and its incidence is rising
- Major risk factors include hypertension, diabetes, SLE, vasculitis, advanced age, African-American or Hispanic race, low birth weight, family history of CKD, nephrolithiasis, urinary tract infections, and low socioeconomic status

PATIENT PRESENTATION

- GFR of 25–50 may be asymptomatic
- GFR of 10–25: Hypertension, anemia (due to decreased erythropoietin production), fluid retention, hyperkalemia, metabolic acidosis (anion gap), and other electrolyte disturbances
  - Hyperphosphatemia and hypocalcemia can cause secondary hyperparathyroidism, resulting in bone pain
- GFR $<$10 (end-stage renal disease) presents with signs and symptoms of uremia: Anorexia, nausea, vomiting, weight loss, metabolic encephalopathy (poor attention, slowing on EEG, asterixis), pruritis, peripheral neuropathy, pericarditis, and bleeding

DIFFERENTIAL DX

- Acute renal failure
- Diabetic nephropathy
- Hypertensive nephrosclerosis
- Autoimmune diseases (e.g., SLE, scleroderma, Wegener's, Good-pasture's)
- Paraproteinemias (e.g., multiple myeloma, amyloidosis)
- Polycystic kidney disease
- IgA nephropathy
- Thin basement membrane disease
- Urinary tract obstruction
- Urinary tract infection
- Renal artery stenosis
- Reflux nephropathy
- Toxic effects of drugs

DIAGNOSTIC EVALUATION

- Serum creatinine is used as a rough indicator of kidney function
  - There are several estimates of GFR, for example: $[(140 - age) \times (weight\ in\ kg)] / 72 \times P_{Cr}$
  - Normal GFR is >90 at age 40 (serum creatinine = 0.8–1.2)
  - Mild CKD: GFR = 50–90 (creatinine = 1.0–2.5)
  - Moderate CKD: GFR = 25–50 (creatinine = 1.2–4)
  - Severe CKD: GFR = 10–25 (creatinine = 2–8)
  - End-stage renal disease: GFR <10 (creatinine = 4–15)
- Differentiate CKD from acute, reversible renal failure by persistence over time (>3 months) and failure to respond to hydration, specific treatments, discontinuation of medications, and other attempts at treatment
- In general, all patients require urinalysis
  - Urine protein-to-creatinine ratio can be used to measure proteinuria, which is a reflection of glomerular injury; patients with any degree of proteinuria should be seen by a nephrologist
  - Hematuria, proteinuria, and red blood cell casts suggest acute glomerulonephritis
- Renal imaging (ultrasound is the best initial test) and renal biopsy are often indicated to determine the etiology
- Follow complete blood counts, electrolytes, calcium, parathyroid hormone level, and other laboratory testing as necessary (e.g., ANCA, anti-GBM antibody, ANA, C3 and C4, rheumatoid factor), and correct abnormalities as necessary

TREATMENT & MANAGEMENT

- The underlying etiology dictates therapy
  - Control blood pressure to less than 130/75; use ACE inhibitors or angiotensin receptor blockers in maximum-tolerated doses in diabetic patients or patients with proteinuria
  - Control blood glucose in diabetic patients
  - Assess and treat reversible factors, including adverse drug effects, obstruction, infection, and fluid imbalance
  - Treat specific diseases as appropriate (e.g., cytotoxic agents for SLE, Goodpasture's syndrome, and Wegener's granulomatosis; steroids for IgA nephropathy and multiple myeloma)
- Dietary therapy includes fluid and sodium restriction to prevent secondary hypertension, moderate protein restriction, and phosphate and potassium restriction
- Treat anemia with iron replacement and recombinant erythropoietin to a target hemoglobin level of 11–12 g/dL
- Phosphate binders and calcitriol are indicated for phosphate levels >5.5 mg/dL
- Use diuretics judiciously
- Dialysis and renal transplantation may be necessary
- CKD is a major independent risk factor for cardiovascular disease; manage hyperlipidemia, hypertriglyceridemia, hypertension, and other cardiac risk factors aggressively

PROGNOSIS & COMPLICATIONS

- Early referral to a nephrologist is essential
- The rate of decrease of GFR can be reduced or even halted with aggressive blood pressure control using ACE inhibitors or angiotensin receptor blockers in diabetic and nondiabetic renal disease with proteinuria
- Plan for creation of an AV fistula for dialysis approximately 6–12 months before the projected date of end-stage renal disease, and educate the patient about all dialysis and transplantation options
- End-stage renal disease requiring dialysis is associated with annual mortality of >20%
- Volume overload and congestive heart failure are common
- Fatal hyperkalemia can occur

Urinary Tract Infections (UTI)

INTRODUCTION

- Cystitis is lower urinary tract inflammation or infection
- Pyelonephritis is upper tract inflammation or infection and a common cause of sepsis
- Pyuria indicates the presence of inflammatory cells in the urine by dipstick or microscopy; it is usually infectious and may or may not be symptomatic
- Uncomplicated UTIs (upper or lower tract) occur in patients with normal bladder function and normal host defenses, nearly always in healthy, sexually active, young women
- Complicated UTIs (upper or lower tract) imply a physiologic or structural abnormality of the urinary tract (e.g., incontinence, obstruction) or abnormal host defenses
  - UTIs in men, elderly patients, and diabetics should be assumed to be complicated UTIs

ETIOLOGY, EPIDEMIOLOGY, & RISK FACTORS

- Nearly all urinary tract infections are ascending
  - Vaginal colonization initially occurs by a urinary pathogen, usually from a colonic source
  - Introduction of bacteria then occurs during intercourse or catheterization
  - Bacteria with virulence factors attach to bladder epithelium, multiply, cause inflammation
- Nearly all uncomplicated UTIs are caused by uropathogenic *E. coli* or *S. saprophyticus*
- Complicated UTIs may be caused by many gram-negative organisms (often polymicrobial)
- Gram-positive organisms other than *S. saprophyticus* rarely cause UTIs; however, they may be present in polymicrobial UTIs or in the elderly (e.g., enterococcus)
- Recurrent UTI is defined as more than 3 symptomatic UTIs in a year
  - Recurrences are rarely relapses; most are reinfections
- Nearly all UTIs in patients younger than 60 occur in women due to their short urethra
- UTIs in men remain less common than in women at any age; however, incidence increases in older men secondary to changes in the prostate
- Spermicides and prior antibiotic use predispose to UTI
- Any catheter use, including condom catheters, may lead to UTI, usually within 1 week
- Recurrent UTIs that occur within a few months may not be associated with sexual activity
- Any cause of abnormal bladder function predisposes to complicated UTIs

PATIENT PRESENTATION

- Dysuria
- Frequency
- Urgency
- Suprapubic or lower back discomfort
- Change in odor of urine
- Hematuria
- Nocturia
- Nausea
- Vomiting
- Fatigue
- Cystitis is rarely a cause of fever; always evaluate for other diagnoses if fever is present
- Pyelonephritis is a clinical diagnosis characterized by fever, flank pain or tenderness, and urinary tract infection

DIFFERENTIAL DX

- Vaginitis (esp. *Candida*)
- Urethritis
  - Sexually transmitted diseases
  - Irritation due to sexual manipulation
  - Chemical irritation (e.g., bubble bath)
- Interstitial cystitis
- Pregnancy
- Pelvic inflammatory disease
- Nephrolithiasis
- Diverticulosis
- Urinary incontinence
- Bladder cancer
- Renal cyst
- Renal carcinoma
- Vaginal foreign body
- Prostatitis
- Atrophic vaginitis

DIAGNOSTIC EVALUATION

- Bacteriuria refers to bacteria in the urine, as detected by dipstick, microscopy, or culture
  - Asymptomatic bacteriuria is common in the elderly, catheterized patients, diabetics, and those with bladder abnormalities; nonetheless, UTI is rare in asymptomatic patients
  - In the presence of symptoms, bacteriuria >102/mL is significant
  - Polymicrobial bacteriuria (>1 species of bacteria) does *not* reliably indicate contamination
- Urinalysis may reveal bacteriuria, WBCs, hematuria, elevated leukocyte esterase, nitrites
- Dipsticks are a specific and sensitive measure of pyuria and hematuria
- Midstream specimens are usually adequate (clean catch is usually unnecessary)
  - Urine culture is indicated for complicated UTIs but not for uncomplicated UTIs
- If urine culture is done, always evaluate sensitivities as resistance is increasingly common
- If cultures are positive in the absence of symptoms, it is usually asymptomatic bacteriuria, and there is no benefit from antibiotic treatment (exceptions to this include pregnancy and prophylactic treatment prior to traumatic urologic procedures such as cystoscopy)
- Recurrent UTI is very rarely due to treatable conditions or anatomic disorders, and diagnostic evaluation should be guided only by clinical suspicion of an underlying disorder
  - Colonization with a uropathogenic strain of *E. coli* with reintroduction of the organism into the bladder after sexual intercourse is more likely than functional disorder
- Imaging is unnecessary for uncomplicated pyelonephritis
  - CT scan is indicated if there is no response within 48 hours and for complicated pyelonephritis

TREATMENT & MANAGEMENT

- Cystitis is usually treated with 3 days of antibiotics for uncomplicated UTI
  - Renal-excreted quinolones (e.g., levofloxacin, ciprofloxacin) have the best cure rate
  - Trimethoprim-sulfamethoxazole may be used if community resistance levels are known to be less than 10–15% or the organism is known to be sensitive
  - All other oral antibiotics are inferior for cystitis, including beta-lactam antibiotics
  - Single-dose regimens fail in at least 20% of uncomplicated UTIs
  - Treatment duration of 7–10 days is safest for complicated UTIs
  - Men should be treated for at least 14 days with a fluoroquinolone, and longer if symptoms of prostatitis are present
  - Phenazopyridine (Pyridium), hydration, or acidification *does not* improve outcomes
- Pyelonephritis is treated for 7–14 days
  - Use broad-spectrum IV antibiotics targeted at gram-negatives (e.g., third-generation cephalosporins, piperacillin-tazobactam, ampicillin/gentamicin) for urosepsis
  - Uncomplicated pyelonephritis can be treated with outpatient oral fluoroquinolones
- Recurrent UTI can be managed by a patient-initiated 3-day course of trimethoprim-sulfamethoxazole or a fluoroquinolone upon onset of symptoms (safest and most cost effective) or a single postcoital dose

PROGNOSIS & COMPLICATIONS

- Asymptomatic patients do not require a follow-up culture or urinalysis
- Symptomatic patients should have a follow-up culture
- Most failures with adequate treatment are due to reinfection, rather than relapse
  - True relapses after short-course therapy should be treated with 2 weeks of culture-directed antibiotics
  - True relapses after a 2-week course of therapy may require further investigation; some authorities would treat for 4–6 weeks (especially men) before consideration of further workup
- Sequelae from treated UTIs are extremely rare

Epididymitis and Orchitis

INTRODUCTION

- Epididymitis (inflammation of the epididymis) is a common disease that leads to more than 600,000 physician visits yearly in the U.S.
  - Nonspecific bacterial epididymitis is caused by the typical UTI pathogens
  - Sexually transmitted epididymitis is caused by organisms associated with urethritis
  - Congenital epididymitis is associated with inherited genitourinary anomalies
  - Traumatic epididymitis is uncommon
  - Epididymitis associated with disseminated infections is rare
- Orchitis (inflammation of the testes) is caused by systemic viral or bacterial infections

ETIOLOGY, EPIDEMIOLOGY, & RISK FACTORS

- Sexually transmitted epididymitis is the most common cause in young men
  - Usually caused by *Chlamydia trachomatis* and *Neisseria gonorrhoeae*
  - Rarely associated with underlying urologic pathology
  - Urethral discharge may not be apparent
  - Responsible for 20% of urologic hospitalizations in military populations
  - Men who are the insertive partner during anal intercourse likely have enteric pathogens
- Nonspecific bacterial epididymitis is the most common cause in men older than 35
  - Caused by gram-negative bacilli (*E. coli*, *Klebsiella pneumoniae*, or *Pseudomonas*) or gram-positive cocci (staphylococci or streptococci)
  - Associated with underlying urologic pathology, recent genitourinary tract manipulation (e.g., catheterization, surgery), or acute bacterial prostatitis
- Orchitis is most commonly caused by viral infections (e.g., mumps, coxsackie B virus, lymphocytic choriomeningitis virus)
  - Bacterial infection is less common; when it does occur, it is caused by the same pathogens as nonspecific bacterial epididymitis
  - AIDS patients may have a broad range of bacterial, viral, and fungal pathogens

PATIENT PRESENTATION

- Patients with epididymitis or orchitis typically complain of painful swelling of the scrotum
  - May have acute (1–2 days) or gradual onset
  - Usually unilateral (orchitis may have bilateral or sequential swelling)
- Epididymitis is often accompanied by dysuria or irritative lower urinary tract symptoms
  - May have urethral discharge (discharge may be apparent on inspection or "stripping" of the urethra)
  - Many only have nonspecific findings (e.g., fever)
  - Swelling may be noted primarily in the posterior aspect of the scrotum
  - Early in the course, swelling may be localized to 1 portion of the epididymis; later, involvement of the ipsilateral testis is frequent, producing an epididymo-orchitis
  - Hydrocele may occur

DIFFERENTIAL DX

- Testicular torsion
- Testicular abscess
- Testicular tumor
- Incarcerated hernia
- Unusual infections
  - Tuberculosis
  - Fungal (blastomycosis) epididymitis or orchitis
- Malignancy
- Varicocele
- Hydrocele
- Trauma

DIAGNOSTIC EVALUATION

- History and physical examination
  - Patients with early epididymitis have swelling limited to the tale of the epididymis; in contrast, patients with testicular torsion typically present with a high-riding, horizontal testicle
- Nonspecific bacterial epididymitis requires urinalysis and culture
  - Consider evaluation for structural urologic pathology
- Sexually transmitted epididymitis
  - Gram stain and culture to assess for urethritis
  - Counseling and testing for other pathogens (e.g., syphilis, HIV)
  - Evaluation and testing of sexual partners
- Testicular ultrasound or MRI may be indicated to differentiate epididymitis from testicular torsion
- Orchitis is a clinical diagnosis
- Prehn's sign: Elevating the affected testicle and epididymis helps to relieve the pain of epididymitis

TREATMENT & MANAGEMENT

- Empiric therapy is usually indicated before culture results are available
- Nonspecific bacterial epididymitis: Initial treatment with agents appropriate for both gram-negative rods and gram-positive cocci (e.g., levofloxacin, amoxicillin/clavulanate); then modify based on urine culture and sensitivity results
  - Consider evaluation for structural urologic pathology
- Sexually transmitted epididymitis: Antibiotics appropriate for both chlamydial and gonococcal infections (e.g., levofloxacin for 10 days OR single-dose ceftriaxone plus doxycycline for 10 days)
  - Patients should be evaluated for other sexually transmitted diseases
  - Evaluate and treat sex partners of patients with proven or suspected sexually transmitted epididymitis if contact was within 60 days
- Viral orchitis is treated symptomatically; bacterial orchitis may initially require broad-spectrum IV antibiotics, such as piperacillin/tazobactam, a fluoroquinolone (e.g., levofloxacin), or a third- or fourth-generation cephalosporin
- Nonspecific measures are often helpful, such as bed rest, scrotal elevation, analgesics, and local ice packs

PROGNOSIS & COMPLICATIONS

- Expect improvement of epididymitis within 3 days of treatment; if signs and symptoms do not subside within 3 days, re-evaluate the diagnosis and/or choice of therapy
- Orchitis resolves more slowly and may require up to a month in severe cases
- Complications include testicular infarction, scrotal abscess, pyocele of the scrotum, chronic draining scrotal sinus, chronic epididymitis, and testicular atrophy and infertility
- Persistent swelling and tenderness after completion of therapy suggest the need for comprehensive evaluation (i.e., for abscess, infarction, testicular cancer, tuberculous epididymitis, or fungal epididymitis)
- Surgery may be necessary for management of complications

Endocrine

Polyuria

INTRODUCTION

- Polyuria is defined as a urine output greater than 3 L/d
- The output of a large volume of dilute urine leads to extracellular dehydration, which stimulates the thirst centers to influence increased fluid intake
- Differentiate polyuria from urinary frequency and nocturia

ETIOLOGY, EPIDEMIOLOGY, & RISK FACTORS

- Diabetes insipidus is a syndrome in which the kidneys are unable to concentrate the urine
  - Caused by either a lack of vasopressin (antidiuretic hormone) release from the pituitary gland (central diabetes insipidus) or an inability to respond to vasopressin at the kidneys (nephrogenic diabetes insipidus)
  - Central diabetes insipidus may occur due to pituitary tumors, head trauma, neurosurgery, and infiltrative diseases (e.g., sarcoidosis, Langerhans cell histiocytosis)
  - Nephrogenic diabetes insipidus may occur due to hypercalcemia, hypokalemia, medications (e.g., lithium, tetracyclines, amphotericin, aminoglycosides), amyloidosis, or Sjögren's syndrome; may be familial
  - In pregnancy, destruction of vasopressin can occur due to placental release of vasopressinase
  - 50% of cases are idiopathic

PATIENT PRESENTATION

- Nocturia
- Polydipsia
- Dehydration if lack access to water
- Hypotension if severe dehydration

DIFFERENTIAL DX

- Uncontrolled diabetes mellitus
- Central diabetes insipidus
- Nephrogenic diabetes insipidus
- Primary polydipsia (psychogenic)
- Diuretics
- Resolving episode of acute renal failure
- Chronic lithium use

DIAGNOSTIC EVALUATION

- History and physical examination
  - Check medications, including herbal and over-the-counter drugs
- Corroborate history with caretakers or family, if available
- Initial laboratory studies include serum and urine fasting glucose, creatinine, electrolytes, osmolality, and serum BUN
- A water deprivation test is used to assess for diabetes insipidus
  - Overnight water restriction followed by injection of vasopressin
  - Normal response is an increase in urine concentration during the water restriction with no response to the vasopressin injection
  - Nephrogenic diabetes insipidus: No increase in urine concentration during water restriction and no response to vasopressin injection
  - Central diabetes insipidus: No increase in urine concentration during water restriction, but positive response to vasopressin injection
  - Primary polydipsia: Serum and urine osmolarity are decreased prior to the test and increase during the water deprivation test
- Evaluate for diabetes mellitus if indicated

TREATMENT & MANAGEMENT

- In the ambulatory setting, the goal of management is to reduce the symptoms of polyuria and polydipsia and treat the underlying cause
- Central diabetes insipidus: Intranasal or oral desmopressin, which is a synthetic analog of vasopressin
  - Must measure serum osmolarity and sodium levels regularly
- Nephrogenic diabetes insipidus: Treat the underlying etiology
  - Thiazide diuretics and dietary salt restriction can be used to decrease the solute load to the kidney and keep a mild sodium depletion so that there is increased proximal tubular resorption
- Primary polydipsia: Limit water intake; however, this can be particularly difficult in cases of psychogenic polydipsia
- Diabetes mellitus: Treat as appropriate
- Hypercalcemia and hypokalemia must be corrected, and the underlying cause should be identified and treated
- Eliminate causative medications, if possible
- Other useful medications may include chlorpropamide (an oral hypoglycemic medication that has antidiuretic effects), a low-sodium diet, and indomethacin

PROGNOSIS & COMPLICATIONS

- Prognosis is good if the underlying cause is treated appropriately
- Patients without an intact thirst center or without access to water (e.g., immobile patients) can develop severe hyperosmolality and dehydration, which may result in hypotension, acute tubular necrosis, shock, seizures, coma, and cerebral infarcts

Thyroid Nodule and Cancer

INTRODUCTION

- Thyroid nodules are common, particularly among women, and in most cases are benign; however, it is imperative to identify those nodules that are likely to be malignant
- The clinical spectrum ranges from an incidental, asymptomatic, small, solitary nodule to a large, partly intrathoracic nodule that causes pressure symptoms
- The most common diagnoses are colloid nodules, cysts, and thyroiditis (80% of cases); benign follicular neoplasms (10–15% of cases); and thyroid carcinoma (5% of cases)
- Previous head and neck radiation is a strong risk factor for all thyroid cancers
- Thyroid nodules are much more common in women (5:1 female:male ratio)

ETIOLOGY, EPIDEMIOLOGY, & RISK FACTORS

- Benign nodules may develop secondary to postsurgical scarring, secondary to radioiodine therapy for hyperthyroidism, or due to the failure of one of the thyroid lobes to develop during development
- The frequency of thyroid nodules increases linearly with age and with decreasing iodine intake
  - As many as 1.5% of adolescents have palpable thyroid nodules
- Nodules have been reported in as many as 4–7% of adults
- Only 1 in 20 clinically identified nodules is malignant
  - This corresponds to 2–4 cases per 100,000 people per year, constituting 1% of all cancers and 0.5% of all cancer deaths
- Papillary carcinoma is most common (75% of cases) and easily curable
- Follicular carcinoma (10%) is common in iodine-deficient areas and is often curable
- Medullary carcinoma (10%) is a cancer of the calcitonin-producing C cells
  - May be associated with MEN II syndromes
- 80% are sporadic; 20% are familial
- Anaplastic carcinoma (5%) is a poorly differentiated, aggressive tumor with poor prognosis

PATIENT PRESENTATION

- Often presents as a solitary thyroid nodule
  - Occasionally (particularly in children), a careful physical exam will detect enlarged cervical lymph nodes as the first indication of disease
- Distant metastasis in lung or bone is only rarely detected as the first sign of cancer
- Recent nodule growth, fixation of the nodule to adjacent structures, dysphagia, obstruction, vocal cord paralysis or hoarseness, or firm surrounding lymph nodes suggest malignancy
- Papillary and follicular carcinomas are generally asymptomatic but may present with change in voice, dysphagia or odynophagia, and adenopathy
- Anaplastic carcinoma presents as a rapidly growing neck mass

DIFFERENTIAL DX

- Benign neoplasm: Follicular adenoma, colloid nodule, dermoid cyst, lipoma, teratoma, Hurthle cell, papillary adenoma
- Malignant neoplasm: Thyroid carcinomas (papillary, follicular, medullary, anaplastic), sarcomas, lymphoma, neck metastases
- Thyroid cyst
- Thyroiditis
- Infection
- Granulomatous disease (e.g., sarcoidosis)
- Nonthyroid lesions (e.g., lymphadenopathy, aneurysm, thyroglossal duct cyst, parathyroid cyst, parathyroid adenoma, laryngocele, cystic hygroma)

DIAGNOSTIC EVALUATION

- The diagnostic challenge is to distinguish benign from malignant nodules
- Laboratory testing includes TSH, calcitonin, and thyroid hormone levels
  - If TSH is elevated, evaluate serum antithyroperoxidase antibody to confirm Hashimoto's thyroiditis
  - Calcitonin levels may be elevated in medullary carcinoma
- Neck ultrasound can accurately detect nonpalpable nodules, can distinguish between solid and cystic lesions, and may be used to aspirate cystic lesions
- Fine-needle aspiration is the best diagnostic test (95% accuracy)
- Radioactive iodine (^{123}) uptake scan may be used to distinguish malignant from benign nodules but is generally reserved for cases when fine-needle aspiration reveals a follicular nodule or to identify whether a nodule is functioning in a hyperthyroid patient
  - Most malignant lesions are "cold" (i.e., no uptake of iodine); however, only 15% of "cold" nodules are malignant
- "Hot" nodules (i.e., those that take up iodine) are almost never malignant

TREATMENT & MANAGEMENT

- Thyroidectomy is the primary treatment for all thyroid cancers (except anaplastic carcinoma), followed by postoperative radioactive ^{131}I ablation of remaining thyroid tissue and potential metastases
  - Thyroid hormone replacement therapy will be necessary following surgery
- Anaplastic cancers may be treated with radiation and radioactive ^{131}I, but neither is particularly effective
- Benign nodules can be treated with thyroxine to suppress TSH stimulation of the thyroid gland; the nodule should be rebiopsied or excised it if grows or changes
  - Nodule growth during thyroxine therapy is a strong indication for surgery

PROGNOSIS & COMPLICATIONS

- Papillary carcinoma has a better than 90% cure rate; follicular carcinoma has 70–80% cure rate; medullary carcinoma has 50–80% cure rate; anaplastic carcinoma is uniformly fatal within 6 months
- Papillary carcinoma tends to spread via lymphatics to the cervical lymph nodes; follicular carcinoma tends to spread hematogenously to distant organs; medullary carcinoma spreads by both lymphatics and bloodstream
- Complications of surgery include recurrent laryngeal nerve or superior laryngeal nerve injuries, hypoparathyroidism, hematoma, seroma, infection, pneumothorax, thyrotoxic storm, and tracheal or esophageal injury

Hypoglycemia

INTRODUCTION

- Defined as a plasma glucose level less than 45–50 mg/dL
- Hypoglycemia is a common problem in diabetic patients
- If untreated, low plasma glucose levels can result in diminished glucose delivery to the brain, which may cause irreversible neurologic dysfunction
- Hypoglycemia can cause significant morbidity and can be lethal if severe and prolonged
- Education of diabetic patients to coordinate the timing of hypoglycemic administration, diet, and exercise is the key to preventing repeated episodes

ETIOLOGY, EPIDEMIOLOGY, & RISK FACTORS

- Glucose is an obligate metabolic fuel for the brain
- The delicate balance of blood glucose level requires dynamic regulation of glucose influx into the circulation; the balance of glucose production in the liver and uptake and utilization in peripheral tissues are regulated by a complex network of hormones, neural pathways, and metabolic signals
- As glucose levels enter the hypoglycemic range, release of glucagon, growth hormone, and epinephrine occurs, which rapidly mobilizes liver glycogen to provide fuel
  - Elevated epinephrine levels cause the characteristic symptoms of hypoglycemia
- Hypoglycemia can be caused by diminished glucose production and/or increased glucose utilization
- Reactive (postprandial) hypoglycemia can occur 2–4 hours after a meal due to delayed and exaggerated insulin release
  - Common after gastric surgery when there is rapid emptying of ingested food, causing overstimulation of vagal reflexes and a mismatch of insulin and glucose levels
  - May be a precursor to type 2 diabetes mellitus

PATIENT PRESENTATION

- Autonomic symptoms include sweating, palpitations, tachycardia, shakiness, and anxiety
- Neuroglycopenic symptoms include weakness, tiredness, or dizziness; difficulty with concentration; confusion; blurred vision; and (in extreme cases) coma and death
  - Reactive hypoglycemia does not cause glucose levels to drop low enough to induce severe neuroglycopenic symptoms
- Whipple's triad for diagnosis of hypoglycemia: Symptoms or signs of hypoglycemia, blood glucose less than 45–50 mg/dL, and reversal of symptoms with glucose administration
- Patients with long-standing type 1 diabetes may have hypoglycemic unawareness until very low glucose levels

DIFFERENTIAL DX

- Diabetic medications (insulin, sulfonylureas) are the most common cause
- Other medications (e.g., salicylates, sulfonamides, tetracyclines, warfarin, MAO inhibitors, phenothiazines)
- Alcohol may cause hypoglycemia by impairing gluconeogenesis
- Hypothyroidism
- Sepsis or severe infection
- Renal failure
- Pituitary or adrenal insufficiency (e.g., Addison's disease)
- Insulinoma or islet cell hyperplasia
- Reactive hypoglycemia

DIAGNOSTIC EVALUATION

- Detailed history should include medications; timing of hypoglycemia relative to medications, meals, or exercise; alcohol intake; history of diabetes, liver or renal disease, or gastric surgery; family history of diabetes or MEN syndromes; signs or symptoms of hormonal excess or deficiencies (e.g., hypopituitarism); nutritional state; and recent illness or infection
- Physical exam should evaluate for signs of adrenal insufficiency (e.g., hypokalemia, hypotension) or sepsis (e.g., hypotension, fever, mental status changes)
- Laboratory studies should be performed when the blood glucose value is below 50 mg/dL and may include serum blood glucose, C-peptide, sulfonylurea levels, cortisol, and insulin levels to assess for factious hypoglycemia, insulinoma, or adrenal insufficiency
- Assess liver and renal function
- Consider workup for infection (e.g., blood, urine, sputum cultures, and possibly lumbar puncture in unclear cases)
- Measure C-peptide and insulin levels prior to glucose infusion
  - Serum insulin is elevated by insulinomas (insulin:glucose ratio >0.3) and sulfonylurea or exogenous insulin administration
  - C-peptide is produced during endogenous insulin production; thus, it is decreased following exogenous insulin use and increased in cases of insulinoma or sulfonylurea use
- CT scan or MRI may be necessary to evaluate for insulinoma
- Administer an oral glucose tolerance test if reactive hypoglycemia is suspected

TREATMENT & MANAGEMENT

- Treatment includes immediate relief of symptoms and then correction of the underlying cause
- Glucose therapy (to target glucose level of >100 mg/dL)
  - Alert patients may be repleted with oral glucose (e.g., juice, glucose tablets)
  - Patients with altered consciousness require infusion of intravenous dextrose solution
  - Frequently recheck blood glucose
  - Thiamine must be given with glucose in any suspected case of alcohol abuse or nutritional deficiency to avoid Wernicke's encephalopathy
- Glucagon may be used to increase glucose release from the liver if unable to obtain IV access and the patient cannot tolerate oral glucose
- Octreotide may be used to inhibit insulin release in cases of sulfonylurea-induced hypoglycemia
- If suspect adrenal insufficiency, administer IV hydrocortisone and measure cortisol level
- Patients with reactive hypoglycemia may benefit from carbohydrate restriction and small, frequent meals
  - Because exercise burns carbohydrates and increases sensitivity to insulin, patients with fasting hypoglycemia should avoid significant physical activity
- Patients with sulfonylurea overdose require hospital admission due to the long half-life of most agents

PROGNOSIS & COMPLICATIONS

- Most patients improve immediately with restoration of normal blood glucose level
- Endocrinology consultation may be warranted if the etiology is not discovered following a thorough evaluation and in diabetic patients with frequent hypoglycemic episodes
- If untreated, hypoglycemia can lead to severe neuroglycopenia and possibly death
- If the underlying cause is identified and curable, prognosis is excellent
- Reactive hypoglycemia generally spontaneously improves over time, and long-term prognosis is very good
- Surgical resection is the treatment of choice for insulinomas

Hirsutism

INTRODUCTION

- Hirsutism is excessive growth of androgen-dependent terminal hairs (stiff, coarse, dark hair) along a male distribution in women
- Usually results as a response to excess androgens; in most cases, excess androgen production occurs secondary to anovulation
- Polycystic ovarian syndrome (PCOS) is the most common etiology, although rare causes should be ruled out
- Differentiate from hypertrichosis, which refers to diffusely increased non-androgen-dependent total body hair and is reversible
- Some degree of hirsutism is estimated to affect 5–15% of all women

ETIOLOGY, EPIDEMIOLOGY, & RISK FACTORS

- Adrenal or ovarian overproduction of androgens can occur due to PCOS, adrenal or ovarian tumors, congenital adrenal hyperplasia, hyperprolactinemia, and Cushing's syndrome
- 70–80% of women with androgen excess present with hirsutism
- Hirsutism is estimated to affect 5–15% of all women
  - One-third of women ages 14–45 have excessive upper lip hair
  - 6–9% have unwanted chin or sideburn hair
- There is strong familial predilection for hirsutism
- Idiopathic hirsutism may occur
  - Usually not related to excess androgens
  - May be due to increased action of androgens at hair follicles

PATIENT PRESENTATION

- Male body hair distribution
  - Face: Mustache, beard, sideburns
  - Body: Chest, circumareolar, linea alba, abdominal trigone, inner thighs
- Other manifestations of excess androgens/virilization:
  - Breast atrophy
  - Frontal balding
  - Acne
  - Deepening voice
  - Clitoromegaly
  - Change in normal female body habitus; (increased musculature, absence of female contours)
  - Acanthosis nigricans (velvety, thickened, hyperpigmented skin) in the axilla and back of neck
  - Menstrual irregularities and hirsutism are associated with PCOS

DIFFERENTIAL DX

- Hypertrichosis
  - Often related to medications (e.g., steroids, phenytoin, diazoxide, cyclosporine, minoxidil)
  - May be associated with hypothyroidism, anorexia, or malnutrition
- Endogenous androgen overproduction: Tumors (pituitary, adrenal, ovarian), congenital adrenal hyperplasia, Cushing's syndrome, androgenized ovary syndrome
- Idiopathic hirsutism
- Normal hair growth for race and ethnicity

DIAGNOSTIC EVALUATION

- History should include time course of symptoms, menstrual history, and medications
  - Progressive worsening, late age of onset, or abrupt onset of hirsutism suggests a tumor
- Physical examination should confirm and document the extent of hirsutism, rule out hypertrichosis, assess for virilization, and assess for abdominal or ovarian masses
- Laboratory studies are generally reserved for women with severe cases, irregular menses, abrupt or late onset, rapid progression, or signs of virilization
  - Serum testosterone level of 50–150 ng/dL suggests an endocrine disorder; levels greater than 200 ng/dL require imaging studies to assess for an androgen-producing tumor
  - LH/FSH ratio >3 may suggest polycystic ovarian syndrome
  - DHEA-S level should be measured if progressive symptoms, irregular menstrual cycles, or signs of virilization (levels >700 µg/dL suggest adrenal hyperplasia or tumor)
  - 17-OH progesterone <300 ng/dL or suppressible rules out adrenal hyperplasia
  - Prolactin and TSH should be measured if menstrual cycles are irregular
- Imaging studies are indicated if a tumor is suspected
  - Abdominal CT scan to rule out an adrenal tumor
  - Pelvic ultrasound or CT scan to rule out an ovarian tumor
- Endometrial biopsy may be indicated to evaluate for endometrial hyperplasia if periods are irregular and there is concern for PCOS

TREATMENT & MANAGEMENT

- Treat the underlying cause to prevent growth of terminal hair (in most cases, the cause is hyperandrogenism secondary to anovulation)
  - Combination low-dose estrogen and nonandrogenic progestin oral contraceptive pills are effective in more than 60% of women; they will inhibit adrenal and ovarian androgen production, stimulate production of sex hormone-binding globulin by the liver (which reduces free testosterone), and diminish terminal hair growth
  - Spironolactone (antiandrogen therapy) blocks the binding of testosterone to its receptors
- Remove terminal hair via waxing, depilatories, electrolysis, or laser treatment
- Gonadotropin-releasing hormone (GnRH) agonists (e.g., leuprolide) in combination with an oral contraceptive pill or estrogen may be used if other therapies fail
- Topical eflornithine hydrochloride cream (13.9%) is FDA approved for unwanted facial hair; acts by inhibiting hair growth, and requires 8 weeks to reach peak effectiveness
- All currently available medications for hirsutism must be stopped if pregnancy is desired
- Dexamethasone will reduce virilization caused by adrenal hyperplasia

PROGNOSIS & COMPLICATIONS

- Hair removal and oral contraceptive use generally provide good results
- Idiopathic hirsutism and PCOS are usually not reversible; however, if untreated, a gradual increase in terminal hair growth may occur with age
- There is no cure for virilization due to adrenal hyperplasia; however, it can usually be controlled with ongoing dexamethasone treatment
- Patients with virilization due to a cancerous tumor have a better prognosis with early diagnosis and treatment
- Therapy is usually continued indefinitely
- PCOS is associated with increased risk of cardiovascular disease, obesity, insulin resistance, infertility, and endometrial hyperplasia

Gynecomastia

INTRODUCTION

- Gynecomastia, or breast swelling, refers to a noninflammatory enlargement of the male breast; it is defined histologically as a benign proliferation of the glandular tissue of the male breast and clinically by the presence of a mass extending concentrically from the nipple
- Common in infancy, adolescence, and in middle-aged or older adult males
- Differentiate gynecomastia from lipomastia (pseudogynecomastia), which is swelling of the breast due to fatty tissue
- May be unilateral or bilateral

ETIOLOGY, EPIDEMIOLOGY, & RISK FACTORS

- Caused by altered balance of estrogen and testosterone
  - There is typically a decrease in androgen production, an increase in estrogen production, or increased availability of estrogen precursors for peripheral conversion to estrogen
  - Other rare mechanisms include androgen receptor blockade and increased binding of androgen to sex hormone-binding globulin in the liver
- Gynecomastia is common in infancy, adolescence, and older adult males
  - 60–90% of infants have transient gynecomastia due to the high estrogen levels during pregnancy
  - Prevalence during puberty is as high as 60% of boys
  - Up to half of older men are affected
- Half of men on chronic dialysis have gynecomastia

PATIENT PRESENTATION

- Gynecomastia can usually be detected when the size of the glandular tissue exceeds 0.5 cm in diameter
- A ridge of symmetrical glandular tissue near the nipple-areolar complex can be felt; in cases of pseudogynecomastia, no ridge will be felt
- Usually asymptomatic, but may be painful or tender
- Signs of breast cancer may include rubbery or firm mass, concentric or asymmetric, skin dimpling, nipple retraction, discharge, and axillary lymphadenopathy

DIFFERENTIAL DX

- Gynecomastia of puberty
- Persistent postpubertal or elderly gynecomastia
- Medications (e.g., estrogens, antiandrogens, spironolactone, nifedipine, digitalis, isoniazid, phenytoin, griseofulvin, cimetidine) or drugs (marijuana)
- Liver disease (e.g., cirrhosis, hepatitis, hemochromatosis)
- Chronic renal insufficiency
- Hypogonadism (e.g., Klinefelter's syndrome, enzymatic defects, testicular trauma or infection)
- Neoplasms (breast, testicular, adrenal, liver, lung, carcinoid)
- Thyroid disease
- Pituitary disease
- Obesity
- Chest wall trauma

DIAGNOSTIC EVALUATION

- History and physical examination, including genital exam
  - Past medical history, family history, developmental and growth history, and medication history (including over-the-counter, herbal, and illegal drugs) are important
- If the patient is an adolescent with normal physical examination, the diagnosis is likely pubertal gynecomastia; gradual improvement with age supports this diagnosis
- Assess for signs and symptoms of liver disease, kidney disease, hyperthyroidism, and hypogonadism
- If gynecomastia is of recent onset, painful, or tender, initial laboratory evaluation may include beta-human chorionic gonadotropin, luteinizing hormone (LH), testosterone, TSH, estradiol, liver function tests, BUN/creatinine, prolactin, and DHEA-S
- Mammogram may be indicated to evaluate for cancer
- Ultrasound may distinguish normal glandular tissue from worrisome solid lesions
- Biopsy may be indicated
- Karyotyping may be indicated if suspect Klinefelter's syndrome

TREATMENT & MANAGEMENT

- Most cases regress spontaneously without treatment
- Weight loss is advisable in obese patients
- Discontinue offending medications, if possible
- Three types of medical therapy are available for elderly patients with severe pain, tenderness, or embarrassment: Androgens (e.g., testosterone, dihydrotestosterone, danazol), antiestrogens (e.g., clomiphene, tamoxifen), and aromatase inhibitors (e.g., testolactone)
- Surgical therapy (e.g., liposuction, direct surgical excision) may be indicated if there is no response to medical therapy
- Treat underlying medical conditions when possible
- Some patients may benefit from psychological counseling

PROGNOSIS & COMPLICATIONS

- Gynecomastia is usually transient and has a very good prognosis without intervention
- 85–95% of cases regress within 6 months
- Complications of surgical therapy include sloughing of tissue, contour irregularity, hematoma, seroma formation, and permanent numbness of the nipple-areolar area

Diabetic Ketoacidosis

INTRODUCTION

- Diabetes ketoacidosis (DKA) is an acute complication of diabetes mellitus characterized by hyperglycemia, acidosis, and production of ketones
- It primarily occurs in type 1 diabetes, with an incidence of 4–8 cases per 1000 person-years
- DKA was uniformly fatal until the discovery of insulin; now, mortality is less than 10%
- The mainstays of treatment are aggressive fluid repletion, correction of electrolyte and acid-base abnormalities, correction of hyperglycemia with insulin administration, and treatment of the underlying etiology (e.g., infection, ischemia)
- New-onset diabetics account for 30% of cases
- Episodes of DKA account for nearly 25% of health care expenditure for type 1 diabetics

ETIOLOGY, EPIDEMIOLOGY, & RISK FACTORS

- DKA occurs when circulating insulin is inadequate or when there is an increased insulin demand (e.g., infection; ischemia; increased catecholamine state, such as illicit drug use or extreme stress)
  - In general, DKA requires the presence of insulin insufficiency, dehydration, and stress
  - The most common precipitating factor is infection (e.g., pneumonia, cellulitis, urinary tract infection)
  - Omission or undertreatment with insulin is a frequent precipitating factor
  - In rare cases of DKA in patients with type 2 diabetes, the cause is usually infection, ischemia, or medications (e.g., steroids, clozapine)
- Lack of insulin combined with increased secretion of counterregulatory hormones (catecholamines, glucagon, and growth hormone) causes lipolysis with generation of ketones
- Ketones are acidic; they deplete body stores of bicarbonate by a buffering mechanism, resulting in potentially severe metabolic acidosis
  - Increased lactate (especially in cases of ischemia) also contributes to the acidosis
- The hyperosmolar state leads to osmotic diuresis with subsequent severe dehydration
- Accounts for 1–2% of all primary diabetes-related hospital admissions and 50% of diabetes-related admissions in young patients

PATIENT PRESENTATION

- Early signs and symptoms include polyuria, polydipsia, nausea, vomiting, abdominal pain, weakness, and altered mental status
- In cases where there is an underlying infection, patients may present with fever, chills, cough, rales, myalgias, and/or dysuria
- Patients with underlying ischemia may complain of chest pain, dyspnea, diaphoresis, back pain, or cool extremities
- Rapid weight loss in new-onset diabetics
- Signs of volume depletion (e.g., tachycardia, orthostasis, dry mucous membranes)
- The characteristic sweet breath odor of acetone may be observed
- Shallow rapid breathing (Kussmaul respirations) as a compensatory mechanism of expiring CO_2 in response to the acidosis
- Altered mental status secondary to volume depletion and transient cerebral edema

DIFFERENTIAL DX

- Nonketotic hyperosmolar state
- Alcoholic ketoacidosis
- Lactic acidosis
- Acute pancreatitis
- Sepsis
- Uremia
- Ethylene glycol poisoning
- Methanol poisoning
- Salicylate poisoning
- Paraldehyde ingestion

DIAGNOSTIC EVALUATION

- Initial laboratory testing includes urinalysis, serum chemistries, acetone level, and arterial blood gas (ABG)
  - Urinalysis is usually positive for glucose and ketones; look for signs of urinary tract infection (e.g., pyuria, nitrates, leukocyte esterase)
  - Blood glucose is usually greater than 250 mg/dL
  - Anion gap is elevated (DKA represents the "D" in the "MUDPILES" mnemonic for anion gap metabolic acidosis)
  - Serum potassium is initially high or normal due to the extracellular shift of potassium in exchange for hydrogen ions; however, total body potassium level is invariably low
  - Serum ketones (most labs can only measure serum acetone) are elevated
  - Serum sodium may also be low secondary to hyperglycemia; there is a 1.6-mEq reduction in sodium for each 100-mg/dL increase in serum glucose
  - White blood cell count may be elevated due to infection, stress, or dehydration
- Cardiac enzymes are often indicated, especially in elderly diabetic patients
- Plasma and urine osmolality are elevated
- Urine and blood cultures and chest X-ray should also be obtained if infection is possible
- Electrocardiogram (EKG) is always indicated to evaluate for ischemia and electrolyte abnormalities (e.g., flattened T waves and U waves in hypokalemia)
- Head CT scan and/or lumbar puncture may be indicated if there are marked changes in mental status or if mental status does not resolve promptly with rehydration

TREATMENT & MANAGEMENT

- Most cases should be managed in a monitored hospital setting
- Ensure large-bore IV access, cardiac monitoring, and supplemental oxygen administration
- Patients typically have a fluid deficit of 100 mL/kg and sodium deficit of 7–10 mEq/kg
  - Administer normal saline at 1 L/h for the first hour, 500 mL/h for the next 4 hours, then 250 mL/h (usually give total of 4–8 L in 24 hours)
  - When serum glucose decreases to 250 mg/dL, change fluids to D5 in half-normal saline (D_5 1/2NS) at 100–200 mL/h, and carefully monitor glucose level
- Administer IV insulin as a 10- to 15-unit bolus, followed by an insulin drip
  - Always start IV fluids along with insulin to prevent circulatory collapse
  - Serum glucose should be decreased at a rate of about 50–75 mg/dL per hour
  - Convert to subcutaneous, short-acting insulin when the anion gap closes; overlap the insulin drip and the subcutaneous injection by 30 minutes
- Aggressive IV potassium repletion is essential because insulin therapy can cause profound hypokalemia due to intracellular shifts; once the potassium level falls below 5.5 mEq/L, add 20–40 mEq/L of potassium into the IV fluids (make sure the patient is urinating first)
- Serum chemistries should be checked every 2 hours to monitor electrolytes and ensure the anion gap is closing; fingersticks should be checked every hour while on insulin drip
- Bicarbonate repletion is rarely indicated; consider if pH <7.1, bicarbonate <5, severe hyperkalemia, and/or severe cardiac or respiratory dysfunction

PROGNOSIS & COMPLICATIONS

- Patients are often initially admitted to an intensive care setting for close monitoring
- Complications include cerebral edema (due to overly rapid correction of hyperglycemia), lactic acidosis (due to prolonged shock), hypoxemia, dehydration, cardiac arrhythmias (due to electrolyte disturbances), and pulmonary edema (due to aggressive fluid administration)
- Cerebral edema is the most serious complication; immediate imaging is indicated if abrupt mental status changes occur; mannitol is the mainstay of treatment
- Prognosis is very good for young patients who are closely monitored in an intensive care setting; prognosis worsens for those who are older, have serious infections, or are treated outside of a monitored setting
  - Coma, oliguria, and hypothermia are poor prognostic signs

Type 2 Diabetes Mellitus

INTRODUCTION

- A chronic metabolic disorder that results in hyperglycemia due to impaired insulin secretion, insulin resistance, and increased hepatic glucose production; glucose is toxic to nerve cells (resulting in neuropathy), blood vessels (resulting in heart disease, kidney disease, vascular disease, and hypertension), retinal cells (resulting in blindness), and other cell types
- Affects 10% of the adult population
- A major cause of death and disability; the costs of treating diabetes and its associated complications surpass $100 billion yearly
- Nearly two-thirds of diabetics die of coronary heart disease

ETIOLOGY, EPIDEMIOLOGY, & RISK FACTORS

- There are strong genetic and environmental factors in the development of diabetes
  - Likely, genetic factors are aggravated by poor diet, obesity, sedentary lifestyle, and aging
- It is unclear whether insulin resistance or insulin secretion initiates the cascade that leads to diabetes
  - Hepatic resistance to insulin and increased basal hepatic glucose production is excessive despite elevated insulin levels
- 16 million people have type 2 diabetes in the United States, and an additional 13 million have impaired glucose tolerance
  - There has been a dramatic increase throughout the world during the past 2 decades
  - Prevalence of diabetes has risen by 25–35% in the United States over the past 12–14 years
- Factors implicated in the epidemic include obesity, decreased physical activity, and changes in food consumption
- Diabetes occurs as part of a complex cardiometabolic syndrome that includes dyslipidemia, hypertension, obesity, microalbuminuria, and accelerated atherosclerosis

PATIENT PRESENTATION

- Typically goes undiagnosed for many years since hyperglycemia develops gradually and patients may be asymptomatic initially
- Classic symptoms are polyuria, polydipsia, polyphagia, recurrent blurred vision, paresthesias, and fatigue
- Frequent infections (urinary tract infections, osteomyelitis, cellulitis, otitis media, vaginitis)
- End-organ symptoms occur after long-term, poorly controlled disease:
  - Retinopathy: Blindness, cataracts
  - Nephropathy: Glomerulosclerosis, nephrotic syndrome, renal failure, secondary hypertension
  - Autonomic neuropathy: Orthostatic hypotension, gastroparesis, urinary retention, neurogenic bladder, impotence, arrhythmias
  - Peripheral neuropathy: Decreased sensation, Charcot joints

DIFFERENTIAL DX

- Impaired glucose tolerance
- Type 1 diabetes
- Polycystic ovarian syndrome
- Insulin resistance syndrome
- Gestational diabetes
- Pancreatic disease (pancreatitis, tumor, infection)
- Systemic disease resulting in pancreatic insufficiency (e.g., amyloidosis, hemochromatosis, cystic fibrosis, hormonal changes)

DIAGNOSTIC EVALUATION

- The American Dietetic Association criteria for diagnosis includes:
  - Symptoms of diabetes (e.g., polydipsia, polyuria, weight loss) plus a random blood glucose concentration >200 mg/dL *or*
  - Fasting blood glucose >126 mg/dL after an overnight fast *or*
  - 2-hour blood glucose >200 mg/dL during an oral (75 g) glucose tolerance test
- Fasting blood glucose test is generally considered the best diagnostic test
  - Blood glucose <110 mg/dL is normal
  - Blood glucose >126 mg/dL is considered diagnostic for diabetes
  - Blood glucose of 110–125 mg/dL is considered impaired fasting glucose (IFG); these patients may benefit from an oral glucose tolerance test, particularly in men with erectile dysfunction, women who have delivered infants greater than 9 pounds in birthweight, and women with recurrent vaginal yeast infections
- In the absence of unequivocal hyperglycemia, criteria should be reconfirmed by repeat testing on a different day; the ADA does not recommend using hemoglobin A1c levels for diagnosis
- Screen all patients over 45 every 3 years; screen earlier if risk factors are present
- Test for end-organ damage, as necessary (e.g., microalbuminuria, stress testing, ophthalmologic examinations)

TREATMENT & MANAGEMENT

- Optimal care includes achieving physiologic control of blood glucose with target hemoglobin A1c level less than 7%, preprandial glucose of 110 mg/dL or lower, and postprandial glucose of 140 mg/dL or lower
- Treatment should integrate dietary changes, exercise, weight loss techniques, smoking cessation, and medical therapy
- Insulin management and/or oral hypoglycemic medications (e.g., sulfonylureas, meglitinides, biguanides, thiazolidinediones, alpha-glucosidase inhibitors) to achieve normal or near-normal glucose and hemoglobin A1c levels
- Aggressive control of conventional and conditional risk factors, with quarterly or semiannual testing
  - Treat elevated cholesterol to a target of 70 mg/dL
  - Treat systolic blood pressure to a target of 120 mg/dL
  - Aspirin, statins, and ACE inhibitors have been shown to decrease the risk of future cardiovascular events
- Annual surveillance of diabetic complications includes dilated funduscopic examination by an ophthalmologist, extremity monofilament exam, screening for microalbuminuria, and complete physical examination
- Flu shots should be administered yearly, and pneumonia vaccinations should be administered every 5 years

PROGNOSIS & COMPLICATIONS

- Hyperosmolar nonketotic acidosis can occur with marked hyperglycemia, hyperosmolarity, and arterial pH >7.3
- Diabetic ketoacidosis is a state of uncontrolled catabolism with metabolic acidosis, hyperglycemia, and the presence of ketones in the blood and urine
- Hypoglycemia due to medication overdose is common
- Chronic microvascular complications include retinopathy, nephropathy, and neuropathy
- Chronic macrovascular complications include MI, stroke, and peripheral vascular disease
- Diabetic retinopathy and nephropathy are the leading causes of blindness and end-stage renal disease, respectively, in the United States
- Neuropathy, vascular disease, and infection predispose to foot injury and amputation

Hyperthyroidism & Thyroid Storm

INTRODUCTION

- Oversecretion of thyroid hormone can occur due to nodular hyperplasia of thyroid, damage to thyroid (e.g., De Quervain's thyroiditis, lymphocytic thyroiditis), or diffuse overproduction of thyroid hormone (e.g., Graves' disease, in which autoantibodies to the thyroid-stimulating hormone [TSH] receptor stimulate excessive thyroid hormone production)
- Graves' disease is the most common cause overall
- Primary hyperthyroidism occurs due to intrinsic dysfunction (overfunction) of the thyroid gland itself
- Secondary hyperthyroidism (TSH-dependent hyperthyroidism) is due to overstimulation of the thyroid gland by excess TSH production

ETIOLOGY, EPIDEMIOLOGY, & RISK FACTORS

- Thyroid-stimulating hormone (TSH) controls thyroid hormone production and release
  - The primary synthesized form of thyroid hormone is T4, which undergoes peripheral conversion to the more active T3
  - Both are bound to carrier proteins, although only the unbound form is biochemically active
- Thyroid hormone affects all organ systems and is responsible for increasing the metabolic rate, heart rate and contractility, and muscle and central nervous system excitability
- Hyperthyroidism: More common in females; most commonly occurs during ages 20–50
  - More than half of cases are due to Graves' disease
- Thyroid storm (thyrotoxicosis) is an acute exaggeration of the usual symptoms of hyperthyroidism involving many organ systems: Thermoregulatory (high fever), central nervous system (delirium, psychosis, stupor, coma), gastrointestinal (nausea, vomiting, abdominal pain, jaundice), cardiovascular (palpitations, tachycardia, CHF, atrial fibrillation)
- Thyroid storm is most commonly precipitated by infection; other precipitants include thyroid surgery, diabetic ketoacidosis, hyperosmolar coma, hypoglycemia, radioactive iodide treatment, pulmonary embolus, thyroid hormone overdose, large iodine load (e.g., amiodarone drip), withdrawal of antithyroid medications, use of iodinated contrast medium, stroke, stress, and toxemia of pregnancy

PATIENT PRESENTATION

- General symptoms include diaphoresis, weight loss, heat intolerance, and fever
- Cardiovascular: Palpitations, tachycardia, wide pulse pressure, PVCs, atrial fibrillation, heart block, CHF, circulatory collapse
  - Hyperthyroidism must be considered in any patient with new-onset atrial fibrillation
- CNS: Restlessness, anxiety, poor concentration, fatigue, agitation, tremor, mania, psychosis, coma
- Gastrointestinal: Diarrhea, nausea, vomiting, abdominal pain
- Pulmonary: Dyspnea
- Muscle weakness
- Exophthalmos (in Graves' disease)
- Goiter may be present
- Oligomenorrhea or amenorrhea occur in women
- Thyroid storm results in exaggerated symptoms of above, plus delirium, seizures, hypertension, and lethargy

DIFFERENTIAL DX

Hyperthyroidism
- Anxiety or mania
- Perimenopause
- Addison's disease
- Anemia
- Congestive heart failure
- Diabetes mellitus
- Anticholinergic toxicity
- Sympathomimetics
- Withdrawal syndromes

Thyroid storm
- Infection
- Sepsis
- Cocaine use
- Psychosis
- Pheochromocytoma
- Neuroleptic malignant syndrome
- Hyperthermia (e.g., heat stroke)

DIAGNOSTIC EVALUATION

- Screen for hyperthyroidism with TSH levels; if abnormal, measure free T4 and T3 levels
  - Overt hyperthyroidism results in decreased TSH and increased free T4 and T3
  - T3 toxicosis: Decreased TSH, increased T3, normal free T4
  - T4 toxicosis: Decreased TSH, increased free T4, normal T3
  - Subclinical hyperthyroidism: Decreased TSH, normal free T4 and T3
- Once a diagnosis of hyperthyroidism is established, determine the underlying etiology
  - Thyroid ultrasound to identify nodules
  - 24-hour thyroid radioiodine uptake scan: High uptake suggests Graves' disease, toxic adenoma, toxic multinodular goiter, iodine-induced disease, or TSH-secreting adenoma; low uptake suggests thyroiditis, amiodarone toxicity (can occur with overdose or therapeutic dose), radiation-induced disease, drug-induced disease, exogenous thyroid hormone ingestion, struma ovarii, or metastatic follicular thyroid cancer
  - If free T4 or T3 levels are elevated, but TSH is normal or high, consider a pituitary MRI to rule out a TSH-secreting adenoma
  - Many cases are observed without further workup
- Thyroid storm is a clinical diagnosis; most patients have pre-existing hyperthyroidism
  - Consider cultures, urinalysis, and chest X-ray to rule out infection
- Electrocardiogram (EKG) to rule out myocardial infarction or arrhythmia

TREATMENT & MANAGEMENT

- Hyperthyroidism due to Grave's disease or thyroid adenoma may require thyroid ablation therapy with radioactive iodine, antithyroid drugs (e.g., methimazole, propothiouricil), or thyroidectomy
- Thyroid storm is treated with supportive therapy, in addition to thyroid-specific treatment
  - Acetaminophen is the antipyretic of choice; aspirin can interfere with protein binding
  - Short-acting beta-blockers (e.g., propranolol) to control adrenergic symptoms
  - Thioamides (e.g., methimazole, propylthiouracil) are used to block de novo thyroid hormone synthesis (propylthiouracil also blocks peripheral conversion of T4 to T3); methimazole is preferred because it has a longer duration of action
  - Iodine-containing solutions (e.g., Lugol's solution, potassium iodide, sodium iodide) are used to block the release of T4 and T3 from the thyroid gland; these should be administered at least 1 hour after thioamides so that they are not used as a substrate for de novo hormone synthesis
  - Glucocorticoids may help reduce conversion of T4 to T3, and may directly treat the primary process if thyroid storm is due to Graves' disease
  - Lithium can block release of thyroid hormone but may cause renal and neurologic toxicity
  - Dialysis and plasmapheresis are last resorts if there is no response to other treatments
  - Radioactive iodine ablation therapy or surgery may be necessary for definitive cure

PROGNOSIS & COMPLICATIONS

- Admit patients with hyperthyroidism if they have serious complaints (e.g., chest pain) or risk factors (e.g., history of coronary artery disease)
- Nearly 30% of cases of Graves' disease go into remission within 2 years; therefore, medical management is preferred to surgery
- Thyroid storm is fatal in nearly all untreated patients and even in about 10% of patients who receive appropriate treatment; all patients diagnosed with thyroid storm require intensive care unit admission
  - Complete recovery can take up to 1 week, depending on how long it takes to deplete the excessive circulating levels of thyroid hormones
- Hypoparathyroidism and hypothyroidism can be complications of surgery

Hypothyroidism & Myxedema Coma

INTRODUCTION

- Hypothyroidism is an underdiagnosed condition that is especially common in aging populations
- The clinical signs and symptoms are nonspecific, so screening with thyroid-stimulating hormone (TSH) levels is important in anyone suspected of having decreased thyroid function
- The thyroid hormones (T4 and T3) are important for many metabolic functions, including bone development, cardiac chronotropic activity, muscle development, and menstruation
- Myxedema refers to swelling of the skin and soft tissues
- Myxedema coma is a severe, life-threatening decompensation of a hypothyroid patient with mental status changes, hypotension, hypothermia, and myxedematous facies

ETIOLOGY, EPIDEMIOLOGY, & RISK FACTORS

- Primary hypothyroidism occurs due to intrinsic thyroid gland dysfunction and accounts for 95% of all cases of hypothyroidism
  - Etiologies include chronic autoimmune thyroiditis (Hashimoto's disease), inadequate iodine intake, radiation exposure to the neck, post thyroidectomy, post radioactive iodine ablation of the thyroid, "downswing" phase of thyroiditis, infiltrative disease (e.g., sarcoidosis, amyloidosis, leukemia), and medications (e.g., lithium, amiodarone)
  - Inadequate iodine intake is rare in developed countries
- Secondary hypothyroidism occurs due to inadequate stimulation of the thyroid gland by the pituitary gland or hypothalamus
- Myxedema coma is most common (nearly 90% of cases) in elderly women during the winter months
  - Mortality rate can approach 30–60% depending on comorbid illnesses
  - Advanced age, bradycardia, and persistent hypotension portend a worse prognosis
  - Precipitants of myxedema coma include sepsis or infection, myocardial infarction, stroke, hypothermia, surgery, trauma, burns, hypoglycemia, hyponatremia, hemorrhage, medications (e.g., beta-blockers, sedatives, narcotics, phenothiazine, amiodarone), and noncompliance with thyroid medications

PATIENT PRESENTATION

- The presentation of hypothyroidism is varied and can affect nearly any organ system
- Fatigue, lethargy, muscle weakness, weight gain, cold intolerance, and hoarseness are most common
- Neurologic: Depression, poor memory, confusion, delayed relaxation of deep tendon reflexes, ataxia
- Cardiac: Bradycardia, distant heart sounds, pericardial effusion
- Gastrointestinal: Constipation, ileus
- Dermatologic: Dry skin, facial swelling, ptosis, macroglossia, periorbital edema, hair loss
- Nonpitting lower extremity edema
- Myxedema coma can present with bradycardia, hypotension, hypothermia (temperature is usually lower than 35.5°C), hypoventilation, and severely altered mental status, which may result in coma

DIFFERENTIAL DX

- Sepsis
- Depression
- Adrenal crisis
- Congestive heart failure
- Hypoglycemia
- Stroke
- Hypothermia
- Drug effect or drug overdose
- Meningitis
- Anemia
- Obesity

DIAGNOSTIC EVALUATION

- Primary hypothyroidism is demonstrated by elevated thyroid-stimulating hormone (TSH) and decreased free T4 (elevated TSH and normal T4 may suggest subclinical hypothyroidism)
  - Secondary hypothyroidism also presents with decreased T4 but with normal or low TSH, which reflects decreased ability of the pituitary gland or hypothalamus to stimulate production of thyroid hormone
  - Hyperlipidemia and hyponatremia may occur
  - In cases of Hashimoto's disease, serum thyroperoxidase antibodies may be detectable
- Thyroid ultrasound may be indicated to assess for nodules
- Fine-needle aspiration biopsy may be indicated to rule out malignancy
- Myxedema coma presents with significantly elevated TSH, decreased free and total T4 and T3, and increased T3 uptake
  - Complete blood count may reveal leukopenia and normochromic, normocytic anemia; some patients also have pernicious anemia with high mean corpuscular volume (MCV)
  - Electrolytes may reveal hyponatremia, hypoglycemia, and increased creatine kinase
  - Serum cortisol is often decreased due to hypothyroid-induced adrenal suppression
  - Arterial blood gas may reveal respiratory acidosis due to intercostal muscle weakness
  - Further testing to evaluate the precipitating cause includes blood and urine cultures to rule out infection; head CT scan and lumbar puncture to rule out hemorrhage, stroke, and infection; cardiac enzymes to rule out myocardial infarction; and renal and liver function tests

TREATMENT & MANAGEMENT

- Hypothyroidism should be treated with oral T4 supplementation (100 µg)
  - It may take weeks for the medication to take effect
  - Begin with a lower dose in the elderly and patients with coronary artery disease (25–50 µg)
  - Pregnant patients may require higher doses
  - Adjust the dose of T4 by monitoring clinical improvement, TSH levels, and T4 levels
  - Monitor patients for signs and symptoms of overtreatment, including tachycardia, palpitations, nervousness, tiredness, headache, excitability, sleeplessness, tremors, or angina
- Myxedema coma must be treated emergently
  - Initiate IV fluids to correct blood pressure and hypoglycemia, supplemental oxygen, and cardiac monitoring for arrhythmias
  - IV thyroid hormone must be administered immediately; T4 (levothyroxine) has better cardiac safety than T3, which may cause arrhythmias or myocardial infarction in large doses
  - Administer IV hydrocortisone prior to thyroid hormone to treat adrenal insufficiency, which may occur along with hypothyroidism
  - Treat hypothermia by passive rewarming (e.g., warming blankets, warm IV fluids); active rewarming (e.g., body cavity irrigation with warm fluid) may cause hypotension due to reversal of cold-induced vasospasm
  - Consider empiric antibiotics because infection is a common precipitating cause
  - Intubation may be required

PROGNOSIS & COMPLICATIONS

- Thyroid hormone replacement can precipitate adrenal crises; always consider and exclude adrenal insufficiency in the absence of an elevated TSH level
- Aggressive replacement of thyroid hormone may compromise cardiac function in patients with existing cardiac disease
- Undertreatment leads to disease progression with gradual worsening of symptoms; however, excessive doses of thyroid hormone may lead to subtle but important side effects (e.g., bone demineralization)
- Myxedema coma has up to 80% mortality; patients with myxedema coma and those who require intravenous thyroid replacement therapy should be admitted to the intensive care unit

Hyperparathyroidism

INTRODUCTION

- Hyperparathyroidism is characterized by excess or inappropriate secretion of parathyroid hormone (PTH)
- PTH is responsible for regulation of calcium and phosphate homeostasis
- PTH increases blood calcium by 3 mechanisms: Increased calcium reabsorption in the kidneys; increased production of vitamin D, which leads to increased intestinal absorption of calcium; and increased calcium release from bone resorption
- Untreated hyperparathyroidism can lead to nephrolithiasis, chronic renal insufficiency, and osteopenia

ETIOLOGY, EPIDEMIOLOGY, & RISK FACTORS

- PTH mediates calcium homeostasis
  - Serum ionized calcium level must be maintained in a narrow range for proper functioning of the many intracellular and extracellular processes mediated by calcium ions
- PTH is secreted in response to a drop in serum calcium level
  - Within minutes, serum PTH levels increase
  - The most immediate action of the increased PTH occurs in bone, where calcium and phosphate are released from skeletal stores
  - Within minutes, the distal tubular reabsorption of calcium is increased
  - Increased intestinal absorption of calcium mediated by vitamin D occurs within days
- Primary hyperparathyroidism is caused by parathyroid adenoma (90% of cases), parathyroid hyperplasia, or parathyroid carcinoma (2%)
  - Most cases occur in women older than 45
  - Prior head and neck irradiation is a strong risk factor
- Secondary hyperparathyroidism is caused by overstimulation of the parathyroid glands due to chronically decreased serum calcium, usually secondary to chronic renal failure
  - In contrast to cases of primary hyperparathyroidism, the parathyroid glands are normal
- Hyperparathyroidism may occur as part of multiple endocrine neoplasia (MEN) syndrome

PATIENT PRESENTATION

- Most cases are relatively asymptomatic; fatigue and other nonspecific symptoms may be present
- "*Stones, bones, abdominal groans, and psychic overtones*" is the classic presentation of hypercalcemia; however, these are not common in clinical practice
  - Stones: Nephrolithiasis
  - Bones (osteitis fibrosa cystica): Bone pain, fractures, osteoporosis
  - Groans: Abdominal pain, nausea, vomiting, constipation, anorexia, peptic ulcers, pancreatitis
  - Psychic: Psychosis, depression, fatigue, anxiety
- Rarely, patients present in a parathyroid crisis characterized by altered consciousness, osteopenia, nephrolithiasis, and gastrointestinal complaints
  - Usually precipitated by concurrent illness and decreased fluid intake or increased fluid losses, which leads to hemoconcentration and an acute rise in the serum calcium level

DIFFERENTIAL DX

- Other causes of hypercalcemia
- Pseudohyperparathyroidism due to ectopic PTH released by squamous cell lung carcinoma
- Hyperthyroidism
- Malignancies
- Bony metastases
- Immobilization (e.g., Paget's disease)
- Sarcoidosis
- Granulomatous disease (e.g., tuberculosis)
- Excess vitamins A or D
- Milk-alkali syndrome
- Familial hypocalciuric hypercalcemia
- Drugs (e.g., lithium, thiazides, isotretinoin, tamoxifen, calcium-containing antacids)

DIAGNOSTIC EVALUATION

- History and physical examination
  - Some patients are discovered to have hyperparathyroidism during evaluation for osteopenia, osteoporosis, or nephrolithiasis
- Serum calcium level greater than 10.5 mg/dL in combination with an elevated PTH level is diagnostic of primary hyperparathyroidism
  - In the setting a concomitant vitamin D deficiency, calcium level may be normal
  - In the setting of hypercalcemia, PTH levels should be suppressed; thus, a normal PTH level in a patient with hypercalcemia represents an inappropriate elevation
- Urinary calcium excretion can be assessed by 24-hour urine collection
  - About half of patients with primary hypercalcemia will have hypercalciuria
  - If urine calcium is greater than 400 mg, early surgical intervention should be considered due to the increased risk of stones
  - Low urine calcium suggests familial hypocalciuric hypocalcemia
- Vitamin D levels may be elevated in primary hyperparathyroidism due to PTH-induced conversion of calcidiol to calcitriol; however, the finding of increased calcitriol is not diagnostic because it may just be a result of vitamin D intoxication
- Ultrasound or CT scan of the parathyroids may be indicated

TREATMENT & MANAGEMENT

- Severe hypercalcemia (calcium >13 mg/dL, or symptoms) requires immediate intervention
  - IV rehydration with large volumes of normal saline followed by loop diuretics once the patient is adequately resuscitated to augment renal calcium excretion
  - Bisphosphonates can also be used
- Parathyroidectomy is the treatment of choice; it is highly effective and has low morbidity
  - A 2002 National Institutes of Health workshop recommended surgery for the following patients: Serum calcium >1 mg/dL above the upper limits of normal, hypercalciuria of >400 mg/d, creatinine clearance that is 30% or more lower than age-matched controls, T-score of less than −2.5, younger patients (under age 50), and patients who may be lost to follow-up
- If surgery is not an option, medical management includes avoidance of drugs (e.g., lithium, thiazide diuretics) that can worsen hypercalcemia, physical activity to minimize bone resorption, adequate hydration to prevent stone formation, and moderate calcium and vitamin D intake to prevent further stimulation of PTH
- Bisphosphonates should be given to patients with osteopenia or osteoporosis
  - Monitor serum calcium twice yearly and serum creatinine and bone density annually

PROGNOSIS & COMPLICATIONS

- Untreated, primary hyperparathyroidism can lead to osteopenia or, in severe cases, osteitis fibrosis cystica (bone marrow fibrosis and expansion of the osteoid surfaces)
- The osteopenia seen in hyperparathyroidism is a result of demineralization; it is largely reversible after parathyroidectomy and is also treatable with bisphosphonates
- Surgical parathyroidectomy is curative and has a low complication rate
  - It may be complicated by transient hypocalcemia or prolonged "hungry bone" syndrome (abrupt decrease in PTH leads to a marked mismatch of bone formation and bone resorption, resulting in systemic hypocalcemia, hypophosphatemia, and hypomagnesemia due to unchecked bone formation; treated with supplemental calcium and vitamin D)

Osteoporosis

INTRODUCTION

- Osteoporosis is characterized by decreased bone density and microarchitectural deterioration of bone tissue (i.e., poor bone quality)
- Lower peak bone mass and accelerated bone loss after menopause leads to increased risks of osteoporosis in women compared to men
- An estimated 1.3 million osteoporotic fractures occur annually in the United States that are associated with significant mortality, morbidity, and economic burden
- Annual costs associated with osteoporotic fractures exceed $17 billion

ETIOLOGY, EPIDEMIOLOGY, & RISK FACTORS

- The World Health Organization definition is based on bone mineral density (the T-score is the number of standard deviations below or above the mean bone density for healthy, young, female adults)
  - Normal: T-score greater than -1.0
  - Low bone mass (osteopenia): T-score less then -1.0 but greater than -2.5
  - Osteoporosis: T-score of -2.5 or less
  - Severe (established) osteoporosis: T-score of -2.5 or less in the presence of one or more fragility fractures
- Half of all postmenopausal women will experience an osteoporosis-related fracture
- Nonmodifiable risk factors include age, female sex, Caucasian or Asian race, small body frame, family history, surgical menopause, history of hyperthyroidism or parathyroidism, and hypogonadism
- Modifiable risk factors include smoking, alcohol abuse, calcium or vitamin D deficiency, lifetime of inactivity, recurrent falls, medications (e.g., anticonvulsants, steroids, chemotherapy, lithium), and possibly high caffeine intake
- Prevalence of osteoporosis in the United States: 13–18% of women over 50; 3–6% of men

PATIENT PRESENTATION

- Usually asymptomatic, initial presentation may be a vertebral, wrist, or hip fracture
- Loss of height of more than 1 inch should increase suspicion for osteoporosis
- Thoracic kyphotic posturing is often seen and may indicate multiple vertebral fractures
- Back pain may indicate vertebral compression fractures

DIFFERENTIAL DX

- Osteopenia
- Osteomalacia
- Malignancy
- Multiple myeloma
- Paget's disease
- Renal dystrophy
- Hyperparathyroidism
- Ischemic bone disease

DIAGNOSTIC EVALUATION

- Decreased bone mass is the most important predictor of fracture risk
  - The National Osteoporosis Foundation recommends bone mineral density testing in all women over age 65, in women less than 65 with one or more risk factors (excluding race, gender, and postmenopausal state), and in any postmenopausal woman who presents with fracture
- Hip and spine dual-energy X-ray absorptiometry (DEXA) scan is the preferred test for bone mineral density
- Optional lab tests in healthy women to rule out secondary causes of osteoporosis may include 24-hour urinary calcium measurement; serum calcium, parathyroid hormone, and 25-hydroxyvitamin D measurements; TSH for patients on thyroid replacement medication; or urinary N-telopeptide (a marker of bone resorption)

TREATMENT & MANAGEMENT

- Adequate dietary calcium supplementation (1000–1200 mg/d) and vitamin D supplementation (400–1000 U/d) are required in all patients
- Adequate physical activity is essential, especially weight-bearing activity; physical activity helps to directly increase bone density, strengthen muscles, improve balance, and prevent falls
- Avoid tobacco and limit alcohol use
- Available pharmacologic agents include bisphosphonates (e.g., alendronate, risedronate), raloxifene, estrogen, calcitonin, and parathyroid hormone
  - Estrogen supplementation should be used cautiously because it may be associated with increased risks of cancer, heart attack, stroke, and venous thromboembolism
  - Parathyroid hormone supplementation is the only treatment that stimulates bone formation; however, safety and efficacy has not been demonstrated beyond 2 years
  - Bisphosphonates appear to reduce the incidence of vertebral and nonvertebral fractures by 30–50%
  - Calcitonin reduces risk of vertebral fractures by up to 20%
  - Raloxifene reduces risk of vertebral fractures by 40%

PROGNOSIS & COMPLICATIONS

- Low bone mass is the most important risk factor for predicting first fracture
- Relative risk for fracture roughly doubles for each standard deviation decrease in bone mineral density
- Osteoporosis-related hip fractures are associated with a 20% excess mortality in the year following the fracture
- Treatment of osteoporosis with bisphosphonates results in a 30–50% reduction in risk for fractures, depending on site and prior fracture history

Cushing's Syndrome

INTRODUCTION

- A syndrome of hyperfunctioning of the adrenal cortex, resulting in hypersecretion of cortisol
- May also be caused by ingestion of cortisol-like drugs (e.g., steroids); indeed, the most common cause of Cushing's syndrome is exogenous use of steroids for weeks to months
- Cushing's syndrome is suggested by the characteristic symptoms and signs; however, none are pathognomonic
- *Cushing's disease* is hypercortisolism due to a pituitary tumor

ETIOLOGY, EPIDEMIOLOGY, & RISK FACTORS

- Cortisol acts as an insulin antagonist, causing increased blood glucose, protein catabolism, and lipolysis; it also has mild aldosterone-like effects, causing sodium retention and water diuresis
- Estimated to affect 10–15 million people yearly
- 80% of cases are categorized as ACTH dependent (e.g., Cushing's disease, ACTH-releasing pituitary tumor, ectopic ACTH production [such as small-cell lung carcinoma], ectopic CRH production)
- The remaining cases are ACTH independent (e.g., adrenal adenoma, adrenal carcinoma, macronodular hyperplasia, micronodular hyperplasia)

PATIENT PRESENTATION

- Moon face
- "Buffalo hump" (increased adipose tissue in the neck and trunk)
- Central obesity
- Purple abdominal striae
- Diabetes
- Muscle weakness and fatigue
- Easy bruising, thin skin
- Hirsutism
- Oligomenorrhea or amenorrhea
- Hyperpigmentation
- Irritability, anxiety, or depression may occur
- Hyperglycemia
- Hypertension
- Osteoporosis

DIFFERENTIAL DX

- Obesity
- Diabetes mellitus
- Hypertension
- Hypercortisolism due to alcohol use
- Pituitary tumors
- Adrenal tumors
- Multiple endocrine neoplasia type I
- Familial Cushing's syndrome
- Lung cancer
- Pseudo-Cushing's (chronic alcoholism, depression, and obesity can mask as Cushing's syndrome)

DIAGNOSTIC EVALUATION

- 24-hour urinary cortisol level
  - Levels greater than 300 μg/d suggest Cushing's syndrome
- Levels of 90–300 μg/d should prompt dexamethasone suppression testing (below)
- Laboratory testing may include morning and evening plasma cortisol levels, plasma ACTH levels, complete blood counts, and chemistries
- Dexamethasone suppression tests: Dexamethasone will suppress adrenal release of cortisol in normal patients but not Cushing's patients
  - Overnight suppression test should be the initial test: 1 mg at midnight should decrease AM cortisol to less than 5 μg/dL
  - Lose-dose suppression test should be done if overnight test yields cortisol greater than 5 (μg/dL: Administer 0.5 mg every 6 hours for 2 days; elevated blood or urine cortisol confirms the diagnosis of Cushing's syndrome
  - High-dose suppression test may be used to establish the etiology of Cushing's syndrome: Administer 2 mg every 6 hours for 2–3 days; cortisol suppression occurs in Cushing's disease (pituitary tumor) but not in other forms of Cushing's syndrome
- Cortisol-releasing hormone (CRH) stimulation test can be used to distinguish pituitary adenoma (increase in ACTH and cortisol) from ectopic ACTH production (increase rarely seen) or cortisol-secreting adrenal tumors (increase not seen)
- Further assessment for malignancies may include chest X-ray; CT scans of the adrenals, head, and chest; or pituitary MRI

TREATMENT & MANAGEMENT

- In cases of steroid overuse, begin tapering of steroids as rapidly as possible
  - A stress dose of steroids may be necessary in acutely ill patients to prevent Addisonian crisis
- Diet should be high in protein; potassium, calcium, vitamin D, and estrogen supplementation may be indicated
- Resection of tumors, as necessary
- Ketoconazole, mitotane, or metapyrone may be indicated; these drugs inhibit adrenal steroidogenesis
- Monitor and treat blood pressure and glucose as necessary

PROGNOSIS & COMPLICATIONS

- Complications include osteoporosis, immunosuppression, diabetes, hirsutism, metastases of malignant tumors, and uncontrolled hypertension

Obesity

INTRODUCTION

- Obesity is defined as having a body mass index (BMI) greater than 30
- Morbid obesity is defined as having a BMI greater than 40
- Over 20% of Americans are obese, and the number is steadily rising
- Obesity-related deaths jumped 33% between 1990 and 2000; they currently stand at approximately 400,000 per year and may become the #1 cause of preventable death in the United States
- 80% of obese adolescents become obese adults

ETIOLOGY, EPIDEMIOLOGY, & RISK FACTORS

- Most obesity is due to consuming more calories than are used over a long period of time
- Portion sizes have doubled over the last 20 years, and physical activity, in general, has decreased secondary to many factors (e.g., safety concerns, neighborhood design, home videos, longer work hours)
- Some believe that current obesity has been caused by a 150 calorie/day average increase in consumption
- There is likely some genetic component, as well as environmental triggers
- Research is ongoing for obesity genes; several markers have been identified
- Family influence on eating habits and exercising are critical, especially in those that were obese during adolescence
- There are several disease states that have obesity as a component (e.g., polycystic ovary syndrome, Prader-Willi, growth hormone deficiency)
- Depression causes many to overeat and become less active

PATIENT PRESENTATION

- Many have acanthosis nigricans (skin with deepened creases and increased pigment seen around the neck and in armpits; may also be seen in other skin folds) as a sign of insulin resistance
- Can present with decreased exercise tolerance, elevated blood pressures, dyslipidemia, insulin resistance, dysthymia or depression, gallstones, arthritis of the knees, or obstructive sleep apnea
- Some can present with binge eating disorders
- Many bulimics are overweight

DIFFERENTIAL DX

- Cushing's disease
- Turner's syndrome
- Hypothyroidism
- Drug-induced (e.g., antipsychotics, antidepressants, antiepileptics, steroids, sulfonylureas, serotonin antagonists, Megace)
- Polycystic ovarian syndrome
- Pseudohypoparathyroidism
- Smoking cessation
- Hypothalamic dysfunction
- Congenital diseases (e.g., Prader-Willi, Laurence-Moon-Biedl, Alstrom-Hallgren, Cohen syndrome, Carpenter syndrome, leptin receptor deficiency)
- Eating disorders

DIAGNOSTIC EVALUATION

- Complete history and physical examination, including special attention to medications, alternative medications, diet history, risk factors for cardiovascular disease, and family history of thyroid and cardiac disease, cancers, and asthma
  - Body mass index (BMI) = [weight (kg) / height (m) / height (m)]
- Psychiatric history important to uncover eating disorders, depression, and history of abuse; many people use food as a medicine
- Laboratory studies may include fasting chemistries to assess glucose and renal function, lipid panel, liver enzymes (screen for hepatic steatosis), fasting insulin level (especially if acanthosis nigricans is present), TSH and free T4, and complete blood count
- Sleep study may be indicated to evaluate for sleep apnea

TREATMENT & MANAGEMENT

- Diet, exercise, and lifestyle modification are the hallmarks of therapy
  - Portion control and caloric density of foods and drinks are important considerations
  - Few weight loss programs have yielded positive long-term results; Weight Watchers has been shown to be helpful
- Bariatric surgery has the best long-term success but is reserved for the morbidly obese (BMI >40) or those with a BMI >35 with risk factors
  - In the United States, the most common procedure is gastric bypass, which results in better weight loss than gastric banding
- Look for and treat cardiometabolic syndrome aggressively
- Cardiac assessment is important; treat hyperlipidemia, hypertension, and diabetes aggressively
- Smoking cessation
- Metformin in cases of PCOS and other hyperinsulinemic states
- Treat sleep apnea as necessary
- Psychiatric referral may be helpful based on history

PROGNOSIS & COMPLICATIONS

- There are many complications related to obesity, including pseudotumor cerebri, increased dementia risk, hypertension, dyslipidemia, disordered breathing, insulin resistance and diabetes mellitus, oligospermia, increased cancer risk (breast, colon, gallbladder, esophagus, cervix, ovary, pancreas, liver, lymphoma), knee osteoarthritis, cholelithiasis, and hepatic steatosis
- Bariatric surgery overall has 1–2% mortality directly related to the procedure and an overall complication rate as high as 30%
- Overall lifespan may be reduced because of obesity-related complications

Gynecology

Abnormal Uterine Bleeding

INTRODUCTION

- Defined as any irregular bleeding during the menstrual cycle
- Varies from complete absence of menses to life-threatening hemorrhage
- Abnormal bleeding patterns include amenorrhea (complete absence of menses), menorrhagia (menses lasting longer than 7 days or bleeding greater than 80 mL), metrorrhagia (irregular but frequent bleeding), menometrorrhagia (prolonged, irregular, and heavy bleeding), polymenorrhea (regular menses with frequency less than 21 days), hypomenorrhea (unusually light menses), and oligomenorrhea (menses frequency of more than 35–40 days)
- Most cases occur in the extremes of reproductive lifespan (menarche and perimenopause) and are usually attributed to dysfunctional uterine bleeding (DUB)

ETIOLOGY, EPIDEMIOLOGY, & RISK FACTORS

- The normal menstrual period lasts 2–7 days, with an average blood loss of 35–150 mL; the interval between menstrual cycles usually lasts 24–35 days
- The menstrual cycle can be divided into two phases: proliferative and secretory
  - During the proliferative phase (prior to ovulation), there is predominance of estrogen
  - During the secretory phase (just after ovulation), estrogen and progesterone are present
- The causes of abnormal uterine bleeding (AUB) can be grouped as idiopathic (dysfunctional uterine bleeding), endocrinopathies, structural lesions, malignant lesions, coagulopathies, pregnancy-related bleeding, and infectious
  - Menorrhagia, metrorrhagia, and polymenorrhea are associated with chronic anovulation, endometrial or cervical cancer, fibroids, endometrial hyperplasia, endometrial polyps, bleeding disorders, and complications of pregnancy
  - Hypomenorrhea is associated with hypogonadotropic hypogonadism (anorexics and athletes), atrophic endometrium, Asherman's syndrome, oral contraceptive pills, hormone replacement therapy, intrauterine adhesions, intrauterine trauma, and outlet obstructions (cervical stenosis or congenital abnormalities)
  - Oligomenorrhea is associated with pregnancy and disruptions of the pituitary-gonadal axis
- Abnormal uterine bleeding accounts for one-third of outpatient gynecologic consultations

PATIENT PRESENTATION

- Amenorrhea (complete absence of menses)
- Menorrhagia (menses lasting longer than 7 days or bleeding greater than 80 mL)
- Metrorrhagia (irregular but frequent bleeding)
- Menometrorrhagia (prolonged, irregular, and heavy bleeding)
- Polymenorrhea (regular menses with frequency less than 21 days)
- Hypomenorrhea (unusually light menses)
- Oligomenorrhea (menses frequency of more than 35–40 days)
- In premenopausal women, pregnancy and malignancy should be considered
- Postmenopausal bleeding is usually associated with vaginal mucosa atrophy, but endometrial carcinoma must be considered

DIFFERENTIAL DX

- Anovulation
- Atrophic endometrium
- Pregnancy
- Premalignant lesions or malignancies (e.g., endometrial carcinoma or hyperplasia, cervical or vaginal cancer)
- Benign lesions (e.g., polyps, ovarian cysts, leiomyomata)
- Cervicitis
- Vaginitis
- Endometritis
- Trauma or foreign object
- Medical disease (e.g., liver, kidney, thyroid)
- Drugs (e.g., oral contraceptives, estrogen replacement therapy, anticoagulants)

DIAGNOSTIC EVALUATION

- Initial evaluation includes history and physical examination, pregnancy testing (serum beta-human chorionic gonadotropin), hormonal tests, and Pap smear
  - History should evaluate timing and quantity of bleeding, menstrual history (e.g., menarche, recent periods, associated symptoms), and family history of bleeding disorders
  - Physical exam should rule out vaginal and cervical causes of bleeding and evaluate for uterine and adnexal masses
  - Hormonal tests include prolactin, TSH, LH, and FSH
  - Pap smear to screen for cervical cancer
  - Consider CBC, PT, PTT, bleeding time to assess for coagulopathy
- Further testing may be indicated based on clinical findings
  - Pelvic ultrasound to assess for polyps or fibroids
  - Hysterosalpingogram to assess for intrauterine defects
  - Sonohystogram to assess for polyps or submucosal fibroids
  - Endometrial biopsy (especially in women older than 35) to screen for endometrial hyperplasia and cancer; if unable to obtain an endometrial biopsy, a hysteroscopy may be used to directly visualize the intrauterine cavity

TREATMENT & MANAGEMENT

- Women with uncontrollable bleeding may require hospitalization, high-dose intravenous or oral estrogen, and volume resuscitation
  - A 30-mL balloon Foley catheter can tamponade bleeding temporarily
- Medical treatment is effective in most cases
  - Oral contraceptive pills are often an effective first-line treatment for anovulatory bleeding, menorrhagia, metrorrhagia, and polymenorrhea
  - Progestin therapy can be used to treat anovulatory bleeding if estrogen is contraindicated (e.g., patients with endometrial hyperplasia)
  - Provera therapy for 10 days to treat menorrhagia
- Hysteroscopy may be used to remove fibroids and polyps
  - If hysteroscopy fails, endometrial ablation and resection of fibroids and polyps by laser, electrocautery, or heated roller may be necessary
- Dilatation and curettage may be diagnostic and therapeutic for dysfunctional bleeding
- Hysterectomy is the definitive treatment for cases refractory to all other treatments

PROGNOSIS & COMPLICATIONS

- Adolescents have an excellent prognosis; most outgrow the problem within 3–5 years of menarche
- Patients on oral contraceptives rarely have recurrent episodes
- For patients with abnormal bleeding related to systemic disease, prognosis depends on the underlying illness (e.g., thyroid disorders have an excellent prognosis with correction of the underlying cause and/or hormone therapy, successful therapy of PCOS is related to the amount of weight loss achieved)
- Anemia is the most common complication
- Most women do not require surgical treatment
- In perimenopausal women, endometrial carcinoma or hyperplasia must be investigated

Amenorrhea

INTRODUCTION

- Complete absence of menstrual bleeding
- Amenorrhea is a normal feature in prepubertal, pregnant, and postmenopausal females
- Primary amenorrhea is defined as lack of menses by age 14 without secondary sexual characteristics or lack of menses by age 16 with or without secondary sexual characteristics
- Secondary amenorrhea is defined as the eventual cessation of menses for 6 consecutive months or 3 cycles in a previously menstruating woman

ETIOLOGY, EPIDEMIOLOGY, & RISK FACTORS

- Amenorrhea can be a result of disorders at the level of the anterior pituitary, hypothalamus, ovary, or outflow tract (uterus or vagina)
- The most common and nonpathologic cause of amenorrhea is pregnancy
- Etiologies of primary amenorrhea include congenital abnormalities (e.g., imperforate hymen, uterine or vaginal agenesis), hormonal aberrations (e.g., androgen insensitivity, Savage's syndrome), chromosomal abnormalities (e.g., Turner's syndrome, Swyer's syndrome), and hypothalamic-pituitary disorders (e.g., Kallmann's syndrome, trauma)
- Etiologies of secondary amenorrhea include pregnancy, anatomic abnormalities (e.g., Asherman's syndrome, cervical stenosis), ovarian dysfunction or premature ovarian failure, prolactinomas and hyperprolactinemia, and central nervous system or hypothalamic disorders (e.g., anorexia nervosa, excessive exercise, Sheehan's syndrome)

PATIENT PRESENTATION

- Note the timing and course of amenorrhea
- Note the presence of symptoms of pregnancy (nausea, vomiting, breast tenderness)
- Note weight changes, calculate body mass index (BMI), dietary history
- Note presence of stressors, depression, fatigue
- Note development of secondary sexual characteristics
- Review medications
- Note heat or cold intolerance
- Assess for hirsutism, acne, or galactorrhea
- Note history of radiation exposure

DIFFERENTIAL DX

- Pregnancy
- Lactation
- Medications
- Gonadal dysgenesis
- Chromosomal abnormality
- Vaginal atresia or agenesis
- Transverse vaginal septum
- Imperforate hymen
- Hypogonadotropism
- Hypopituitarism
- Anovulation
- Asherman's syndrome
- Cervical stenosis
- Cushing's syndrome
- Pituitary tumor/infarct
- Thyroid disease

DIAGNOSTIC EVALUATION

- History and physical examination
  - Menstrual history, medical and surgical history, and review of medications
  - Perform a detailed physical exam including Tanner staging and pelvic exam
  - Assess for signs of outflow tract abnormalities: Imperforate hymen (hematocele) or transverse vaginal septum
- Initial laboratory testing includes pregnancy test, TSH, prolactin, FSH, and LH
  - Low FSH and LH suggest hypothalamic or pituitary disorder
  - High FSH and LH suggest ovarian failure
- Progestin challenge test to assess for the presence of estrogen and an adequate outflow tract
  - Withdrawal bleeding within 2–7 days confirms the presence of endogenous estrogen, appropriate endometrial response, and an intact outflow tract and suggests a diagnosis of anovulation
- If uterus and/or breasts are absent, order karyotype analysis followed by testosterone and serum FSH levels
- Evaluate for stress, weight loss, and/or eating disorders
- Consider DHEA-S, CT scan or MRI of the head, and/or chromosomal analysis based on clinical suspicion

TREATMENT & MANAGEMENT

- Management depends on the underlying etiology
- Ovarian dysfunction: Oral contraceptive pills
- Ovarian failure: Hormone replacement therapy
- Asherman's syndrome: Hysteroscopic lysis of adhesions followed by hormone therapy
- Pituitary microadenoma or hyperprolactinemia: Excision or medical treatment with bromocriptine
- Pituitary macroadenoma: Surgical resection
- Hypothalamic dysfunction: Correct the underlying cause and induce ovulation with gonadotropins
- Congenital abnormalities: Plastic surgery to allow outflow of menses or to create a functional vagina
- Androgen insensitivity: Testes should be surgically excised due to risk of testicular cancer
- Chronic anovulation: Correct any contributing factors (e.g., stress, excessive weight loss, disordered eating)

PROGNOSIS & COMPLICATIONS

- Overall, the prognosis is good depending on the etiology; in most cases, symptoms and conditions related to amenorrhea are reversible and treatable
- In cases of secondary amenorrhea, medication, lifestyle change, and/or surgery generally provide good outcomes
- Chromosomal abnormalities are unlikely to be corrected by any intervention
- Complications include psychological distress or crisis and failure of proper bone growth and/or osteoporosis

Breast Mass

INTRODUCTION

- The occurrence of a new palpable breast mass or a breast lesion on mammography is a common problem in clinical practice; although breast lumps are a serious concern due to the risk of cancer, most breast lumps and other breast complaints are of benign origin
- Multiple methods are available to differentiate benign from malignant breast lesions, including clinical examination, mammography, ultrasound, fine-needle aspiration, and needle core or open breast biopsy
- 75% of women diagnosed with breast cancer have advanced age as their only risk factor
- Clinical breast examination is important; however, most breast masses should be radiographically examined, and solid lesions require biopsy to rule out malignancy

ETIOLOGY, EPIDEMIOLOGY, & RISK FACTORS

- Benign disorders are more frequent than cancer up until age 75
- The most common benign breast masses are cysts and fibroadenomas
  - Gross cystic disease is found in approximately 7% of adult women in the U.S., most frequently during the fourth decade and perimenopause; they arise from dilatation or obstruction of the collecting ducts
  - Fibroadenomas are the most common benign tumor in young women, with median age at diagnosis of 30 years; they arise from proliferation of periductal stromal connective tissue within the lobules of the breast; growth is stimulated by exogenous estrogen or progesterone, lactation, and pregnancy
- Breast cancer usually originates from the epithelial cells that line the ductal system
  - Affects 1 in 8 women
  - Risk factors include family history of breast cancer, BRCA gene mutations, advancing age, personal history of breast cancer or atypia, early menarche or late menopause, nulliparity, hormone therapy, obesity, diet and lifestyle
- Breast abscess: Commonly caused by *Staphylococcus aureus* or streptococci

PATIENT PRESENTATION

- Breast may be tender or painful
- Normal physiologic nodularity (often incorrectly called fibrocystic disease, it is less likely to have clear borders, is often cord-like, and often changes with menstrual cycle) can be difficult to distinguish from a discreet mass
- Nipple discharge is rarely associated with a mass; bloody discharge is usually benign (95%) but requires evaluation
- Breast cancer typically results in a painless, palpable mass or asymptomatic lesion on mammogram
- Breast cyst may be painful and may vary in size with menses
- Breast abscess is a painful, nonmobile mass with rapid onset; may have overlying blanching erythema, fevers, or chills
- Fibroadenoma: Painless, mobile mass

DIFFERENTIAL DX

- Normal physiologic nodularity
- Fibroadenoma
- Cyst
- Abscess
- Primary breast cancer
- Phyllodes tumor
- Metastatic disease to the breast
- Papilloma
- Nodular breast tissue
- Galactocele
- Fat necrosis
- Radial scar
- Intramammary node
- Trauma

DIAGNOSTIC EVALUATION

- History and physical examination
  - Collect historical information to establish baseline risk, including age, menstrual status, parity, family history, previous biopsy results, and exogenous hormone use
  - Clinical breast examination should document approximate size, site, mobility, and texture, as well as associated skin retraction, erythema, or adenopathy
  - Benign features include smooth, well-demarcated, and mobile lesions
  - Malignant features include hard, irregular, and fixed lesions; bloody nipple discharge; skin dimpling; and nipple retraction
- Further diagnostic evaluation depends on age
  - Under age 35: Ultrasound or fine-needle aspiration to determine whether the lesion is cystic or solid
  - Over age 35: Diagnostic mammography should be done first; if the lesion is benign appearing or not seen on mammogram, then ultrasound is indicated to determine whether it is cystic or solid
- Biopsy of masses, nonpalpable lesions, or suspicious calcifications on mammogram may be indicated: Fine-needle aspiration extracts cells for cytologic examination to distinguish benign versus malignant; core-needle biopsy of solid lesions or complex cysts extracts tissue and provides a definitive diagnosis; excisional biopsy is definitive and may be curative if the full lesion is removed
- Perform cytologic exam of any nipple discharge

TREATMENT & MANAGEMENT

- Cystic masses may be treated by observation with repeat clinical breast exam in 3–6 months or may be aspirated by a therapeutic fine-needle aspiration or a core-needle biopsy under ultrasound guidance
  - Aspiration is indicated for complex cysts, simple cysts in postmenopausal woman, or symptomatic cysts (pain or anxiety)
  - Send fluid to cytology if bloody or complex
- All solid masses require tissue diagnosis via fine-needle aspiration biopsy, core-needle biopsy under ultrasound guidance, or excisional biopsy
- Fibroadenomas require surgical excision for diagnosis and treatment
- Fibrocystic changes can be treated with caffeine avoidance, vitamin E, aspiration of large or painful cysts, and medical therapies (e.g., danazol, oral contraceptives) for pain relief
  - Routine follow-up is sufficient unless cytologic atypia is present
- Breast cancer requires consultation with an oncologist for definitive surgical and/or oncologic treatment
- Galactocele: Needle aspiration
- Abscess: Antibiotics, incision and drainage, and possibly excision

PROGNOSIS & COMPLICATIONS

- Cystic masses require follow-up 4–6 weeks after aspiration to ensure no reaccumulation
  - Recheck every 6 months thereafter, and perform biopsy if reaccumulation occurs
- Solid masses require a tissue diagnosis
  - If fibroadenoma is smaller than 1 cm, follow clinically every 6 months
- Enlarging masses require surgical excision, even if benign
- Early-stage breast cancer (I and II) has a favorable prognosis, with 10-year survival of 80% and 60%, respectively; recurrences are most common within the first years but may continue thereafter, necessitating close follow-up
- Frequent follow-up (every 3–6 months) is warranted if an examination is particularly difficult in order to maintain familiarity and confirm stability

Vaginal Discharge

INTRODUCTION

- Vaginal discharge is a common primary care complaint and one of the most common reasons for gynecologic visits
- It is often accompanied by concerns about the presence of a sexually transmitted disease
- Whenever one sexually transmitted disease is identified, a search for all other STDs is indicated in an effort to treat the individual patient as well as to prevent spread to others

ETIOLOGY, EPIDEMIOLOGY, & RISK FACTORS

- The most common causes of vaginal discharge are candidiasis ("yeast" infection), bacterial vaginosis, and trichomoniasis
  - Bacterial vaginosis is an overgrowth of normal vaginal flora, including *Gardnerella vaginalis*, nonfragilis *Bacteroides*, *Mobiluncus*, *Mycoplasma hominis*, and other anaerobes
  - Candidiasis is caused by *Candida albicans*, *Candida glabrata*, and *Candida tropicalis*; etiologies of candidal overgrowth include antibiotic use, diabetes, pregnancy, and immunocompromise
  - Trichomoniasis is caused by *Trichomonas vaginalis*, a motile, single-cell parasite; risk factors include multiple sexual partners, history of previous sexually transmitted infections, and coinfection with other sexually transmitted infections
- Accounts for about 10 million office visits yearly
- In women with vaginal symptoms, 40–50% have bacterial vaginosis, 20–25% have vaginal candidiasis, 15–20% have trichomoniasis, and many remain undiagnosed

PATIENT PRESENTATION

- Symptoms include odor, irritation, dyspareunia, bleeding, or pruritus
- Discharges are characterized by color (clear, white, green, gray, or yellow), consistency (thin, thick, or curd-like), and amount (more or less than usual)
- Signs include erythema, excoriation, or discharge on the perineum or introitus
- *Candida* may present with extremely intense and often unbearable itching

DIFFERENTIAL DX

- Bacterial vaginosis
- Vaginal candidiasis
- Trichomoniasis
- Gonorrhea
- Chlamydia
- Herpes simplex
- Allergic reactions to chemical irritants, latex, or semen
- Mechanical irritation
- Atrophic vaginitis (in post-menopausal women)
- Normal vaginal or cervical discharge

DIAGNOSTIC EVALUATION

- A focused history and physical examination are crucial, including a complete sexual and exposure history and full abdominal and pelvic examination
- Evaluate the appearance, pH, odor, and microscopic exam of the discharge (see chart)

	pH	Discharge	Odor	Microscopy
Trichomonas	>4.5	yellow-green, copious	present	motile, flagellated
Bacterial vaginosis	>4.5	white-grey	fishy	clue cells
Candida	<4.5	white, curd-like	none	pseudohyphae
Gonorrhea/chlamydia		mucopurulent	varies	PMNs
Atrophic vaginitis		thin, gray, watery	none	few epithelial cells

- Initial labs may include complete blood count, urinalysis, urine culture, pregnancy test, and gonorrhea and chlamydia cultures
- Test for and treat other STDs when any STD is found (e.g., HIV, hepatitis, syphilis)

TREATMENT & MANAGEMENT

- Bacterial vaginosis: Oral metronidazole for 7 days, metronidazole vaginal gel for 5 days, clindamycin for 7 days, or 2% clindamycin vaginal cream for 7 days
- Trichomonas: Oral metronidazole (single-dose or 7-day course)
  - Treat sexual partner(s), as well
- Candidiasis: Fluconazole, itraconazole, or intravaginal azoles
  - If recurrent, screen for diabetes mellitus
  - Recurrent candidiasis can be treated with 6-month suppression therapy
- Avoid alcohol consumption during treatment with metronidazole and for 24 hours thereafter
- If no pathologic condition is identified, "watchful waiting" may be employed
- Resources include the CDC National Prevention Information Network (info@cdcnpin.org or www.cdcnpin.org) and the American Social Health Association (www.ashastd.org or std-hivnet@ashastd.org)

PROGNOSIS & COMPLICATIONS

- Prognosis is usually good after treatment
- To prevent further yeast and bacterial vaginosis infections, patients should avoid tight-fitting synthetic-fiber clothes, wear cotton underwear, wipe from front-to-back, do not douche or use feminine hygiene sprays, and avoid vaginal deodorants, sanitary pads, tampons, and bubble baths
- To prevent trichomoniasis, condoms should be used, and sexual partners should be treated
- Bacterial vaginosis and trichomoniasis during pregnancy are associated with adverse pregnancy outcomes, including premature rupture of membranes, preterm labor, preterm birth, and postpartum endometritis
- Bacterial vaginosis can increase susceptibility to HIV and pelvic inflammatory disease

Evaluation of Abnormal Pap Smear

INTRODUCTION

- Several million screening Pap smears are performed annually in the U.S.; approximately 3–5% are abnormal, although the prevalence varies broadly depending on risk factors
- Pap smears are typically reported using the Bethesda System, which requires evaluation of specimen adequacy, general categorization, interpretation, and results
- Pap smears are named for a Greek physician, George Papanicolaou, who described a method of cytologic evaluation of cervical cells to screen for cervical cancer
- Pap smears are recommended every year for all women above 21 years of age and younger women who are sexually active; some groups recommend screening every 3 years in low-risk women; women with hysterectomy for benign disease do not need continued Pap smears

ETIOLOGY, EPIDEMIOLOGY, & RISK FACTORS

- The preadolescent cervix is covered by columnar epithelium but eventually becomes squamous endothelium in the mature cervix; the squamocolumnar junction (the transformation zone) is most susceptible to human papillomavirus (HPV) and other infections
- Squamous cell carcinoma accounts for 90% of cervical cancers; adenocarcinoma accounts for 10%
  - The primary risk factor for squamous cell carcinoma is HPV infection, which is transmitted by sexual contact
  - Condoms do not completely protect against HPV due to scrotal-labial transmission
  - HPV types 16, 18, and 31 are more likely to have oncogenic potential
  - The main risk factor for adenocarcinoma is diethylstilbestrol (DES) exposure in utero
- Other epidemiologic factors that may increase the risk of developing abnormal cervical cells include sexual intercourse at an early age, multiple sexual partners, cigarette smoking, STDs, and immunodeficiency
- Screening Pap smears are believed to decrease cervical cancer rates by 60–90%

PATIENT PRESENTATION

- Abnormal pap smear findings include:
  - ASC-US (atypical squamous cells of undetermined significance) may represent reactive or reparative changes secondary to inflammation
  - ASC-H (atypical squamous cells, cannot exclude HSIL)
  - LSIL (low-grade squamous intra-epithelial lesion, or CIN I) is often due to a transient HPV infection
  - HSIL (high-grade squamous intraepithelial lesion, or CIN II/III) is associated with HPV persistence and higher risk for progression to carcinoma
  - AGUS (atypical glandular cells of undetermined significance) has a greater risk of underlying neoplasia
  - Squamous cell carcinoma

DIFFERENTIAL DX

- Postmenopausal cellular alterations (e.g., prominent perinuclear halos, nuclear hyperchromasia, variation in nuclear size, multinucleation)
  - Often misclassified as koilocytotic atypia
- Metaplasia (a process whereby the columnar epithelium is replaced by squamous epithelium)
- Cervical infection (e.g., HPV, gonorrhea, chlamydia, herpes simplex virus, *Trichomonas*)
- Cervical polyp
- Cervical, vaginal, or vulvar trauma
- Vaginal foreign body
- Nabothian cyst

DIAGNOSTIC EVALUATION

- An abnormal pap smear is not a diagnosis in itself and requires further testing
- ASC-US finding: Repeat pap smear in 4–6 months
  - Colposcopy is indicated if repeat Pap smear shows ASC-US
  - If a liquid-based Pap smear is used, perform HPV testing on the original specimen; all women who test positive for HPV should be referred for colposcopy
  - Colposcopy is also recommended for immunosuppressed patients with ASC-US, including all women with HIV
- ASC-H, LSIL, and HSIL findings: Perform colposcopy with directed biopsy
- AGUS finding: Perform colposcopy with directed biopsies and endocervical curettage to rule out endometrial pathology
- Diagnostic conization should be performed in cases of unsatisfactory colposcopy, uncertainty regarding the presence of invasive disease, lesions of the endocervical canal, cells on cytologic examination not adequately explained by biopsy specimens, biopsy that suggests microinvasion, or abnormal endocervical glandular cells

TREATMENT & MANAGEMENT

- Confirmed HSIL cells require excision or destruction to prevent progression to cancer
- Small lesions confined to the exocervix in which biopsies have ruled out invasive disease can be destroyed by cryotherapy, laser vaporization, or loop excision
- Larger lesions that involve the endocervix must be excised via conization (can be performed as a diagnostic procedure for the reasons listed above or as a therapeutic procedure) to remove a cone-shaped wedge of the cervix, the transformation zone, and all or a portion of the endocervical canal
- Treatment for a Pap smear that is confirmed as squamous cell carcinoma may involve conization for small lesions in situ or a radical hysterectomy with adjuvant therapy for more extensive disease
- Management of dysplasia changes rapidly, so be sure to consult the most recent guidelines
- Treat infection as appropriate:
  - *Trichomonas* or bacterial vaginosis: Oral metronidazole; intravaginal clotrimazole if pregnant or unable to use metronidazole
  - Gonorrhea: Oral azithromycin or IM ceftriaxone
  - Chlamydia: Oral azithromycin or doxycycline
  - *Candida*: Clotrimazole vaginal cream or oral fluconazole

PROGNOSIS & COMPLICATIONS

- LSIL: The majority of lesions will either spontaneously regress or persist unchanged
- HSIL: The risk of progression to invasive cancer without treatment is 6% within 3 years and as high as 70% by 12 years
- Success rate of conization is better than 90%
- Cervical surgery is a risk factor for cervical incompetence and cervical stenosis; however, these complications are rare
- Most cervical cancer occurs in unscreened or underscreened women or those who have an abnormal Pap smear and do not follow-up on treatment recommendations
- Complications of conization include vaginal discharge (up to 6 weeks), pain, infection, and occasionally an incompetent cervix, which may lead to pregnancy complications

Menopause

INTRODUCTION

- Menopause is the permanent cessation of menstrual flow due to ovarian failure, depletion of all primary ovarian follicles, and decreased levels of circulating estrogen
- Defined as 12 months after the final menses
- Perimenopause begins 2–8 years before menopause and lasts about a year after the last menstrual period; it is characterized by normal ovulatory cycles interspersed with anovulatory cycles of varying length and is often associated with vasomotor symptoms ("hot flashes") and irregular menses

ETIOLOGY, EPIDEMIOLOGY, & RISK FACTORS

- There is a corresponding decrease of estradiol, estrone, and inhibin production from the ovaries, resulting in increased pituitary FSH and LH production via the hypothalamic-pituitary axis
- Absence of menses occurs due to the failure of endometrial lining production in the absence of adequate estrogen and progesterone production
- Menopause is genetically programmed and is not related to race, socioeconomic status, body mass index, height, age at menarche, number of pregnancies, or use of hormones
- Cigarette smoking decreases the age at menopause by an average of 2 years, presumably by decreasing blood flow to the reproductive organs
- Mean age of onset in the United States is 51 years; the average age at menopause has increased from 40 to 51 years of age during the past century

PATIENT PRESENTATION

- Irregular menstrual cycles (perimenopause) or lack of menses
- Hot flashes are the most common post-menopausal complaint; characterized by 3- to 4-minute episodes of reddening and warmth of the skin over the head, neck, and chest
  - Coincides with surges of LH
  - Insomnia secondary to nocturnal hot flashes
- Bone loss increases after menopause and may result in osteopenia or osteoporosis
- Vaginal dryness, atrophic vaginitis
- Urinary urge incontinence
- Increased facial hair may occur
- Increased body fat and body weight, with a shift of fat from peripheral to central distribution
- Thinning of the skin and increased wrinkling
- Increasing loss of teeth (due to estrogen deficiency)

DIFFERENTIAL DX

- Premature ovarian failure (menopause before 40 years old)
- Late menopause (after 55 years old)
- Surgical menopause
- Amenorrhea due to pregnancy or endocrine abnormality
- Pregnancy
- Hypothyroidism
- Hyperprolactinemia
- Ovarian neoplasm
- Asherman's syndrome
- Adrenal dysfunction
- Polycystic ovarian syndrome
- Hypothalamic dysfunction
- Pituitary microadenoma
- Uterine outflow obstruction
- Medications (including chemotherapy)

DIAGNOSTIC EVALUATION

- Generally no workup is needed because menopause is a normal physiologic event
- If the diagnosis is in question, evaluation may include pregnancy testing, FSH (elevated in menopause), LH, prolactin, and TSH
- Screening for osteoporosis with a bone density assessment is advisable for women at increased risk (e.g., lean women, family history of osteoporosis, Caucasians, Asians, and those with inadequate calcium intake and/or long-term steroid use)
- Endometrial sampling and/or pelvic ultrasound may be used to evaluate postmenopausal bleeding

TREATMENT & MANAGEMENT

- No treatment is required for normal menopause
- Oral contraceptives can be continued through perimenopause for reduction of vasomotor symptoms and control of dysfunctional uterine bleeding
  - Prescribe only to nonsmokers and women without risk factors for coronary artery disease
  - In smokers with irregular menses, progestin may be used to induce monthly withdrawal bleed to regulate menses
- Hormone replacement therapy may be useful for short-term symptomatic treatment of hot flashes
- Some patients may find natural supplements effective for the symptoms of menopause (e.g., dong quai, black cohosh, soy products)
- Additional medications for severe hot flashes include selective serotonin reuptake inhibitors and clonidine
- Vaginal dryness may be treated with topical (vaginal) estrogen creams
- Ensure adequate calcium (1500 mg/d) and vitamin D (400–1000 U/d) intake
- Kegel exercises may be useful for urinary incontinence

PROGNOSIS & COMPLICATIONS

- Complications of menopause include osteopenia or osteoporosis, increased cardiovascular risk, weight gain, urinary urge incontinence, and atrophic vaginitis
- Osteoporosis, which results from estrogen deficiency, should be aggressively treated with medications to prevent hip fractures, which are associated with a 20% mortality rate within the first year, and vertebral fractures, which are painful and cause significant morbidity
- Hot flashes tend to decrease over time, regardless of whether or not they are treated

Infertility

- The failure to conceive after 1 year of regular unprotected intercourse; affects 1 in 6 couples and is more common with increasing age
- Most clinicians initiate a workup at 6 months for women 35 or older
- Fecundity is the probability of pregnancy in 1 menstrual cycle; normal fecundity is 20% at each cycle, 50% at 3 months, and 85% at 1 year
- An age-related decrease in fecundity begins at age 35 and is exacerbated after age 40
- 1% of live births in the United States in 2002 were conceived through assisted reproductive techniques

ETIOLOGY, EPIDEMIOLOGY, & RISK FACTORS

- Female factors account for 30–40% of cases
  - Peritoneal factors (40%): Pelvic adhesions from prior surgery, endometriosis, chronic pelvic inflammatory disease
  - Ovulatory factors (15–20%): Polycystic ovarian syndrome, thyroid dysfunction, premature ovarian failure
  - Uterine-tubal factors (30%): Tubal occlusion, fibroids, endometriosis
  - Cervical factors (5–10%): Structural abnormalities, mucous abnormalities
- Male factors account for about 20% of cases
  - Endocrine disorders: Pituitary/hypothalamic dysfunction, adrenal hyperplasia, thyroid disease, testosterone deficiency
  - Abnormal spermatogenesis: Mumps orchitis, varicocele, cryptorchidism
  - Abnormal motility: Antisperm antibodies, immotile cilia syndrome
  - Sexual dysfunction: Retrograde ejaculation, impotence, ductal obstruction
- Male and females factors combined account for about 20% of cases
- The rest of cases are unexplained

PATIENT PRESENTATION

- Male infertility: May present with lack of sexual hair growth, gynecomastia, varicocele, scars of prior surgery (e.g., hernia repair) or trauma to the genitals, or hypogonadism
- Female infertility: May present with dysmenorrhea or cyclic pelvic pain, dyspareunia, and menstrual irregularity outside the normal range (22–35 days); hirsutism, obesity, galactorrhea, or signs of virilization; recurrent pregnancy loss, heavy bleeding, and pain; signs of thyroid disease; or may have history of prior gynecologic procedures (e.g., cryotherapy, conization, cervical dilations)

DIFFERENTIAL DX

- Sexual dysfunction
- Andropause
- Recurrent implantation failure: Poor embryo transfer technique, uterine cavity lesion, hydrosalpinx, fibroids, and endometriosis
- Celiac disease (more common in infertile males and females)
- Subclinical bulimia nervosa
- Male occupational heat exposure increases time to achieve pregnancy

DIAGNOSTIC EVALUATION

- Complete medical history and physical examination looking for risk factors that could impact fertility
- Tests for male infertility may include semen analysis (e.g., sperm count, volume, motility, morphology, pH, and white blood cell count) and endocrine tests (e.g., FSH, testosterone, TSH, prolactin)
  - Less common tests include postejaculatory urinalysis (if semen volume <1.0 mL) to assess for retrograde ejaculation and postcoital testing to examine the interaction between sperm and the cervical mucus
- Tests for female infertility include basal body temperature charts, FSH on day 21 of menstrual cycle, urine LH surge, TSH, prolactin, and cervical culture
  - In women 35 or older, test for FSH on day 3 of the menstrual cycle to assess ovarian reserve
  - Hysterosalpingogram may be indicated to evaluate the uterine cavity and fallopian tubes
  - Peritoneal examination via laparoscopy may be indicated if there is a history of increasing dysmenorrhea
- No apparent cause for infertility is found in 15–20% of couples

TREATMENT & MANAGEMENT

Male infertility
- Correct endocrine disorders
- Limit intercourse to once every 2 days
- Repair anatomic defects (e.g., varicocele), if present
- Washed sperm for intrauterine insemination
- Intracytoplasmic sperm injection
- Refractory cases may attempt artificial insemination with donor sperm

Female infertility
- Intrauterine insemination
- Ovulation induction with clomiphene citrate or gonadotropins
- In vitro fertilization (IVF) or gamete intrafallopian transfer (GIFT) and gonadotropins
- Refractory cases may attempt egg or embryo donation, gestational surrogacy, or adoption
- Group psychotherapy may improve pregnancy rate

PROGNOSIS & COMPLICATIONS

- Correction of endocrine disorders generally restores fertility
- Surgical ligation of varicoceles restores fertility in 50% of cases
- Clomiphene is associated with multiple pregnancy (8–10%) and ovarian cysts (5–10%)
- Gonadotropin therapy is associated with multiple pregnancy (33%) and ovarian hyperstimulation syndrome (1%)
- IVF is associated with multiple pregnancy (38%), ovarian hyperstimulation (5%), increased pregnancy losses (25%), and ectopic pregnancy (5%)
- Pregnancy rate in unexplained, untreated infertility cases approaches 60% over 3–5 years

Polycystic Ovary Syndrome

INTRODUCTION

- A syndrome of androgen excess, possibly due to excess luteinizing hormone (LH) stimulation of the ovaries
- Presents with the classic clinical triad of hirsutism, anovulation, and obesity
- Polycystic ovaries each contain at least 8 small (2–8 mm) follicles
- Approximately 4–6% of women have PCOS; it may be the most common endocrinopathy in reproductive-aged women

ETIOLOGY, EPIDEMIOLOGY, & RISK FACTORS

- Etiology is unknown
  - Proposed theories include excess trophic hormones (LH or ACTH) amplified by disturbances in intrinsic (inhibin and/or follistatin) or extrinsic (insulin or insulin-like growth factor) regulatory peptides
- Patients have insulin resistance and compensatory hyperinsulinemia and hyperandrogenism; the abnormal insulin function causes the cascade of diverse syndrome presentations and the ultimate morbidity in these patients
- Chronic oligo- or anovulation occurs due to functional ovarian hyperandrogenism (80%) and/or functional adrenal hyperandrogenism (50%)

PATIENT PRESENTATION

- Menstrual irregularity: Oligo- or anovulation, amenorrhea, irregular bleeding
- Evidence of hyperandrogenism: Hirsutism, acne, or alopecia
- Obesity
  - Obesity-related sleep disorders (e.g., sleep apnea) may occur
- Impaired glucose tolerance or diabetes mellitus
- Infertility
- Premature pubarche and precocious puberty
- Acanthosis nigricans (due to insulin resistance)

DIFFERENTIAL DX

- Congenital adrenal hyperplasia
- Hyperprolactinemia
- Cushing's syndrome
- Acromegaly
- Ovarian tumors (e.g., Sertoli-Leydig cell tumors)
- Ovarian steroidogenic block (e.g., aromatase deficiency)
- Adrenal tumors
- Drugs (e.g., danazol, oral contraceptive pills containing androgenic progestins)
- Hyperthecosis
- Severe insulin resistance syndromes
- Hypothyroidism

DIAGNOSTIC EVALUATION

- Diagnosis depends on clinical and/or biochemical evidence of hyperandrogenism
- Ultrasound may reveal polycystic ovaries (80–100%); however, the isolated finding of polycystic ovaries (without hyperandrogenism) is very common and does not constitute the disease
- Laboratory studies include elevated LH:FSH ratio >3, exaggerated pulsatile LH levels, elevated androgens (androstenedione and testosterone), low serum steroidal hormone-binding globulin (which results in elevated free testosterone levels), and fasting blood glucose and insulin levels
- Lipid panel is recommended
- TSH, prolactin, and 17-hydroxyprogesterone should all be normal; if not, consider other diagnoses

TREATMENT & MANAGEMENT

- Administer oral contraceptives to regulate the menstrual cycle and for endometrial protection
  - Progesterone can be used if oral contraceptives are contraindicated
- Improve insulin resistance via weight loss and insulin-sensitizing drugs (e.g., metformin, pioglitazone); as little as 5% weight loss can result in normalization of menses, increased fertility, and decreased hirsutism
- Treat hirsutism via hair removal by shaving, depilatories, electrolysis, or laser treatment; additionally, oral contraceptives and antiandrogenic medications (e.g., spironolactone, finasteride) may also decrease hirsutism
- In patients who desire pregnancy, initial choices include clomiphene or metformin to induce ovulation
  - Persistent cases may be treated with assisted reproductive technologies (e.g., in vitro fertilization)
  - If pregnancy is achieved, there is a high incidence of gestational diabetes

PROGNOSIS & COMPLICATIONS

- The syndrome is not curable; however, with proper diagnosis and treatment, including weight loss and diet, most symptoms can be adequately controlled or eliminated
- In most women, pregnancy can be achieved with appropriate medical interventions
- Associated complications include sterility, diabetes (glucose levels should be checked regularly), negative self-image, increased risk of endometrial hyperplasia and endometrial cancer due to oligo-ovulation, and increased risk of cardiac disease
- Prognosis for fertility, decreased hirsutism, and decreased glucose intolerance is improved if weight loss is achieved

Rheumatology

Fever

INTRODUCTION

- Fever is a nonspecific response to a variety of environmental and internal factors
- Among the most frequent emergency room and ambulatory presentations; however, most fevers are of short duration and resolve without specific therapy
- Normal temperature is 36–37.8°C, with circadian rhythmicity (daily variation of 1°C)
  - Body temperatures are lowest in the early morning and highest in the late afternoon
- Temperature is measured either orally, rectally, axillary, or tympanic (oral temperatures measured after intake of hot/cold beverages, smoking, or hyperventilation may be inaccurate)
- Most fevers are induced by polypeptide molecules called endogenous pyrogens, which are produced in response to infection, injury, inflammation, or antigenic challenge

ETIOLOGY, EPIDEMIOLOGY, & RISK FACTORS

- Fever is usually due to an infectious etiology; however, inflammatory, neoplastic, and immunologically mediated diseases may cause fever as their primary clinical presentation
  - Almost any infection can cause fever
  - Respiratory, urinary, GI, and skin/soft tissue infections are the most common causes
  - Exogenous pyrogens (e.g., microorganisms, toxins) cause fever by inducing the host to produce endogenous pyrogens, a heterogeneous collection of cytokines that include interleukin-1 (IL-1), interleukin-6 (IL-6), tumor necrosis factor (TNF), interferon-α and -β
- Noninfectious etiologies of fever:
  - Tissue ischemia or infarction: Venous thromboembolism, myocardial infarction, stroke, hematoma, subarachnoid hemorrhage, intramuscular injections, intestinal infarction, renal infarction, splenic infarction, pancreatitis, atheroembolic syndrome, heterotopic ossification
  - Postoperative or postprocedure: Major surgery, endoscopy, transfusion reaction, infusion-related phlebitis or chemical injury, atelectasis
  - Allergy and inflammation: Drugs (e.g., antibiotics, antineoplastic agents, anticonvulsants), autoimmune disorders, gout/pseudogout, malignancy, fecal impaction, Dressler's syndrome
  - Autonomic and endocrine dysfunction: Central nervous system or spinal cord dysfunction, delirium tremens, neuroleptic malignant syndrome, thyrotoxicosis, Addison's disease

PATIENT PRESENTATION

- Verify the temperature: Oral measurement is preferred but may be influenced by eating, drinking, smoking, mouth breathing, and hyperventilation; if uncertain, evaluate rectal temperature (especially in the elderly), but note that rectal temperatures are generally 1°C higher than oral readings (axillary temperatures are notoriously inaccurate and should not be used)
- Review history and current medical condition
- Evaluate for prosthetic devices, IV lines, catheters, and wounds, and inspect for signs of inflammation surrounding them
- Evaluate for a recent change in medications, medical procedures, blood transfusions, and exposure to persons with communicable diseases
- Further evaluation based on systems involved
- Inspect the skin carefully

DIFFERENTIAL DX

Infection
- Viral (e.g., influenza, URI, acute HIV, CMV, EBV)
- Bacterial (e.g., UTI, otitis media, pneumonia, meningitis, dental abscess, pharyngitis, sinusitis, hepatic abscess)
- Fungal (e.g., candidiasis)
- Parasitic

Noninfectious etiologies
- Tissue ischemia or infarction
- Neoplasm
- Allergy
- Inflammation
- Autonomic dysfunction
- Endocrine dysfunction
- Drugs (e.g., aspirin, isoniazid, antibiotics, drug allergy)

DIAGNOSTIC EVALUATION

- The history and physical examination guides further workup
  - Evaluate the current illness, chronology of symptoms, details of the fever (e.g., remitting/relapsing, duration), and associated symptoms
  - Evaluate past medical history, with attention to immune status
  - A careful epidemiologic and risk factor history is important in raising the suspicion for specific diagnoses, including immunosuppression, sick contacts, employment history, exposures (e.g., animal, water, soil), sexual history, recent travel (including pretravel vaccinations and precautions, known endemic areas), and new medications
  - Physical examination should include a careful search to identify clues to the diagnosis (e.g., skin rash, lymphadenopathy, hepatosplenomegaly, embolic phenomena, clinical signs of meningitis or focal neurologic signs, joint effusion or tenderness over the spine, signs of pneumonia, costovertebral angle tenderness)
- Judicious use of laboratory and radiologic testing
  - Initial tests may include complete blood count with differential, electrolytes, urinalysis and culture, blood cultures, and CRP or ESR measurement
  - Chest and sinus X-ray in patients with respiratory symptoms
- Further investigations may include CT scans of the chest, abdomen, and pelvis; WBC scans; rheumatologic tests, such as ANA and ferritin; and workup for malignancy
- If deep venous thrombosis is suspected clinically or based on high risk, Doppler studies of the lower extremities should be done without delay

TREATMENT & MANAGEMENT

- Attempt to treat the etiology, rather than the fever: Only extreme fevers (temperature greater than 106°F) are in themselves potentially harmful; in contrast, "treating" the fever with antipyretics can be potentially harmful
  - Specific therapies to reduce temperature are not always warranted; consider treating a fever if the patient is symptomatic, especially if there is a history of cardiopulmonary disease (these patients may be more susceptible to the increased metabolic demands of fever)
  - Antipyretics (e.g., aspirin, NSAIDs, acetaminophen) are the mainstay of therapy for temperature reduction; always consider potential toxicities (e.g., hepatic or renal failure)
  - Corticosteroids and NSAIDs may confuse the diagnostic search, mask important clues, and result in partially treated illness that relapses
- Empiric therapy is not necessary unless the patient is hemodynamically unstable or is immunocompromised

PROGNOSIS & COMPLICATIONS

- Prognosis depends on the underlying etiology
- High fevers usually have an obvious source, whereas low-grade fevers may elude attempts at diagnosis
- Death is rarely a complication of fever but could occur as a result of untreated pathology
- Serious complications (e.g., sepsis) could occur if bacterial infections go untreated
- A persistent high core temperature can lead to cardiac, pulmonary, and CNS collapse
- Be cautious regarding antibiotic administration if there is not a definite source of infection

Osteoarthritis

INTRODUCTION

- A noninflammatory "wear-and-tear" disease of the articular surface, resulting in a slowly progressive destruction of the articular cartilage
- Also known as degenerative joint disease
- By age 40, 90% of the population has X-ray evidence of osteoarthritic changes, although most are asymptomatic

ETIOLOGY, EPIDEMIOLOGY, & RISK FACTORS

- Trauma leads to the release of degradative factors and inadequate repair by chondrocytes
- Synthesis and secretion of matrix-degrading enzymes (e.g., stromelysin, collagenase, metalloproteinases) by chondrocytes is markedly increased in these patients
- Softening, ulceration, and focal disintegration of articular cartilage occurs, leading to formation of bone and cartilage at the joint margins
- Some inflammation does occur, which is associated with immune complex deposition in the extracellular matrix of the articular cartilage
- Distinguish idiopathic osteoarthritis from secondary osteoarthritis
  - Idiopathic disease is usually associated with a family history and may be related to hereditary defects of collagen; more common in the hands and fingers
  - Secondary disease may occur due to acute or repetitive trauma, joint hypermobility, congenital hip dysplasia, Legg-Calve-Perthes disease, and other causes; more common in load-bearing joints, such as the knees and hips
- Prevalence increases with increasing age
- Obesity is a major risk factor for osteoarthritis of the knees and hips
- Sports participation and certain occupations may predispose to osteoarthritis

PATIENT PRESENTATION

- Deep, gnawing joint pain that increases with activity and often subsides with rest
- Morning stiffness less than 30 minutes
- The most involved joints are the hip, knee, DIP, PIP, 1st MTP, 1st CMC, and AC joints, and the discs and facet joints of the spine
- Joint swelling
- Joint deformities may be present, especially in the hands, including Heberden's nodes (DIP) and Bouchard's nodes (PIP)
- Bony enlargement
- Decreased and painful range of motion
- Crepitus
- Tenderness to palpation

DIFFERENTIAL DX

- Inflammatory arthritides (e.g., systemic lupus erythematosus, rheumatoid arthritis)
- Avascular necrosis
- Gouty arthritis
- Calcium pyrophosphate arthropathy
- Spondyloarthropathies
- Osteonecrosis
- Neuropathic joint related to endocrine disease
- Septic arthritis
- Reiter's syndrome
- Musculoskeletal disorders (e.g., tendonitis, bursitis)
- Polymyalgia rheumatica
- Hemochromatosis
- Trauma

DIAGNOSTIC EVALUATION

- History and physical examination
  - History of trauma, sports participation (wear-and-tear), obesity, poor conditioning, or meniscal tear may be present
  - Physical findings of crepitus, decreased range of motion, and bony enlargement are common
- X-ray of the involved joint may reveal joint space narrowing, subchondral sclerosis, osteophyte formation, or subchondral cysts
- Synovial fluid analysis reveals few WBCs, less than 25% PMNs, no crystals, and normal viscosity
- Tests of inflammation (e.g., ESR, CRP) are usually normal
- Rheumatoid factor titers are less than 1:40
- If suspect septic arthritis, assess a complete blood count and blood culture
- Other tests may be indicated to identify an inflammatory arthritides (e.g., antinuclear antibodies, anti-ds-DNA)

TREATMENT & MANAGEMENT

- No therapeutic intervention has been shown to prevent the development of osteoarthritis, slow the progression of damage in joints that are already involved, or reverse pathologic changes
- Exercise and physical therapy
- Weight loss in obese patients
- Topical capsaicin is often effective for mild to moderate pain
- Acetaminophen or NSAIDs for pain
- Intra-articular steroids for severe pain
  - Generally not given more frequently than every 4–6 months
- Viscosupplementation with hyaluronic acid injections may preserve and/or replenish articular cartilage and has been shown to decrease pain for 6 months
- Glucosamine and chondroitin sulfate may be useful, although evidence is mixed
- Surgical intervention may be necessary for advanced disease, which may include joint replacement

PROGNOSIS & COMPLICATIONS

- Insidious onset with chronic and sometimes debilitating sequelae
- Symptoms can be treated, but the progression of the disease is unaffected
- Ultimately, many patients with advanced disease will require surgical treatment
- The results of surgical intervention are usually very good and allow patients to return to all or most activities of daily living
- Can result in a significant decrease in quality of life, decreased activity, and loss of independence in the elderly
- Medication-induced complications may occur (e.g., gastrointestinal bleeding due to NSAIDs)

Fibromyalgia

INTRODUCTION

- A noninflammatory syndrome of chronic, generalized muscular pain and arthralgias
- Formerly known as fibrositis; however, this term is a misnomer because there are no signs of inflammation
- Widespread muscular involvement occurs with multiple, bilateral, fibromyalgia-specific "tender points"
- Can be associated with multiple vague systemic complaints, such as chronic fatigue
- The current definition of fibromyalgia stresses the presence of widespread pain for greater than 3 months in an axial distribution on the right and left sides of the body above and below the waist

ETIOLOGY, EPIDEMIOLOGY, & RISK FACTORS

- The etiology is unknown
- May involve abnormal nociceptive pain processing, upregulation of pain sensation, or a maladaptive behavior to stress
- May be related to viral disease, psychiatric factors, sleep disorders, or hypothyroidism
- Prevalence of 2% in the U.S. population
- Females are affected much more than males
- Can affect adolescents and elderly
- Caucasians are most affected
- Men tend to have less severe pain and fewer tender points
- The average age of presentation is the early 30s
- Patients with fibromyalgia are at higher risk for chronic fatigue syndrome and irritable bowel syndrome, and vice versa

PATIENT PRESENTATION

- Widespread pain and fatigue
- Arthralgias with subjective joint swelling
- Feeling of weakness or diffuse muscle aching
- Light touch may elicit severe pain
- Headache
- Vestibular symptoms (e.g., dizziness)
- Chronic pelvic pain or vulvodynia may be present
- Symptoms of poor sleep
- Cognitive impairment
- Noncardiac chest pain may occur

DIFFERENTIAL DX

- Chronic fatigue syndrome
- Polymyositis
- Rheumatoid arthritis
- Myofascial pain syndrome
- Polymyalgia rheumatica
- Systemic lupus erythematosus
- Ankylosing spondylitis
- Hypothyroidism
- Viral syndrome
- Lyme disease
- Depression
- Parathyroid disorders
- Metabolic myopathy
- Drug-induced myalgias (e.g., statins)
- Chronic viral disease
- Vitamin B_{12} deficiency
- Multiple sclerosis
- Cervical myelopathy

DIAGNOSTIC EVALUATION

- History and physical examination
- A diagnosis of exclusion
- 11 of 18 characteristic tender points must be present for diagnosis
  - These areas become painful even with mild pressure (i.e., enough pressure to blanch a fingernail)
  - Tender points (all bilateral) include the occiput at the insertions of the trapezius, the trapezius at the midpoint of the upper border, the sternal insertion of the second rib, the lateral epicondyles of the elbow, medial portion of knees, outer potion of the hips at the greater trochanter, the upper and outer gluteal quadrants, and the supraspinatus above the scapular spine near the medial border
- X-rays of the spine or other joints may be indicated to rule out other disease
- Routine lab testing (ESR, rheumatoid factor, ANA, CBC, liver function tests, thyroid function tests, chemistries, creatine phosphokinase, urinalysis) should be performed but will usually be normal
- EMG and EEG may be warranted

TREATMENT & MANAGEMENT

- Patient education and reassurance
- Stress management techniques, massage, relaxation exercises, and biofeedback may be useful
- Exercise, physical therapy, and cardiovascular fitness
- Aspirin and NSAIDs can be used; avoid opioids and steroids
- 1% lidocaine injections into tender points may be indicated in cases of severe pain
- Tricyclic antidepressants and selective serotonin reuptake inhibitors (SSRIs) can be effective
- Treat sleep disturbances as necessary, including evaluation and treatment of sleep apnea
  - Foam or egg-crate mattress can be used for night pain
- Psychiatric evaluation may be warranted
- Avoid smoking, which can exacerbate pain

PROGNOSIS & COMPLICATIONS

- The disease follows a chronic course with exacerbations and remissions that can be improved by judicious exercise, stress reduction, and possibly pharmacologic agents
- Good prognosis if the patient is willing to apply treatment suggestions
- Disability is not encouraged but may be necessary in severe cases not responsive to treatment
- The work environment may need to be modified to fit limitations

Temporal Arteritis

INTRODUCTION

- Temporal arteritis is an immune-mediated vasculitis characterized by granulomatous infiltrates of medium- to large-sized arteries
- The classic picture of temporal arteritis is an elderly patient complaining of a new onset of unilateral headache, visual loss, and myalgias
- Symptoms occur due to vessel wall inflammation with resulting lumen occlusion and tissue ischemia; presenting symptoms include headache, jaw claudication, amaurosis fugax, and irreversible blindness
- About half of affected patients have concurrent symptoms of polymyalgia rheumatica

ETIOLOGY, EPIDEMIOLOGY, & RISK FACTORS

- An inflammatory condition of unknown cause that affects all layers of the walls (intima and inner part of the media) of the medium- to large-sized arteries, resulting in thickening, obstruction and ischemia
- Most often affects the temporal artery, choroidal artery (which supplies the optic disc), and the extracranial carotid artery, resulting in optic nerve damage (can lead to blindness if untreated); masseter muscles (results in jaw claudication); and posterior circulation of the central nervous system
- Involvement of the aortic arch branches, particularly the subclavian and axillary arteries, can cause arm claudication, while aortic infiltration can lead to aortic dilation and aneurysms
- Granulomatous infiltrates in the arterial wall, including giant cells and lymphocytes, may be demonstrated on microscopy
- Temporal arteritis is one of three entities that are a part of giant cell arteritis; the others are polymyalgia rheumatica and aortic arch syndrome
- Females are more commonly affected
- Age is the most important risk factor, with an increasing incidence starting at 50
  - Rarely affects persons under 50
- In persons over 50, the prevalence is approximately 200 per 100,000 persons

PATIENT PRESENTATION

- New onset headache
  - Typically occurs in the temporal areas, but may be frontal or occipital or generalized
  - The pain is pulsatile or pressure-like
- Jaw claudication with chewing
- Arthralgias, myalgias
- Transient monocular blindness or sudden loss of vision occurs in 25–50% of patients
  - If vision is lost in one eye, there is greater than 50% likelihood of visual loss in the other eye within 1 month
  - Ophthalmoparesis may occur
- Arm claudication may occur
- Proximal muscle aches and morning stiffness if polymyalgia rheumatica is present
- Low-grade fever
- Constitutional symptoms (e.g., low-grade fever, malaise, anorexia, weight loss)

DIFFERENTIAL DX

- Migraine
- Tension headache
- Cluster headache
- Cervical arthritis
- Myofascial pain syndrome
- Intracranial mass headache
- Central retinal artery obstruction
- Anterior ischemic optic neuropathy
- Fibromyalgia
- Amyloidosis
- Arteriovenous fistula
- Atherosclerotic disease of the temporal arteries
- Other causes of vasculitis
- Systemic infections
- Transient ischemic attack
- Trigeminal neuralgia

DIAGNOSTIC EVALUATION

- History and physical examination
  - Patients with polymyalgia rheumatica may present with decreased range of motion of the shoulders, neck, and hips
- Laboratory testing includes complete blood count (may show leukocytosis and/or normocytic anemia) and ESR (elevated in 90% of patients but may be falsely lowered in patients taking corticosteroids, aspirin, or NSAIDs)
  - Other lab abnormalities may include increased acute-phase reactants (e.g., C-reactive protein, fibrinogen), anemia of chronic disease, thrombocytosis, and elevated liver enzymes
- Biopsy of the superficial temporal artery is diagnostic
  - If the biopsy is negative but temporal arteritis is still suspected, a biopsy of the contralateral temporal artery should be done
- The presence of 3 or more of the following criteria has been shown to have better than 95% sensitivity and nearly 80% specificity for temporal arteritis: age at onset over 50 years, new onset of headache, temporal artery abnormalities, erythrocyte sedimentation greater than 50 mm/h, and positive temporal artery biopsy

TREATMENT & MANAGEMENT

- Corticosteroids are the mainstay of treatment
  - Prednisone should be started in high doses (80 mg/d) in suspected cases, even before a biopsy is performed (results of the biopsy will not be altered by steroid therapy of up to 2 weeks)
  - Do not delay steroids; failure to start steroids early in the course of the disease can result in permanent vision loss
  - Gradually taper the steroid dose after 1–2 months to a maintenance dose of 7.5–10 mg/d once the patient becomes asymptomatic and the ESR decreases to about 25 mm/h
- Cyclophosphamide and methotrexate may be used in steroid-intolerant patients
- Treatment should be maintained for 18 months to 2 years

PROGNOSIS & COMPLICATIONS

- The disease is generally adequately controlled with steroids; corticosteroids are usually tolerated well despite the advanced age of patients
- Relapse is common if steroids are discontinued too soon
- Untreated, it can lead to blindness: 50% of patients will lose sight in one or both eyes
- Once blindness occurs, it is often permanent; however, if therapy is started after unilateral vision loss, the other eye is protected
- ESR and C-reactive protein levels may be used to monitor response to treatment
- After 2 years of treatment, relapses are rare (less than 20% of cases)

Polymyalgia Rheumatica

INTRODUCTION

- A systemic inflammatory syndrome occurring in older people and characterized by pain and stiffness of the neck, shoulder girdle, and pelvic girdle
- Often accompanied by systemic symptoms, such as fatigue and malaise
- Although it is classified as a rheumatic disease, the etiology is unknown

ETIOLOGY, EPIDEMIOLOGY, & RISK FACTORS

- The etiology is unknown
- Autoimmune responses have been postulated, most likely secondary to an infectious process (especially viral); however, no infectious agent has been identified, and no characteristic antibodies have been found
- Pathologic findings are minimal or absent
- Polymyalgia rheumatica may represent a less severe and less localized point in the spectrum of another disease process, such as temporal arteritis
- Possible association with HLA-DR4
- A genetic predisposition is likely
- Affects approximately 1 in 200 people older than 50, with mean age of 70
  - Rare in persons younger than 50
- Affects females twice as often as males
- Most common in whites of northern European descent, but occurs in all ethnic groups
- More prevalent in northern latitudes
- For unclear reasons, termporal arteritis occurs concomitantly in 15–25% of polymyalgia rheumatica patients

PATIENT PRESENTATION

- Muscle pain in the neck, shoulder, and hip regions
  - Usually symmetrical
  - Shoulders are often affected first
- Morning stiffness (often lasting beyond 1 hour)
- Stiffness following inactivity ("gelling phenomenon")
- Constitutional symptoms (e.g., fatigue, malaise, weight loss, low-grade fever)
- Depression
- Symptoms are usually abrupt in onset, with maximal symptoms within 2 weeks of onset
- All patients with complaints of headache, tenderness over the temporal region, pain upon brushing hair, or jaw pain upon chewing need to be evaluated for temporal arteritis

DIFFERENTIAL DX

- Fibromyalgia
- Dermatomyositis
- Polymyositis
- Osteoarthritis
- Rheumatoid arthritis
- Connective tissue diseases (e.g., SLE)
- Occult infection (e.g., endocarditis, osteomyelitis, Lyme disease)
- Malignancy (e.g., multiple myeloma, leukemia, lymphoma)
- Depression
- Hypothyroidism

DIAGNOSTIC EVALUATION

- History and physical examination
  - Affected muscles may be tender to palpation
  - Mild or absent synovitis/tenosynovitis
  - Strength is preserved unless disease is advanced (disuse atrophy)
  - Decreased range of motion of the neck, shoulders, and hips may occur
  - If there is tenderness to palpation over the temporal arteries, test for temporal arteritis
- Several diagnostic criteria have been proposed, including age greater than 65, ESR greater than 40 mm/h, bilateral shoulder pain, less than 2 weeks from onset to maximal symptoms, morning stiffness lasting beyond 1 hour, and depression or weight loss
- Laboratory testing includes complete blood count, liver function tests, rheumatoid factor, antinuclear antibodies, creatine phosphokinase, and C-reactive protein
- Muscle biopsies are normal
- The diagnosis is usually confirmed by dramatic response to corticosteroid therapy

TREATMENT & MANAGEMENT

- Oral corticosteroids are the mainstay of treatment
  - Dramatic improvement usually occurs within 24–72 hours
  - Studies suggest a starting dose of 10–20 mg/d of prednisone; however, if temporal arteritis is suspected, high-dose prednisone (at least 40–60 mg/d) is indicated
  - A slow taper can be attempted once symptoms resolve, usually by increments of 1–2.5 mg/d every 4 weeks until reaching a maintenance dose of 5–7.5 mg/d; the maintenance dose is usually continued for at least 1–2 years and then slowly tapered
  - If relapse occurs, resume treatment at the starting dose of 10–20 mg/d
- For mild cases, consider high-dose NSAIDs; however, this is only effective in 10–20% of cases
- Other immunomodulating therapies are under investigation
- Physical therapy may help improve pain and range of motion and prevent disuse atrophy
- Use symptoms as a guide to steroid tapering
- Consider referral to a rheumatologist if the patient has inadequate response to steroids, contraindication to use of steroids, frequent exacerbations with tapering steroid doses, or relapses

PROGNOSIS & COMPLICATIONS

- Usually a self-limited illness that resolves without sequelae, but can have recurrent exacerbations, especially if steroids are tapered too rapidly
- Average length of disease is 2 years, but the clinical course ranges from several months to 4 years, and relapses are common

Rheumatoid Arthritis

INTRODUCTION

- A chronic inflammatory disease of unknown etiology characterized by synovial proliferation, cartilage destruction, and bony erosion
- Frequent flares occur, and systemic involvement is common
- Appropriate treatment can limit joint destruction, making early diagnosis critical to preserving quality of life

ETIOLOGY, EPIDEMIOLOGY, & RISK FACTORS

- The etiology is unknown
- Progresses in 3 stages:
  - First, there is swelling of the synovial joint lining associated with pain, warmth, and stiffness
  - Next, there is rapid growth and division of cells, leading to synovial thickening
  - Finally, these inflamed cells release enzymes that cause bone and cartilage destruction, loss of joint mobility, and further pain
- Affects up to 1% of the population
- Risk factors include obesity, smoking, and coffee consumption
- Environmental and genetic factors also contribute to the disease
- HLA-DR4 is associated with higher incidence and more aggressive disease
- More prevalent in Native-American populations
- Females are affected more often than males
- Peak onset during ages 20–50
- Higher risk in close family members

PATIENT PRESENTATION

- Early morning stiffness lasting longer than 1 hour
- Symmetrical joint pain and swelling
  - Worse with motion
- Relieved by rest
- Fever, malaise
- Swan-neck deformity: Extended PIP joint, flexed DIP joint
- Boutonniere deformity: Flexed PIP, extended DIP
- Subcutaneous nodules
- Extra-articular manifestations include keratoconjunctivitis, episcleritis, serositis, vasculitis, and pulmonary nodules
- Rheumatoid nodules: Subcutaneous nodules over bony prominences or around joints

DIFFERENTIAL DX

- Parvovirus/rubella arthritis
- Hepatitis C virus infection
- Psoriatic arthritis in a rheumatoid pattern
- Inflammatory bowel disease
- Ankylosing spondylitis
- Relapsing polychondritis
- Sarcoidosis
- Lyme disease
- Systemic lupus erythematosus
- Polyarticular gout
- Dermatomyositis
- Polymyositis
- Whipple's disease
- Syphilis
- Polymyalgia rheumatica
- Fibromyalgia
- Felty's syndrome
- Sjögren's syndrome

DIAGNOSTIC EVALUATION

- Complete history and physical examination
  - Joint examination
  - Assessment of ability to perform activities of daily living
  - Assessment of psychosocial impact
- Initial laboratory tests include CBC with differential, ESR, uric acid, C-reactive protein, urinalysis, rheumatoid factor, and antinuclear antibody testing
- Joint fluid aspiration is diagnostic; reveals greater than 2000 WBCs/μL and more than 75% PMNs, with absence of crystals
- 4 of 7 diagnostic criteria should be present for diagnosis:
  - Morning stiffness lasting more than 1 hour, experienced for more than 6 weeks
  - Symmetrical joint swelling for more than 6 weeks
  - Must involve PIP, MCP, or wrist joint
  - Greater than 3 joints affected for more than 6 weeks
  - Subcutaneous nodules
  - Positive rheumatoid factor (IgM antibody to IgG)
  - X-ray evidence of joint erosion or osteopenia of hand or wrist
- In endemic areas, *Borrelia burgdorferi* should be excluded by enzyme-linked immunosorbent assay (ELISA) testing and Western blot

TREATMENT & MANAGEMENT

- Goals of therapy are to prevent joint destruction, relieve pain and inflammation, maintain range of motion, and maintain independence
- Nonpharmacologic treatment includes rest, hot baths, paraffin wax, and physical and occupational therapy
- Pain relief with NSAIDs or aspirin
- Aggressive early intervention with a disease-modifying antirheumatic drug (DMARD) used alone or in combination with gold compounds, penicillamine, hydroxychloroquine, methotrexate, leflunomide, sulfasalazine, and minocycline
  - Other agents include cyclophosphamide, azathioprine, and cyclosporine A
- New biologic agents probably prevent bone erosions, including etanercept and infliximab (TNF-α receptor antibodies) and anakinra (IL-1 receptor antibody)
- Reconstructive surgery in patients who develop destructive arthropathy

PROGNOSIS & COMPLICATIONS

- There are different patterns of progression; some patients have a slow onset with multiple remissions and relapses, while others have an acute, rapid onset
- Half of patients are disabled within 10 years
- Reconstructive surgery often significantly improves quality of life
- Decreased life expectancy by 3–7 years
- Poor prognosis in white females, rheumatoid factor positive, more than 20 joints affected, elevated ESR, rheumatoid nodules, or joint changes on X-ray
- Complications include permanent joint deformities, carpal tunnel syndrome, extensor tendon rupture, vasculitis, pericardial effusion, and atlantoaxial subluxation

Systemic Lupus Erythematosus

INTRODUCTION

- A chronic inflammatory disease of unknown etiology that is characterized by B-cell hyper-reactivity, complement activation, and T-cell defects
- 90% of cases occur in females
- African-Americans are most commonly affected

ETIOLOGY, EPIDEMIOLOGY, & RISK FACTORS

- Autoantibodies directed against nuclear components, including DNA, mediate the formation of immune complexes
- Circulating immune complexes become deposited in vascular walls of tissues; complement activation at the vessel walls further destroys tissue
- Peak incidence at 15–40 years of age
- Prevalence is approximately 1 in 2000
- Greater incidence and prevalence in African-Americans, African-Caribbeans, and some Native-American tribes
- Increased incidence in close relatives
- Ultraviolet B light and pregnancy can induce flare-ups
- A lupus-like syndrome may occur due to certain drugs, including procainamide, isoniazid, and hydralazine

PATIENT PRESENTATION

The American Association of Rheumatology suggests that at least 4 diagnostic criteria be present for diagnosis:

- Malar ("butterfly") rash
- Discoid (red, raised, scaly) rash
- Photosensitivity (skin rash in response to light)
- Oral ulcers
- Symmetrical migratory arthritis, particularly of the fingers, hands, wrists, or knees
- Serositis (pleuritis or pericarditis)
- Renal disorder (persistent proteinuria >0.5 g/d or cellular casts
- Neurologic disorder (seizures, psychosis)
- Hematologic disorder (hemolytic anemia, leukopenia, lymphopenia, or thrombocytopenia)
- Immunologic disorder (anti-DNA, anti-SM, or antiphospholipid antibodies)
- Positive antinuclear antibody (ANA)

DIFFERENTIAL DX

- Rheumatoid arthritis
- Spondyloarthritis
- Sjögren's syndrome
- Progressive systemic sclerosis
- Dermatomyositis or polymyositis
- Connective tissue diseases
- Acute rheumatic fever
- Serum sickness
- Behçet's disease
- Polyarteritis nodosa
- Infections (e.g., HIV, syphilis, parvovirus B19, rubella, Epstein-Barr virus, toxoplasmosis, tuberculosis, leprosy, schistosomiasis, leishmaniasis)
- Sarcoidosis
- Porphyria
- Lymphoma

DIAGNOSTIC EVALUATION

- Careful history and physical examination
- Initial testing includes complete blood count with differential, metabolic profile, urinalysis, 24-hour urine collection for protein and creatinine clearance
- Test for ANA level; if ANA is positive, further testing for anti-DNA, anti-SM, anti-SSA, anti-SSB, and antiribonucleoprotein antibodies is indicated
- Test for complement levels (C3, C4, CH50)
- If either RPR or PTT are abnormal, test for antiphospholipid antibodies
- Direct and indirect Coombs test and reticulocyte count
- ESR and C-reactive protein
- Chest X-ray and echocardiogram may be indicated if there is cardiac involvement
- Renal biopsy may be indicated
- Pregnancy test in women of child-bearing age

TREATMENT & MANAGEMENT

- Avoid sun exposure and use sunscreens
- NSAIDs for arthritis or serositis
- Severe disease is treated with steroids or immunosuppressive drugs
  - Daily prednisone (<30 mg) for non-life-threatening manifestations
  - High-dose oral or intravenous steroids (1–2 mg/kg/d) for cerebritis, glomerulonephritis, or other life-threatening manifestations
  - Immunosuppressive drugs (e.g., cyclophosphamide, azathioprine, mycophenolate, methotrexate, cyclosporine) may be used in cases of life-threatening disease or steroid sparing
- Intravenous immunoglobulin (IVIG) may be used for acute thrombocytopenia or hemolytic anemia
- Warfarin for anticoagulation in cases of antiphospholipid antibody syndrome
- Dialysis and renal transplantation for renal failure
- Experimental therapies include anti-CD40 ligand antibody and tumor necrosis factor blockade

PROGNOSIS & COMPLICATIONS

- Follows a chronic course with exacerbations and remissions
- Complications include Jacoud's arthropathy (tendon disease and rupture), avascular necrosis of the hip and other joints due to chronic steroid use, thrombosis, vasculitis, glomerulonephritis, pericarditis, pleural effusions, pneumonitis, and complications of NSAIDs and steroids (e.g., gastritis, ulcers, gastrointestinal bleeding, chronic renal failure)
- More than 90% of patients are alive 10 years after diagnosis; 70% survive 20 years
- Indicators of poor prognosis include hypertension, nephritic syndrome, elevated creatinine, anemia, or antiphospholipid antibody syndrome
- The most common causes of death during the initial decade after diagnosis are infections and renal failure; thromboembolic events are the most common cause of death thereafter

Gout and Hyperuricemia

INTRODUCTION

- Gout is a syndrome in which hyperuricemia leads to precipitation of monosodium urate crystals in joints and other tissues, resulting in inflammation, tissue injury, tophi, and arthritis
- The greatest risk factors appear to be certain medications and alcohol consumption
- Unusual presentations may occur in women, young men, and posttransplantation patients on cyclosporine chemotherapy
- Similar disorders include pseudogout (precipitation of calcium pyrophosphate crystals) and other crystal deposition disorders (e.g., calcium hydroxyapatite, calcium oxalate)

ETIOLOGY, EPIDEMIOLOGY, & RISK FACTORS

- Hyperuricemia is defined as serum urate >6.5
- Most cases (90%) occur due to decreased excretion of uric acid (e.g., chronic renal disease, low-volume states, diuretic use)
- The rest of cases occur due to excess production of uric acid (e.g., genetic enzyme defects such as HGPRT deficiency and PRPP synthetase overactivity), increased cell turnover as occurs in leukemias, psoriasis, and hemoglobinopathies
- After 10–20 years of sustained hyperuricemia, clinical gout can develop
  - In posttransplantation patients, gout develops after 2–5 years
- Many drugs alter uric acid metabolism, including thiazides and other diuretics, cyclosporine, aspirin, alcohol, and lead
- Predominantly a disease of men
- Risk factors include family history, age greater than 30, females after menopause (particularly when using thiazides diuretics), alcohol abuse, obesity, and lack of exercise

PATIENT PRESENTATION

- Acute gouty arthritis
  - Repeated attacks of severe joint pain, swelling, and erythema
  - The 1st metatarsophalangeal (MTP) joint is most commonly affected (called podagra)
  - Also commonly involved are the ankle, intertarsal joints, knee, and wrist
  - Fever may be present
- Recurrent oligoarthritis, with each episode initially lasting 5–7 days
- An "intercurrent period" may then occur, during which symptoms of arthritis are absent but uric acid continues to accumulate and tissue deposition continues
- Ultimately, chronic tophaceous gout occurs (usually after 10–20 years), presenting with palpable tophi in subcutaneous tissues, periarticular areas, or bone

DIFFERENTIAL DX

- Acute monoarthritis: Septic arthritis, gonococcal arthritis, Reiter's syndrome (especially in cases of podagra), Lyme disease, trauma, pseudogout, osteoarthritis
- Recurrent monoarthritis: Palindromic rheumatism, spondyloarthropathies, pseudogout, osteoarthritis
- Polyarthritis: Rheumatoid arthritis, psoriatic arthritis, polyseptic arthritis (rare), Reiter's syndrome, osteoarthritis
- Tophi may mimic rheumatoid nodules or rheumatic fever nodules
- Cellulitis

DIAGNOSTIC EVALUATION

- History and physical examination
- Aspiration of synovial fluid or tophi is diagnostic
  - Synovial fluid aspiration reveals negatively birefringent, needle-shaped crystals, up to 60,000 cells/mm^3 with greater than 70% PMNs
  - Aspirate of tophi shows urate crystals (vs. rheumatoid nodules)
- Serum uric acid levels do not always correlate with clinical gout
- 24-hour urine uric acid levels may help distinguish overproduction of uric acid versus underexcretion
  - Urinary uric acid of 400–800 mg/d is normal; elevated levels (>800 mg/d) indicate over-production of uric acid
  - Not useful in patients with renal failure or chronic diuretic use
- X-rays may reveal "punched out" lytic areas with overhanging bony edges (Martel's sign)

TREATMENT & MANAGEMENT

- Discontinue offending drugs, if possible, and attempt to correct contributing lifestyle habits, such as excessive alcohol use, obesity, and lack of exercise
- Acute gouty arthritis can be treated with ice, indomethacin and other NSAIDs, colchicine, or corticosteroids
  - Corticosteroids may be used in severe disease; can be administered orally, IM, IV, or intra-articular
  - Avoid hypouricemic therapy with allopurinol and diuretic use during acute attacks
- Recurrent attacks of acute gout (more than 3 per year) suggest the need for chronic prophylaxis
  - Uricosuric agents (e.g., probenecid, sulfinpyrazone, losartan) decrease renal reabsorp-tion of uric acid and may be effective in underexcretors if tophi are absent and renal function is normal; avoid in patients with a history of renal stones
- Chronic tophaceous gout is treated with allopurinol to decrease the production of uric acid
  - Avoid in patients using azathioprine, 6-mercaptopurine, and trimethoprim

PROGNOSIS & COMPLICATIONS

- Acute attacks are often triggered by trauma, stress, surgery, illness, alcohol, diet, or abrupt changes in uric acid levels
- Tophaceous gout can occur in rare areas, including the conduction system of the heart
- Skin tophi can ulcerate and become infected
- A major cause of morbidity in patients after transplantation, particularly after cardiac transplantation
- Preventive treatment is best via modification of risk factors

Spondyloarthropathy

INTRODUCTION

- A group of inflammatory arthritides with predilection for the sacroiliac joints and entheses (the skeletal attachment of tendons)
- Spondyloarthropathies include ankylosing spondylitis (AS), psoriatic arthritis, enteropathic arthritis, and postinfectious reactive arthritis (Reiter's syndrome)
- Associated with the genetic haplotype HLA-B27
- Extra-articular features are common, including disorders of skin (keratoderma blenorrhagicum), nails, eyes (e.g., iritis), mucosa, and (rarely) the aortic root

ETIOLOGY, EPIDEMIOLOGY, & RISK FACTORS

- These disorders have genetic susceptibilities in common
  - About 90% of affected ankylosing spondylitis patients carry HLA-B27
  - In cases of reactive arthritis, 50–75% of patients carry HLA-B27; in cases of psoriatic arthritis and enteropathic arthritis, HLA-B27 positivity is increased when sacroiliac disease occurs
  - HLA-B27 is found in 7% of the Caucasian population
  - In patients who exhibit the HLA-B27 haplotype, the risk of disease is 10% with a negative family history and 20% with a positive family history
  - There are more than 11 allelic subtypes of HLA-B27
- Infections are thought to be a common trigger
  - In Reiter's syndrome, gastrointestinal and genitourinary infections are most common, including *Chlamydia*, ureaplasma, *Shigella*, *Campylobacter*, and *Clostridium difficile*
- Onset often occurs between the teenage years and middle adulthood
- Males are more commonly affected than females
- Northern European populations, Native-Americans, and South American Indians have the highest prevalence

PATIENT PRESENTATION

- Low back pain associated with at least 1 hour of morning stiffness and improvement with mild to moderate activity
- Limited motion of spine and chest expansion
- Sacroiliitis (tender sacroiliac joints) and large lower extremity joint arthritis
- Enthesopathy: Inflammation, tenderness, swelling, and/or stiffness of entheses (e.g., plantar fascia insertion, Achilles tendon insertion, tibial tubercle, costochondral joints, epicondyles, anterior superior iliac spine, trochanteric insertion)
- AS: Ascending spine stiffness with decreased chest expansion
- Reiter's syndrome: Triad of conjunctivitis, urethritis, and arthritis 2–4 weeks after a gastrointestinal or genitourinary infection
- Enteropathic arthritis: Flare-ups of peripheral arthritis are associated with exacerbations of Crohn's disease or ulcerative colitis

DIFFERENTIAL DX

- Back pain: Mechanical low back pain, osteoarthritis, referred back pain from visceral disease, diffuse idiopathic skeletal hyperostosis, sacroiliac septic arthritis, psoas muscle abscess, discitis, vertebral osteomyelitis (Pott's disease)
- Inflammatory oligoarthritis: Juvenile idiopathic arthritis, gout, septic arthritis, gonococcal arthritis, pseudogout, arthropathy of Whipple's disease, Behçet's disease and other autoimmune arthropathies, rheumatoid arthritis, systemic lupus erythematosus

DIAGNOSTIC EVALUATION

- Primarily a clinical diagnosis based on careful history and physical examination
  - Positive family history of a spondyloarthropathy or psoriasis lends weight to the diagnosis
- X-rays of the sacroiliac joints (Ferguson views taken at a 30-degree cephalad angle) will show sacroiliitis but may take up to 10 years to be diagnostic
  - Bilateral sacroiliitis in AS
  - Unilateral sacroiliitis in Reiter's syndrome, psoriatic arthritis, and enteropathic arthritis
  - Later stage disease may show a "bamboo spine"
- MRI of the sacroiliac joints shows edema and joint effusion
- HLA-B27 testing is not diagnostic but may lend weight to a suspected diagnosis
  - May also be useful for genetic counseling
- Lab changes are generally nonspecific, including elevated ESR or C-reactive protein, anemia of chronic disease, and elevated IgA levels
- In cases of Reiter's syndrome, culture for gastrointestinal or genitourinary organisms may occasionally be useful

TREATMENT & MANAGEMENT

- There is no cure
- Exercise, appropriate rest, and proper sleeping position to avoid neck flexion can improve symptoms
- NSAIDs or intra-articular steroids for pain control and suppression of inflammation
  - Indomethacin is usually more effective than other NSAIDs (avoid in patients with ulcer disease or elevated creatinine)
- Doxycycline for 3 months may be helpful in cases of reactive arthritis or Reiter's syndrome and may also be beneficial in other spondyloarthropathies
- Sulfasalazine has a disease-modifying role in enteropathic, psoriatic, and reactive arthritis
  - Monitor for sulfa toxicity and cytopenias
- Methotrexate is particularly helpful for peripheral joint disease
  - Liver toxicity is a major concern; monitor liver function tests every 1–2 months
- Anti-tumor necrosis factor (anti-TNF) drugs (e.g., etanercept, infliximab, adalimumab) may be useful for cases of AS, psoriatic arthritis, and inflammatory bowel disease
  - These agents appear to make a large impact in patients with severe spondylitis
- Hip replacement and/or surgical correction of deformities may be necessary
- Eye examinations as needed or annually to monitor for uveitis
- Consider echocardiography to assess for aortitis

PROGNOSIS & COMPLICATIONS

- In general, the prognosis of all spondyloarthropathies is good with proper physical therapy, medications, and exercise
- Highly variable prognosis; spontaneous remissions and exacerbations occur, particularly in the early stages of disease
- Morbidity is related to fused joints in the spine
- Complications include severe hip arthritis requiring hip replacement, spinal fractures, uveitis, aortitis, osteoporosis of the spine, secondary amyloidosis, apical pulmonary fibrosis, and complications secondary to chronic NSAID use
- Anti-TNF drugs have significantly improved prognosis in patients with AS
- Enteropathic spondylitis patients are at increased risk for colon cancer

Sjögren's Syndrome

INTRODUCTION

- A chronic autoimmune disease of the exocrine glands
- Destruction of the exocrine glands leads to absence of physiologic secretions and dryness of mucus membranes and conjunctiva, resulting in keratoconjunctivitis sicca, xerostomia, and other manifestations
- Diagnosed by the presence of dry eyes and dry mouth with associated positive autoimmune serologies
- The second most common rheumatic disease

ETIOLOGY, EPIDEMIOLOGY, & RISK FACTORS

- Infiltration of the exocrine glands by lymphocytes, plasma cells, and macrophages occurs, resulting in destruction of the glands, inflammation, and decreased secretions
- May be primary or secondary to a systemic connective tissue disease, such as rheumatoid arthritis, systemic lupus erythematosus, scleroderma, or polymyositis
- The etiology is unknown
- Several genes, including HLA-DR3 and HLA-DR4 loci, are associated with the disease
- Environmental factors, such as viruses, may trigger the disorder in susceptible persons
- The vast majority of cases occur in females
- Lymphoma may occur in cases of longstanding Sjögren's syndrome
- Affects as much as 1% of the population

PATIENT PRESENTATION

- Burning and dryness of the oral mucosa, which may cause sticking of the lips and tongue and increased risk of dental caries
  - Dysphagia occurs secondary to mouth dryness
  - Oral candidiasis can also occur due to mouth dryness; may be associated with angular cheilosis
- Eye dryness causing gritty or sandy discomfort
- Blepharitis with thick mucous eye secretions
- Dry skin
- Dry vaginal mucosa
- Symmetric, nonerosive polyarthralgias affecting the small joints
- Dryness of the respiratory tract causing chronic cough or pulmonary disease due to chronic inflammation
- "Stocking and glove" polyneuropathy may occur due to small-vessel vasculitis
- Bilateral, rubbery parotitis

DIFFERENTIAL DX

- Medication effect (e.g., diuretics, antidepressants, antihistamines)
- Perimenopausal symptoms
- Hypothyroidism
- Postradiation dryness
- Sarcoidosis
- HIV
- Hepatitis C
- Lymphoma
- Amyloidosis
- Tuberculosis
- Hemochromatosis
- Mumps
- Alcoholism
- Dry eyes may be caused by vitamin A deficiency, meibomian gland dysfunction, or drugs (e.g., anticholinergics)

DIAGNOSTIC EVALUATION

- Complete history and physical examination
  - Schirmer's test: Dry eyes are indicated by less than 5 mm of tear production on filter paper that is placed into the patient's lower conjunctival sac for 5 minutes
  - Rose-Bengal test: Rose-Bengal dye is placed into each eye; after blinking, areas of damaged epithelium caused by dryness can be assessed
- Minor salivary gland biopsy is the most specific and sensitive test; will demonstrate lymphocytic infiltration
- Lab values that indicate the possibility of Sjögren's syndrome include positive antinuclear antibodies (ANA), positive rheumatoid factor, and positive SSA or SSB
- Anemia of chronic disease, mild leukopenia, and hypergammaglobulinemia may occur

TREATMENT & MANAGEMENT

- There is no cure; treatment is symptomatic and aimed at improving dry eyes and mouth
- Artificial tears without preservatives are helpful for eye dryness
- Patients require frequent ophthalmologic evaluations (every 6 months to 1 year) to assess for ocular ulcerations; occasionally, punctal plugs must be added if artificial lubrication is insufficient
- Frequent dental visits (every 6 months to 1 year) to assess for dental caries; chewing sugarless gum or sugarless lozenges are helpful, and small sips of water may be useful
- Skin and vaginal lubricants may be used
- Salagen may be used prior to meals and before bedtime
- Treatment of arthritis with NSAIDs or hydroxychloroquine (Plaquenil)
  - Systemic steroids (low-dose prednisone) are generally reserved for severe arthritis or swelling of the glands
- More aggressive therapy with immunosuppressants can be used if systemic symptoms are evident and should prompt a specialist referral

PROGNOSIS & COMPLICATIONS

- The disease progresses over 8–10 years
- Earlier onset and the presence of anti-Ro or anti-La antibodies tend to signify more severe disease
- Complications include corneal ulceration, dental caries, and increased risk of lymphoma
- Systemic manifestations occur in one-third of patients
- Patients with organ system involvement may have a poorer prognosis

Polymyositis

INTRODUCTION

- An inflammatory muscle disease that affects the proximal skeletal muscles of the upper and lower extremities, resulting in bilateral muscle weakness
- Associated skin rash indicates dermatomyositis
- Together, polymyositis and dermatomyositis are the most common acquired causes of muscle weakness
- Characterized by elevated creatine phosphokinase (CK) enzyme levels
- May be associated with other connective tissue diseases, such as systemic lupus erythematosus or scleroderma

ETIOLOGY, EPIDEMIOLOGY, & RISK FACTORS

- An immune-mediated process of unknown etiology
- Environmental factors are thought to trigger the disease in genetically susceptible persons
- Several infectious agents are thought to be the underlying trigger, particularly Coxsackie B virus or *Toxoplasma gondii*
- Antigen-derived T cells attack myofibrils expressing class I major histocompatibility complex (MHC) antigens, causing invasion of myofibrils with CD8-positive mononuclear cells
- Muscle weakness may be a direct result of inflammatory cells causing muscle necrosis and fibrosis or of abnormalities in the contractile process
- Annual incidence of 2–10 new cases per million persons
- May occur in any age group
- Predominantly seen in women

PATIENT PRESENTATION

- Symmetric, bilateral, proximal muscle weakness occurring over a 3- to 6-month period
  - Patients may complain of difficulty combing hair or rising from a seated or prone position
- Myalgia or arthralgia
- Atrophy of the involved muscles
- Neck muscle weakness occurs in half of cases
- Ocular muscles are not involved, but dysphagia may occur due to involvement of the esophageal muscles
- Systemic symptoms may occur, including fatigue, weight loss, fever, malaise, and morning stiffness
- Patients may present acutely with rhabdomyolysis and myoglobinuria
- Pulmonary or cardiac involvement may occur
- Dermatomyositis is often preceded by a heliotropic upper eyelid rash and periorbital edema, macular facial rash, and rash on knuckles

DIFFERENTIAL DX

Muscle weakness with normal CK level
- Motor neuron disease (ALS)
- Myasthenia gravis
- Muscular dystrophy
- Inherited myopathies
- Steroids
- Neoplasm

Weakness with elevated CK
- Hypothyroidism
- Sarcoidosis
- Inclusion body myositis
- Amyloidosis
- Trauma
- Infections (e.g., Epstein-Barr, HIV, influenza, rubella, CMV)
- Drugs (e.g., penicillamine, statins, cocaine, alcohol)

DIAGNOSTIC EVALUATION

- Complete history and physical examination
- Initial laboratory workup will reveal elevations of skeletal muscle-derived enzymes, including total CK level, aldolase, AST, ALT, and LDH
  - Tests for inflammation (e.g., ESR, CRP) may or may not be normal
- Diagnosis is established by an abnormal muscle biopsy
- Electromyography (EMG) is helpful to document a myopathic pattern, which is interpreted as increased insertional activity, fibrillations, sharp positive waves, spontaneous high-frequency discharges, and polyphasic motor unit potentials with low amplitude and short duration
  - EMG is normal in 10% of cases
- MRI with T2-weighted images and fat suppression can detect subtle changes of muscle inflammation, which may prove useful to guide the site of muscle biopsy
- Myositis-specific autoantibodies can be seen, including anti-Jo-1, which may herald the onset of pulmonary involvement

TREATMENT & MANAGEMENT

- Referral to a specialist is warranted to confirm the diagnosis and guide therapy
- Treatment is aimed at increasing muscle strength
- Immunosuppression is the mainstay of therapy
  - Prednisone is administered for 3–6 months until clinical improvement occurs and then is slowly tapered
  - Most patients will improve with steroid therapy; many will achieve complete remission
  - Other immunosuppressive agents include azathioprine and methotrexate; these may be added to steroids if the patient does not respond within 3 months
  - Some patients respond temporarily to intravenous immunoglobulin (IVIG)
- Physical therapy to encourage passive range of motion and prevent contractures
- Bed rest may be indicated during periods of severe inflammation

PROGNOSIS & COMPLICATIONS

- Symptoms progress over weeks to months
- Dermatomyositis has a better prognosis (80% 5-year survival)
- Most deaths occur from pulmonary or cardiac complications, including conduction defects, arrhythmias, dilated cardiomyopathy, interstitial lung disease, and pulmonary dysfunction
- Other complications include joint contractures and subcutaneous calcifications
- There is an increased incidence of melanoma and breast, ovarian, and colon cancers
- Complications from immunosuppressive therapy can occur, including diabetes, osteoporosis, and infections
- Patients with dysphagia are at risk for aspiration
- Disease may recur long after the initial illness

Dermatology

Pruritus

INTRODUCTION

- Pruritus, or itching, is the most common dermatologic complaint
- Pruritus is not itself serious, but it may be a clinical manifestation of an underlying dermatologic or systemic disease (e.g., urticaria, uremia, liver disease); however, identifying the underlying etiology may be difficult, and symptomatic treatment may be all that can be offered initially
- Pruritus can occur with or without a skin rash
  - Skin changes may be induced by scratching

ETIOLOGY, EPIDEMIOLOGY, & RISK FACTORS

- The sensation of itching can originate at any point along the afferent pathway from the skin to the brain: The impulse is transmitted through C fibers that originate superficially in the skin; the dorsal horn of the spinal cord and the spinothalamic tract convey the impulse to the thalamus and the somatosensory cortex
  - Mediators of itch include histamine, serotonin, acetylcholine, leukotrienes, prostaglandins, cytokines, and opioids
- Underlying systemic disease may be present in patients with pruritus without rash
  - Systemic etiologies include hepatobiliary disorders (e.g., cholestasis), chronic renal failure (uremia), hypo- or hyperthyroidism, polycythemia vera, malignancies (e.g., Hodgkin's lymphoma), and HIV
- Pruritus with an associated rash is often related to infection or dermatologic disease
  - Infectious etiologies include fungi (e.g., *Tinea*, candidiasis), viruses (e.g., varicella), bacteria (e.g., *Corynebacterium*), insect vectors (e.g., scabies, lice, flea bits, mosquito bites), and mixed infections (e.g., intertrigo)
  - Noninfectious etiologies include contact dermatitis, atopic dermatitis, eczema, pityriasis rosea, lichen planus, and psoriasis
- The prevalence of itch increases with age

PATIENT PRESENTATION

- Atopic dermatitis (eczema): Dry, scaly, fine papules often with a "sandpaper" texture; may have surrounding erythema or hyperpigmentation
- Contact dermatitis: Lesions may be macular or papular and are often erythematous
- Urticaria (hives): Erythematous, raised wheels with central pallor that often appear on the face or extremities
  - May present with angioedema (swelling of the face, tongue, larynx, or gastrointestinal system)
- Scabies: Areas of papules and excoriated lesions, particularly in the digital web spaces and antecubital and inguinal regions; occasionally, thin, grey or brownish burrows occur, which are very contagious
- Pediculosis (lice): May occur on the trunk, head, or pubic area; the louse or the eggs (nits) appear on the hair shafts

DIFFERENTIAL DX

- Isolated pruritis
- Pruritis secondary to underlying infection, dermatologic disease, or systemic disorder (refer to etiology section)
- Drug reaction (e.g., aspirin, alcohol, morphine, codeine)
- Senescence (pruritis is very common in the elderly)
- Psychogenic (e.g., emotional stress)
- Fiberglass exposure

DIAGNOSTIC EVALUATION

- History and physical examination
  - Note presence of skin lesions that preceded the itching, timing (new vs. recurrent, acute vs. chronic), associated systemic symptoms (e.g., fever, malaise, weight loss, night sweats), evidence of systemic disease (e.g., uremia, liver disease), and pregnancy
  - Note past medical and family history (e.g., asthma, psoriasis) and exposure history (e.g., poison ivy, poison oak, or poison sumac)
  - Complete review of systems may identify underlying disease (e.g., change in bowel habits with colon cancer, cold intolerance with hypothyroidism, abdominal pain with liver disease)
  - Detailed medication history
  - Complete skin examination to determine the presence or absence of primary skin disease and to define the type of rash or specific abnormalities
  - Assess exposure to other individuals (family, friends, contacts) with similar complaints
- Lab testing if pruritis lasts longer than 2 weeks may include complete blood count with differential, liver function tests, renal function tests, and thyroid function tests; other testing may be indicated based on clinical suspicions
- Scrape lesions and perform KOH test if fungal infection is suspected
- Scrape possible burrow site to identify a mite in scabies
- Patch testing may be done if allergic contact dermatitis is suspected
- Punch biopsy may be done to establish a histologic diagnosis
- Consider referral to a dermatologist if the diagnosis remains unclear

TREATMENT & MANAGEMENT

- Symptomatic treatment is often sufficient
  - Avoid hot baths/showers and harsh soaps; bathe with lukewarm water and bath oil; limit the use of soap as much as possible
  - Apply an emollient immediately after bathing; emollients with menthol will provide a cooling sensation, emollients with phenol or camphor will provide an anesthetic effect
  - Oral antihistamines (e.g., hydroxyzine, diphenhydramine) may be used but are sedating (nonsedating antihistamines are not effective in reducing pruritis); benzodiazepines may be used adjunctively if antihistamines are ineffective
  - Low-dose topical corticosteroids may be used for short durations
  - Ultraviolet light therapy may be helpful in some cases
- Oral corticosteroids are a last resort to interrupt the inflammatory cascade; however, a thorough evaluation for a secondary cause of pruritis (e.g., infection) should be pursued prior to beginning oral corticosteroids
- Pruritic lesions may become infected due to excessive scratching and excoriation; antibiotics may be necessary
- Ultimate treatment is aimed at the underlying etiology

PROGNOSIS & COMPLICATIONS

- Although pruritis is not an emergent issue, it can be very uncomfortable and lead to anxiety, depression, and loss of sleep
- Pruritis often resolves on its own or upon elimination of the underlying cause
- If pruritis is persistent after routine interventions, a dermatology and/or allergy referral may be warranted

Urticaria (Hives)

INTRODUCTION

- Urticaria (hives) are well-circumscribed, raised, erythematous, pruritic wheals; they are polymorphic, round, or irregularly shaped with central clearing and range in size from a few millimeters to several centimeters in diameter
- Lesions are transient and typically disappear over a few hours
- Urticarial lesions affect the superficial dermis; in contrast, angioedema involves the deeper dermis and subcutaneous tissues
- Affects up to 25% of the population

ETIOLOGY, EPIDEMIOLOGY, & RISK FACTORS

- Most cases are immunologically mediated
  - Type I reaction (IgE hypersensitivity): Reaction to foods, drugs, Latex, venom, and other allergens results in histamine release from mast cells, local vasodilation and edema, and an inflammatory response with wheals and erythema
  - Type II reaction (cytotoxic antibody): Due to transfusion reaction
  - Type III reaction (antigen-antibody complex): Due to serum sickness
  - Type IV reaction (delayed-type sensitivity): Due to drugs, foods, or animal exposures
  - Other cases involve autoimmune diseases (e.g., vasculitis, thyroiditis, SLE), infections (e.g., *Helicobacter pylori*, viruses), and malignancies (e.g., lymphoma)
- Nonimmune cases may be caused by physical entities (e.g., dermatographism, cold, sun exposure), direct mast cell degranulation caused by certain drugs (e.g., opiates, NSAIDs, vancomycin, radiocontrast media), and foods with high histamine content (e.g., shellfish)
- Acute urticaria (less than 6 weeks) accounts for more than two-thirds of cases
- Chronic urticaria (episodes occurring at least twice weekly for more than 6 weeks) accounts for about 30% of cases
- Up to 50% of patients with urticaria have angioedema
- A family or personal history of atopy may be present

PATIENT PRESENTATION

- Lesions are intensely pruritic, erythematous, and well circumscribed and display central clearing
- Lesions appearing after cold exposure (e.g., ice cube) suggest cold-induced urticaria
- Punctate lesions after exercise or hot showers suggest a cholinergic response
- Lesions appearing within 30 minutes of food, contact, or medication ingestion may suggest the etiology
- Painful urticaria may be a sign of an underlying vasculitis
- Schnitzler's syndrome: Patients with a mono-clonal IgM or IgG with associated fever, bone pain, adenopathy, weight loss, and urticaria
- Dermatographism: Transient wheal produced by pressure on the skin

DIFFERENTIAL DX

- Contact dermatitis
- Lymphangitis
- Atopic dermatitis
- Mastocytosis
- Angioedema
- Hepatitis B
- Insect bite
- Erythema multiforme
- Dermatitis herpetiformis
- Bullous pemphigoid
- Vasculitis
- Cellulitis
- Muckle-Wells syndrome
- Familial cold autoinflammatory syndrome
- Schnitzler's syndrome

DIAGNOSTIC EVALUATION

- A thorough history and physical exam should guide the workup
  - Pay specific attention to potential triggers (e.g., foods, medications, environmental exposures)
- In patients with acute urticaria, no laboratory workup is necessary; however, a symptom diary may be useful
- In patients with chronic urticaria, concerning features of the history and physical examination should prompt a diagnostic evaluation; a complete blood count with a differential cell count and an erythrocyte sedimentation rate (ESR) is a cost-effective screen
  - Additional testing for patients with elevated ESR may include liver function tests, serum protein electrophoresis, hepatitis serologies, complement levels, antinuclear antibodies (ANA), or IgE antibodies
- Consider a punch biopsy if vasculitis is a possibility (e.g., painful urticaria)

TREATMENT & MANAGEMENT

- Identify and remove the offending trigger, if possible
  - Consider an elimination diet to pinpoint suspicious foods
- H1 receptor blockers (e.g., hydroxyzine, diphenhydramine) have the quickest onset and are often the initial choice for symptomatic relief
  - Cyproheptadine has been shown to be helpful for cold-induced urticaria
  - Longer acting agents, such as loratadine, fexofenadine, or desloratadine, may be more convenient for patients
- H2 receptor blockers (e.g., ranitidine, cimetidine) are often helpful in treating urticaria that is refractory to therapy with H1 receptor blockers
- Doxepin has both H1 and H2 receptor blockade properties and may be very effective in treating urticaria
- Corticosteroids do not block mast cell degranulation and, therefore, are often not helpful in treating urticaria; however, a trial of high-dose prednisone tapered to the lowest effective dose may be indicated
- Leukotriene inhibitors may be beneficial as add-on therapy with antihistamines
- An epinephrine pen should be prescribed for any patient who has angioedema associated with urticaria

PROGNOSIS & COMPLICATIONS

- In the vast majority of cases of acute urticaria, symptoms resolve spontaneously within 24 hours or upon removal of the offending agent
- Recent data suggest that almost 50% of patients with chronic urticaria have spontaneous resolution of symptoms in less than 1 year
- Patients with physical urticaria are often refractory to treatment
- Some cases may be lifelong

Hyperhidrosis

INTRODUCTION

- Hyperhidrosis is a disorder characterized by excessive sweating
- May be generalized (entire body) or localized (e.g., palms, soles, forehead)
- May be primary (idiopathic) or secondary to a disease or medication
- This can be an embarrassing problem that patients may not spontaneously report but may be evident on physical examination
- Hyperhidrosis is present in approximately 3% of the population and is most commonly idiopathic

ETIOLOGY, EPIDEMIOLOGY, & RISK FACTORS

- Human sweat (eccrine) glands are sympathetically mediated via noradrenergic fibers that are affected by emotions and by cholinergic fibers that are affected by temperature changes
- Emotionally induced sweating tends to be localized to the palms, soles, and occasionally the forehead
- Axillary sweating appears to be induced by both emotional and thermal sweating
- Generalized hyperhidrosis may be caused by temperature increases (e.g., heat, humidity, exercise, fever), metabolic conditions, neurologic conditions, situations resulting in sympathetic discharge (e.g., intense pain, drug withdrawal states, alcohol intake), or medications (e.g., estrogen, SSRIs, stimulants, antipyretics, meperidine, emetics)
- Localized hyperhidrosis is most commonly idiopathic but may also occur due to heat, olfactory or gustatory stimuli, or neurologic lesions
- Familial hyperhidrosis is common
- Palmoplantar (palms of hands and soles of feet) hyperhidrosis is common
- Usually begins in childhood or adolescence and is more common in females

PATIENT PRESENTATION

- Excessive perspiration or sweating
- Other signs and symptoms may be present depending upon the underlying etiology (e.g., fatigue, decreased reflex relaxation in secondary hyperhidrosis due to hypothyroidism)

DIFFERENTIAL DX

- Emotional upset or stress
- Drug induced
- Exercise
- Defervescence after fever
- Diabetes mellitus
- Hypothyroidism
- Hypopituitarism
- Hypoglycemia
- Familial dysautonomia
- Tumor
- Chédiak-Higashi syndrome
- Pheochromocytoma
- Vitiligo
- Physiologic gustatory sweat
- Spinal cord transection
- Syringomyelia
- Raynaud's phenomenon
- Thoracic sympathetic trunk injury

DIAGNOSTIC EVALUATION

- History and physical examination to distinguish localized versus generalized hyperhidrosis and primary versus secondary disease
- Primary hyperhidrosis can be treated without additional workup; however, if the diagnosis is in doubt, an investigation for a cause should be sought
- If secondary hyperhidrosis is considered, a thorough workup may be necessary to determine the underlying etiology

TREATMENT & MANAGEMENT

- Focal hyperhidrosis can be treated with topical 20% aluminum chloride (Drysol) nightly
  - Must be applied to dry skin because it will react with moisture to create hydrochloric acid, which is very irritating
  - Less effective topical agents include boric acid, anticholinergic medications, tannic acid, resorcinol, potassium permanganate, formaldehyde, and glutaraldehyde
  - Apply just before bedtime for 7–10 nights, and then once weekly for maintenance
- Patients may then use regular daytime applications of baking soda as needed to maintain dryness and limit skin irritation
- Botulinum toxin injections are beneficial but must be repeated regularly
- Iontophoresis (a low electrical current device that alters the permeability of the epidermis) may be effective, but treatment must be repeated regularly
  - Home iontophoresis units now make this treatment more practical
  - May use tap water alone or a combination of tap water, aluminum hydroxide, and an anticholinergic medication
- Generalized hyperhidrosis can be managed by alpha-blockers (e.g., phenoxybenzamine, clonidine), muscarinic blockers (e.g., propantheline, glycopyrrolate), calcium channel blockers (e.g., diltiazem), NSAIDs (e.g., indomethacin), or tranquilizers (e.g., diazepam)
- Regional sympathectomy or excision of axillary sweat glands may be indicated in extreme cases

PROGNOSIS & COMPLICATIONS

- The prognosis for continued hyperhidrosis is poor unless continuous treatment is used; however, aluminum chloride appears to cause atrophy of secretory cells over time, which may decrease the severity of the symptoms
- Serious complications are rare, but embarrassment, skin irritation, itching, and skin breakdown can occur
- Skin infection is a rare complication

Dry Skin

INTRODUCTION

- Xerosis, or dry skin, is extremely common
- Dry skin has a low level of sebum and can be prone to sensitivity
- Low humidity and cold temperatures make winter xerosis a common complaint
- Mild xerosis can cause impaired skin barrier function and allow irritants and allergens to more easily affect the skin
- Most common on the legs, but can affect the entire skin surface
- Can present with severe pruritus without much evidence of a rash
- Nearly all cases are benign
- Simple measures, such as daily emollient use, can make a big difference in patients' lives

ETIOLOGY, EPIDEMIOLOGY, & RISK FACTORS

- Excess water loss from the epidermis results in dehydration of the stratum corneum and cell shrinkage
- The outer keratin layers require 10–20% water concentration to maintain their integrity
- A significant decrease in free fatty acids in the stratum corneum results in transepidermal water loss to 75 times that of healthy skin
- Multiple etiologic factors may coexist, including environmental factors, physiologic factors, nutritional factors, or pre-existing disease
  - Environmental factors include prolonged bathing in hot water, use of harsh soaps, infrequent use of emollients, use of degreasing agents (cleansers), low humidity, and excessive winds
  - Physiologic factors include decreased sebaceous or sweat gland activity, low keratin synthesis, increasing age (which results in decreased rate of skin repair)
  - Nutritional factors include nutritional deficiencies (e.g., zinc, essential fatty acids)
  - Pre-existing diseases that contribute to dry skin include atopy, ichthyosis, thyroid disease, neurologic disorders, and malignancies

PATIENT PRESENTATION

- May be generalized or local
  - Commonly occurs on the anterior shins, extensor arms, and flanks
- The skin may have a parched look due to its inability to retain moisture; chapping, erythema, scaling, and cracking are signs of extremely dehydrated skin
- Excoriations may be present due to excessive rubbing or scratching
- Patients may complain of tightness, chapping, and flaking of the skin, especially at cold temperatures or after bathing
- Seasonality is prominent; many patients present during the winter months, especially in areas where indoor humidity is decreased by heating

DIFFERENTIAL DX

- Allergic contact dermatitis
- Irritant contact dermatitis
- Atopic dermatitis
- Nummular eczema
- Drug induced (e.g., diuretics, antispasmodics, antihistamines)
- Mycosis fungoides
- Inheritable icthyoses
- Nutritional deficiency
- Parapsoriasis

DIAGNOSTIC EVALUATION

- Perform a complete history, including social, family, environmental, and exposure history, as well as past medical history, along with a focused physical examination including thyroid and skin exams
  - Note frequency of bathing, showering, and cleansing and which soaps and cleansers are used
  - Note the types of skin lubricants used and method and frequency of application
  - Dietary history may be revealing
  - Note types of clothing worn (wool may cause irritation)
- If xerosis is severe, of acute onset, or associated with intractable pruritus or other systemic symptoms, consider a complete blood count and thyroid function tests
- Consider HIV testing for patients at risk who have severe xerosis of recent onset
- If the patient fails to respond to conservative therapy, age-appropriate malignancy screening may be indicated
- In patients with underlying hepatic or renal disease causing secondary xerosis, the pruritus can be especially severe

TREATMENT & MANAGEMENT

- During bathing use lukewarm water (hot water can dry out the skin), and limit bathing to no more than 15 minutes once a day to avoid stripping the skin of its natural oils
- Avoid harsh soaps that may dry out the skin, including deodorant soaps; instead, use non-detergent, neutral pH products such as Dove, Oil of Olay Sensitive Skin, Cetaphil, and Aquaphor
  - Liquid skin cleansers containing petrolatum, such as Dove and Olay body washes, are also advisable
- Avoid vigorous use of a washcloths during cleansing; when towel drying, blot or pat dry, rather than rubbing the skin
- Apply oil-based moisturizing emollients (e.g., petroleum jelly ointment, Aquaphor) or creams (e.g., Eucerin, Cetaphil) twice daily; in general, water-based lotions should be avoided
- Lactic acid-containing moisturizers (e.g., AmLactin, Lac-Hydrin) may be used once daily to particularly scaly patches
- Use a humidifier during the winter months
- Drink plenty of water and ensure appropriate intake of essential fatty acids
- Avoid irritating fabrics such as wool; use cotton clothing and cotton bedding
- Topical steroid ointments may be necessary to control pruritis in severe cases

PROGNOSIS & COMPLICATIONS

- Xerosis responds well to therapy; however, if the causative factors are not identified, recurrences are common
- Nonhealing or recalcitrant areas may represent another diagnosis
- Generalized xerosis is rare and should provoke a search for underlying malignancy

Acne Vulgaris

- Acne, the most common of all skin disorders, is an inflammatory disease of pilosebaceous follicles
- It affects 17 million people in the United States, including 85% of adolescents and young adults

ETIOLOGY, EPIDEMIOLOGY, & RISK FACTORS

- There is a genetic predisposition, but the pathogenesis is multifactorial, including sebum secretion and retention under androgen stimulus, overgrowth of *Propionibacterum acnes* bacteria, hyperproliferation of epithelial cells causing obstruction of the pilosebaceous follicles, and inflammation
  - Obstruction of the pilosebaceous follicle leads to retention of sebum, which is an ideal media for growth of *P. acnes* bacteria, and may result in rupture of the follicle
  - Both of these consequences lead to the typical inflammatory reaction of acne
- Cosmetic agents and hair pomades may worsen acne
- Medications that promote acne include steroids, lithium, some antiepileptics, and iodides
  - Testosterone stimulates sebum production; estrogen suppresses it; thus, oral contraceptives may prevent acne
- Congenital adrenal hyperplasia, polycystic ovary syndrome (PCOS), Cushing's disease, and other endocrine disorders associated with excess androgens may trigger acne
- More common in males than in females during adolescence
- More common in women than in men during adulthood
- May be present in newborns due to the influence of maternal hormones; this form of acne resolves but may recur during adrenarche

PATIENT PRESENTATION

- Acne vulgaris is characterized by comedones, papules, pustules, and nodules in areas with increased concentrations of sebaceous glands
  - The face may be the only involved skin surface, but the chest, back, and upper arms are often involved
- Characterized by severity type:
  - I: Noninflammatory comedonal acne: Open ("whitehead") and closed ("blackhead") comedones without inflammatory lesions
  - II: Mild inflammatory acne with inflammatory papules and comedones
  - III: Moderate inflammatory acne: Comedones, inflammatory papules, and pustules
  - IV: Nodulocystic acne: Inflammatory lesions, large nodules >5 mm in diameter, and scarring
- Local symptoms may include pain or tenderness
- Menstruation may worsen acne
- May be pruritic

DIFFERENTIAL DX

- Folliculitis (particularly due to *Pityrosporum*)
- Perioral dermatitis
- Acne rosacea
- Acne conglobata
- Acne fulminans
- Syringomas
- Cellulitis
- Herpes zoster
- Adenoma sebaceum
- Multiple trichoepitheliomas
- Miliaria ("heat rash")
- Erythema infectiosum
- Hidradenitis suppurative
- Pyoderma faciale

DIAGNOSTIC EVALUATION

- Acne is a clinical diagnosis
  - Examination should include the face, chest, and back
  - Comedones are the hallmark: Open ("blackheads") comedones are follicles with dilated, black orifices; closed ("whiteheads") comedones are white papules without surrounding erythema
  - Assess for severe acne: Inflammatory papules, pustules, cysts, nodules, scars, and pits
  - Document the number of comedones, inflammatory lesions, scars, and cysts
  - Assess acne severity (mild, moderate, or severe) based on the number, size, and extent of lesions, as well as the presence or absence of scarring
- Patients with evidence of virilization should have total testosterone and DHEA-S levels evaluated to assess for PCOS or adrenal tumors
- Findings of Cushing's disease should prompt evaluation of a 24-hour urine cortisol
- If acne remains recalcitrant to therapy, consider skin cultures to rule out gram-negative organisms and *Pityrosporum* folliculitis

TREATMENT & MANAGEMENT

- Patient education: Dispel common myths (e.g., acne is *not* caused by dirt or diet), counsel against behaviors that may worsen acne (e.g., picking at lesions, using oil-containing cosmetics/moisturizers), and assess the level of psychological distress
- Instruct patients to use mild cleansers and noncomedogenic moisturizes with sunscreen and avoid excessive irritation or scrubbing of the face
- Topical therapies include benzoyl peroxide, antibiotics, retinoids, and salicylic acid
- Intralesional steroids may be used to transiently decrease inflammation in severe cases
- Systemic therapies include oral antibiotics (e.g., tetracycline, erythromycin, ampicillin) and hormonal therapy (e.g., low-dose oral contraceptives, spironolactone)
- Isotretinoin (Accutane) may be used with caution for severe cystic acne unresponsive to conventional therapy
  - Highly teratogenic and absolutely contraindicated in pregnancy; patients should be warned to use appropriate contraception, and they must submit formal consent
  - May be associated with an increased risk of suicide in adolescents
- Dermatologist referral is warranted for severe acne, refractory disease despite appropriate therapy, consideration of isotretinoin treatment, and management of acne scars
- Other treatments may include dermabrasion, peels, and ablative laser treatments for acne scars

PROGNOSIS & COMPLICATIONS

- The overall prognosis is good; however, acne can result in long-lasting psychosocial impairment and physical scarring
- In male patients, acne generally clears by early adulthood; female patients may have more persistent acne
- Patients should be instructed to use mild cleansers and noncomedogenic moisturizers with sunscreen and avoid excessive irritation or scrubbing of the face
- Comedone extraction may be performed with a comedone extractor
- Dry skin is a complication of many acne drugs

Seborrheic Dermatitis

INTRODUCTION

- Also known as seborrheic eczema, pityriasis capitis, or dandruff, seborrheic dermatitis is a common dermatosis with uncertain pathophysiology
- Characterized by red, flaking, greasy patches of skin
- Often seen in combination with rosacea or acne

ETIOLOGY, EPIDEMIOLOGY, & RISK FACTORS

- No clear etiology has been identified but several hypotheses exist, including overgrowth of *Malassezia* yeast, abnormal immune response to *Malassezia* yeast, or excessive sebum production, which has a permissive growth effect on *Malassezia*
- Most likely, seborrheic dermatitis is a combination of increased sebum, increased yeast, and a resultant inappropriate immune response
- Affects 1–3% of immunocompetent adults and up to 80% of immunocompromised adults
- Can also occur in infants within the first 6 months of life
- Affects males more commonly than females
- Most common in adolescents/young adults and adults over age 50
- Commonly seen in Parkinson's disease, mood disorders, and HIV/AIDS
- May be associated with alcoholic pancreatitis, hepatitis C infection, malignancies, and following PUVA (psoralen plus ultraviolet A light) treatment

PATIENT PRESENTATION

- Usually asymptomatic, but patients may have mild pruritus
- Appears as symmetrical, red, flaking, greasy patches of skin
- Scale may have a bran-like appearance
- Most commonly affects the scalp, eyebrows, nasolabial folds, ears, chest, and flexural areas
- In dark-skinned patients, patches may be hypopigmented and circinate, which is referred to as petaloid seborrheic dermatitis
- Infantile seborrheic dermatitis commonly affects the vertex and is called "cradle cap"
  - Other affected areas in infants include the eyebrows, flexures, and paranasal folds
- Immunocompromised patients demonstrate a thicker scale with increased erythema and seborrhea; the upper extremities are more commonly affected than the face or scalp

DIFFERENTIAL DX

- Sebopsoriasis
- Rosacea
- Malar rash of lupus
- Tinea faciei
- On body: Pityriasis rosea, tinea versicolor
- In intertriginous areas: Erythrasma, inverse psoriasis, candidiasis
- In infants: Atopic dermatitis, Langerhans cell histiocytosis, irritant diaper dermatitis, candidiasis, Leiner's disease, Omenn's syndrome

DIAGNOSTIC EVALUATION

- History and skin examination
- Skin scraping with KOH to rule out tinea infection
- Skin biopsy is usually not necessary for diagnosis but may be wise in severe or persistent cases (especially in infants older than 8 months of age with severe presentation to rule out Langerhans cell histiocytosis)
  - Histologically, spongiform dermatitis is present with dermal edema and occasional "squirting" of granulocytes from the dermal papillae into the epidermis
  - Epidermal proliferation and parakeratosis are also evident
  - In longstanding lesions, there is less spongiosis and more psoriasiform hyperplasia with elongated rete ridges
  - In immunocompromised patients, the histology is slightly different; there is more widespread parakeratosis, keratinocyte necrosis, and leukoexocytosis, and superficial perivascular plasma cells may be seen

TREATMENT & MANAGEMENT

- Good hygiene to prevent accumulation of sebum
- The treatment strategy includes: 1) reduce yeast burden with antifungals; 2) reduce inflammation with steroids, and 3) reduce scale with keratolytic agents
- Topical agents are often used in combination; shampoos can be applied to scalp or to face as a wash
  - Tar shampoo or lotion
  - Benzoyl peroxide
  - Propylene glycol
  - Low-potency topical steroids
  - Zinc pyrithione shampoo or cream
  - Ketoconazole cream or shampoo
  - Ciclopirox shampoo or cream
  - Metronidazole gel
  - Terbinafine 1% solution
- Oral agents (which have potentially severe side effects) are reserved for severe seborrheic dermatitis
  - Ketoconazole for 4 weeks
  - Itraconazole for 7 days
  - Terbinafine for 4 weeks

PROGNOSIS & COMPLICATIONS

- Often has a chronic, recurrent course
- Once the initial flare is under control, a single agent, such as Nizoral shampoo, should be used weekly for maintenance
- Infantile seborrheic dermatitis often resolves by 8 months of age

Atopic Dermatitis

INTRODUCTION

- Atopic dermatitis is a chronic inflammatory disease of the epidermis and dermis
- Atopic dermatitis, contact dermatitis, and seborrheic dermatitis are all members of the eczematous dermatitis family of superficial, erythematous, intensely pruritic skin lesions
- Often associated with a personal or family history of atopy (an inherited predisposition to asthma, allergic rhinitis, conjunctivitis, or atopic eczema)
- The terms "dermatitis" and "eczema" are often used as general terminology for atopic dermatitis
- Uncontrollable itching, which disrupts quality of life, is a prominent feature of the disease

ETIOLOGY, EPIDEMIOLOGY, & RISK FACTORS

- An allergic, pruritic dermatitis induced by specific triggers
- Allergic triggers are evidenced by the finding that 85% of affected patients have elevated serum IgE levels and positive allergy skin tests to a variety of food and inhaled allergens
- The precise immunologic mechanisms are not completely understood
- Allergic diseases are present in 25% of the population, and the incidence is increasing worldwide
- There is a positive family history in the majority of patients
- Affects all races and ages, usually starting during early childhood
  - 60% of affected patients are affected within the first year of life, but remission occurs in 75% of cases by age 15
- There is an increased incidence of atopic dermatitis and other allergic disease in urban areas and developed countries, especially Western societies
- There is a hypothesis that atopic-associated diseases occur in part due to decreased microbial exposure in early life

PATIENT PRESENTATION

- Intense pruritis with erythema, edematous papules, crusting, and excoriation
- Skin becomes chronically dry, hyperkeratotic, and lichenified; may result in exfoliation
- Dry, flaky skin appears over red, inflamed areas, causing intense itching and burning
- Has been called "an itch that rashes" because patients often develop a rash secondary to chronic scratching of pruritic skin areas
- Familiar pattern involvement of flexor surfaces, such as the antecubital and popliteal fossa, neck, wrists, and ankles
- Signs of scratching and rubbing of the affected skin are particularly problematic at night and may interfere with sleep
- In between flares, skin may appear normal or have chronic eczema

DIFFERENTIAL DX

- Allergic contact dermatitis
- Irritant contact dermatitis
- Seborrheic dermatitis
- Cutaneous T-cell lymphoma
- Psoriasiform eruptions
- Pityriasis rubra pilaris
- Scabies
- Glucogonoma syndrome
- Pellagra
- Drug reactions

DIAGNOSTIC EVALUATION

- A clinical diagnosis; testing is rarely needed
- Clinical criteria include the presence of at least 3 major and 3 minor criteria
- Major criteria:
  - Pruritis
  - Chronic or relapsing dermatitis
  - Dermatitis affecting flexural surfaces in adults or face and extensors in infants
  - Personal or family history of cutaneous or respiratory atopy
- Minor criteria:
  - Features of atopic facies (e.g., hypopigmented patches, cheilitis)
  - Sensitivity to typical triggers, including foods (e.g., milk, eggs, peanuts), emotional stress, environmental allergens, and skin irritants (e.g., wool, solvents, sweat)
  - Complications of atopic dermatitis (e.g., cutaneous infections)
  - Others: Early age of onset, dry skin, ichthyosis, hyperlinear palms
- 80% of patients have elevated total serum IgE levels
- Skin prick test and radioallergosorbent test (RAST) for inhalant and food allergens are frequently positive

TREATMENT & MANAGEMENT

- The goal of treatment is to improve symptoms while minimizing exposure to potentially toxic drugs
- Eliminate or mitigate exacerbating factors (e.g., low humidity, emotional stress, dry skin, rapid temperature changes, exposure to solvents/detergents)
- Keep the skin moisturized using emollients applied immediately after bathing
  - Thick creams: Eucerin, Cetaphil, Nutraderm
  - Ointments: Petroleum jelly, Aquaphor, petrolatum
- Mild disease: Low-potency (1% or 2.5%) hydrocortisone cream
- Moderate-severe disease: Medium-potency (0.1%) triamcinolone ointment, topical calcineurin inhibitors (e.g., pimecrolimus, tacrolimus), or oral calcineurin inhibitors (e.g., cyclosporine, tacrolimus)
- Acute flares can be treated with higher potency topical corticosteroids for up to 10 days or short courses of systemic steroids
- Antihistamines are used as an adjunctive therapy for pruritis and eye irritation
  - Sedating antihistamines (e.g., diphenhydramine, hydroxyzine, cyproheptadine) are most effective at night
- Phototherapy, immunosuppressants, and coal tar may be tried
- Dietary modification, including probiotics, may be helpful
- Antibiotics for secondary bacterial infections

PROGNOSIS & COMPLICATIONS

- May improve with time, recur, or remain a chronic disorder
- Exclusive breastfeeding during the initial 6 months of life is associated with decreased incidence and severity
- Local skin infections occur in 30% of patients
  - Secondary bacterial infection with *Staphylococcus aureus*
  - Increased susceptibility to viral infections with molluscum contagiosum and warts
  - Propensity to develop widespread lesions with herpes simplex
  - Fungal infections with *Malassezia furfur*
- Ichthyosis vulgaris: Small scales on the extensor aspects of limbs and back, which may indicate underlying malignancy

Psoriasis

INTRODUCTION

- Psoriasis is a chronic inflammatory disease of the skin that affects nearly 5 million people in the United States (1–2% of the population)
- Peak age of onset is 25–40 for most forms of psoriasis; however, it can occur at any age, including infancy and elderly
- Up to 25% of affected individuals will develop psoriatic arthritis, which can result in permanent joint deformity if left untreated
- Psoriasis can have significant psychosocial and physical impacts
- About 350 deaths occur yearly due to psoriasis and its treatments

ETIOLOGY, EPIDEMIOLOGY, & RISK FACTORS

- A disorder of epidermal hyperproliferation: Psoriatic epithelial cells have a cell cycle one-tenth as long as normal cells, and they take just 1–2 days to migrate to the skin surface from deeper layers in order to be exfoliated (vs. nearly 30 days in normal cells); the rapid lifecycle does not allow these cells to adequately mature; thus, even minor trauma, inflammation, mild sunburn, or humidity can precipitate lesions
- The etiology is multifactorial and has not been completely elucidated; however, a genetic predisposition is involved
  - Up to 75% of patients have a positive family history
  - The most consistently involved gene is HLA-Cw6, which confers 10 times greater risk
  - Psoriatic arthritis is associated with HLA-B27
- There are several types of psoriasis
  - Plaque psoriasis (psoriasis vulgaris) is most common, accounting for 80% of cases
  - Guttate psoriasis is more common in children; may be triggered by streptococcal infection
  - Pustular psoriasis may evolve from longstanding plaque psoriasis
- Exacerbating factors include trauma (Koebner phenomenon), cold and dry climates, stress, smoking, HIV, end of pregnancy, and medications (Plan B contraception, steroid withdrawal, lithium, Plaquenil, NSAIDs, beta-blockers, calcium channel blockers, terbinafine)

PATIENT PRESENTATION

- Plaque psoriasis: Thick, scaling red plaques on the elbows, knees, lower back, gluteal cleft, scalp, palms, and soles; may be extensive
- Guttate psoriasis: "rain droplets" (many small, red, scaling patches, predominantly on the trunk, arms, and legs)
- Inverse psoriasis: Red patches in intertriginous areas (axilla, beneath breasts, umbilicus, groin, genitalia); does not scale like other types
- Erythrodermic psoriasis: Generalized redness and scaling; may be the presenting sign of or may evolve from plaque psoriasis
- Pustular psoriasis: Innumerable tiny pinpoint (sterile) pustules on a red background; may be localized or generalized; may arise in pre-existing plaques; patients may be febrile with severe itch
- Palmar-plantar pustulosis: Many pustules on a red base occurring on the palms and soles
- Nails: Pitted, oils spots, distal onycholysis

DIFFERENTIAL DX

- Eczema
- Tinea infections
- Seborrheic dermatitis
- Lichen planus
- Pityriasis rubra pilaris
- Pityriasis rosea
- Onychomycosis
- Fungal infections (e.g., tinea)
- Cutaneous T-cell lymphoma
- Cutaneous lupus
- Dermatomyositis
- Viral exanthem
- Secondary syphilis
- Folliculitis
- Drug reactions

DIAGNOSTIC EVALUATION

- History and physical examination
  - Note time course of onset, family history, new or changing medications, morning stiffness, arthralgias or arthritis, and preceding illness
  - Evaluate the presentation and distribution of the lesions; nail and scalp changes can be a clue to the diagnosis
  - Removal of a scale produces pinpoint bleeding (Auspitz's sign)
- Skin biopsy is the gold standard for diagnosis
- KOH test and fungal cultures may be indicated to distinguish from fungal infection
- Other testing is based on ruling out other disorders in the differential diagnosis
  - Assess for folliculitis in suspected cases of pustular psoriasis
  - Assess for other causes of erythroderma in suspected cases of erythrodermic psoriasis, including thorough exam for other inflammatory dermatoses, lymphadenopathy, changes of palms and soles, and nail changes, along with CBC with Sézary count and chest X-ray)
- There is no diagnostic test for psoriatic arthritis
  - Joint X-ray shows a "pencil-in-cup" deformity of the digits

TREATMENT & MANAGEMENT

- Treatment is based on the type, extent, distribution, and severity of disease
  - Must weigh individual risk:benefit ratio carefully when considering systemic treatments
  - Limited disease of the hands and feet can be very disabling and may warrant more aggressive treatment despite the small surface area involved
- Topical therapies include medium- to high-potency steroids, calcipotriene, tazarotene (retinoid), tar, or anthralin preparations
  - For thick plaques, salicylic acid and urea preparations may be helpful to reduce scale
- Scalp lesions can be treated with topical steroid shampoos, solutions, or oil preparations, along with tar, anthralin, or salicylic acid shampoos
- Laser treatment can be used for stable recalcitrant plaques
- Phototherapy may be used for more generalized disease: ultraviolet (UV) B, narrow-band UVB, or PUVA (psoralen plus UVA) given 2–3 times per week
  - May combine with oral retinoid, tar, or calcipotriene for increased efficacy
- Systemic treatments include acitretin (oral retinoid), methotrexate, cyclosporine, sulfasalazine, and hydroxyurea (avoid systemic prednisone)
  - Medications under investigation include infliximab, etanercept, efalizumab, and alefacept
- Antibiotics may be indicated in cases of guttate psoriasis following streptococcal infection
- Patients with psoriatic arthritis should be referred to rheumatology
- May have psychosocial impact comparable to other chronic diseases; treat as necessary

PROGNOSIS & COMPLICATIONS

- The clinical course is unpredictable; it tends to wax and wane over lifetime
  - May persist in a localized form or progress to more extensive involvement
- Guttate psoriasis may remit completely or may develop into plaque psoriasis
- Arthritis may result in permanent joint deformity
- Erythrodermic and generalized pustular forms often require hospitalization
  - Dehydration, electrolyte abnormalities, high-output cardiac failure, acute respiratory distress syndrome, and hepatitis have been reported in these patients
- Complications from treatment may include atrophy, striae, telangiectasias, increased risk of skin cancers (PUVA therapy), cytopenia, hepatitis, cirrhosis, nephrotoxicity, opportunistic infections, hypertriglyceridemia (retinoid therapy), and many others

Herpes Zoster

INTRODUCTION

- Varicella zoster virus is the causative agent of varicella (chickenpox) and herpes zoster (shingles); after natural infection with the virus or immunization, the virus remains latent in the sensory dorsal root ganglion cells; herpes zoster represents the reactivation of latent varicella infection
- The activated virus replicates and travels down the sensory nerve to the skin, resulting in severe pain in a dermatomal distribution
- Develops in 20% of healthy adults and 50% of immunocompromised adults
- Herpes zoster has high morbidity and mortality rate in immunocompromised patients
- May occur without cutaneous eruption (zoster sine herpete)

ETIOLOGY, EPIDEMIOLOGY, & RISK FACTORS

- Following initial varicella infection or immunization, the virus invades the dorsal root ganglion where it remains latent until reactivation
- At a later time in select individuals, the virus replicates in the dorsal root ganglion, producing ganglionitis, and then travels down the sensory nerve to the skin
- 98% of adults are seropositive
- A person with a history of varicella infection has a 20% lifetime risk for developing herpes zoster
- Generally affects older adults
- Annual incidence increases with age (2.5 cases per 1000 persons 20–50 years of age, 5 cases per 1000 persons 51–79 years of age, more than 10 cases per 1000 persons older than 80 years of age)
- Multiple risk factors exist, including past history of varicella infection, acute stress, fever, radiation therapy, and immunosuppression
- Postherpetic neuralgia is a painful syndrome that occurs as a result of nerve damage in the affected dermatome
  - Affects 20% of zoster patients
  - Can last months to years and may be debilitating

PATIENT PRESENTATION

- 90% of patients have a prodrome of localized, unilateral, intense pain with pruritis, tenderness, and tingling
  - The intense pain may be misdiagnosed as a myocardial infarction or an acute abdomen
- Painful eruption of grouped vesicles with an erythematous base, usually occurring within a sensory dermatome
- Thoracic dermatomes are most commonly affected, followed by cranial, lumbar, and sacral
- In immunocompromised patients, the eruption may manifest as crusted, verrucous lesions
- Disseminated cutaneous disease may occur outside the primary dermatome and may include visceral involvement
  - The pain of postherpetic neuralgia may be sharp, piercing, throbbing, or stabbing and can result in increased skin sensitivity

DIFFERENTIAL DX

- Herpes simplex eruption
- Vesicular viral exanthem
- Drug eruption
- Localized bacterial infection
- Contact dermatitis
- Scabies
- Insect bites
- Rickettsial pox

DIAGNOSTIC EVALUATION

- A clinical diagnosis based on history and physical examination
- Initial test of choice is the Tzanck smear, which will show multinucleated epithelial giant cells in affected individuals; however, the test cannot differentiate herpes zoster from herpes simplex infection
- Another excellent test is direct fluorescent antibody
  - Quick results are available in most labs (within 6 hours)
  - Preferable to culture due to higher yield
- Viral culture is the most specific test but requires 1–2 days for results
  - Histopathologic appearance is the same for herpes zoster and herpes simplex infection (balloon cells in the epidermis)
- Serology is only useful retrospectively because it is only diagnostic if there is a 4-fold increase in the varicella zoster virus titer
- Polymerase chain reaction (PCR) is the most sensitive test but is not readily available
- Consider HIV testing if the patient has disseminated zoster or is under 50 years of age with no known risk factors

TREATMENT & MANAGEMENT

- Within 72 hours of the first vesicle, antiviral medications should be started
  - Acyclovir, famciclovir, and valacyclovir are FDA-approved options for immunocompetent patients; these medications have been proven to decrease disease duration and pain
  - In general, 7 days of treatment are as effective as 21 days of treatment
- Intravenous acyclovir is used for immunocompromised patients and for those with serious complications
- Postherpetic neuralgia can be treated with famciclovir or valacyclovir; both proven to reduce duration and pain in immunocompetent patients older than 50
  - Analgesics, lidocaine patches, capsaicin, nerve blocks, narcotics, and biofeedback are often used
  - Low-dose tricyclic antidepressants and gabapentin may be effective in patients with pain and sleep disturbance
- A live zoster vaccine (Zostavax) is indicated for individuals older than 60
  - Decreases the incidence of zoster in half
  - For those who develop zoster, the vaccine may decrease the duration of symptomatic illness

PROGNOSIS & COMPLICATIONS

- Early initiation of antiviral therapy can reduce the risk for serious complications
- Most patients have skin healing and pain resolution in 3–4 weeks
- Serious complications include postherpetic neuralgia, secondary bacterial infection, scarring, ophthalmic zoster (occurs in 7% of patients, and 20–70% of these patients will develop associated ocular disease), Ramsay-Hunt syndrome, hepatitis, pneumonitis, neurologic disease (e.g., encephalitis, myelitis, facial paresis, polyradiculitis), and visceral zoster (occurs in 3–15% of immunocompromised patients)
- Postherpetic neuralgia occurs in 10–15% of immunocompromised patients, particularly in the elderly, and carries a high mortality rate

Warts

INTRODUCTION

- Warts (verrucae) are benign, slow-growing, hyperplastic epidermal lesions; they are the most common viral infection of the skin
- Appear as raised, piled-on growths of variable size, most commonly on the skin of the hands or mucus membranes
- Most commonly due to human papillomavirus (HPV)
  - Certain HPV types cause specific types of warts that favor particular anatomic locations (e.g., plantar warts, genital warts)
- Management of warts is based on their clinical appearance, their location, and the immune status of the patient

ETIOLOGY, EPIDEMIOLOGY, & RISK FACTORS

- Warts are found in all age groups but tend to favor adolescents and immunocompromised patients (e.g., HIV patients, chemotherapy patients, transplantation patients)
- More than 80 types of HPV exist
- Infection occurs during casual or intimate contact
- Certain HPV types favor particular anatomic sites:

HPV Types	Type of Wart
1	Palms or plantar surfaces
2, 4	Common
3, 10	Flat
6, 11	Anogenital
16, 18, 31, 33–35	High-risk anogenital, Bowenoid papulosis

- Autoinoculation involves transmission of the HPV virus from one location to another
- Some warts will spontaneously resolve in patients who mount an effective immune response; others require numerous destructive therapies

PATIENT PRESENTATION

- Hyperkeratotic, verrucous, painless, rough papules or plaques on exposed skin surfaces
- Common warts (verruca vulgaris) occur on the hands; they are asymptomatic and usually disappear within 2 years
- Flat warts (verruca plana) are flat-topped papules that occur on the face, hands, and legs; they appear in multiples, possibly hundreds
- Plantar warts (verruca plantaris) are located on the plantar surface of foot, usually as a single wart; they are often tender and classically demonstrate pinpoint bleeding when removed
- Anogenital or venereal warts (condyloma acuminatum) appear as "cauliflower-like" growths on the penis, vulva, vagina, cervix, or perianal region; cervical lesions are often pre-malignant

DIFFERENTIAL DX

- Nevus (mole)
- Cutaneous horn
- Actinic keratosis
- Seborrheic keratosis
- Keratoacanthoma
- Keratosis pilaris
- Lichen planus
- Basal cell carcinoma
- Squamous cell carcinoma
- Corn (clavus)
- Molluscum contagiosum
- Secondary syphilis

DIAGNOSTIC EVALUATION

- Clinical lesions are usually visible by gross inspection
- Subclinical lesions may only be seen by aided examination (e.g., acetic acid soaking) to differentiate from surrounding normal skin
- Biopsy confirms the diagnosis and may also determine the serotype of HPV
  - Histologically, biopsied warts will show papillomatous epidermal changes with a prominent granular cell layer, koilocytes, and dilated blood vessels in the dermis
- HPV typing is not necessary for most warts, unless the risk of cervical cancer associated with labial or cervical HPV types 16, 18, 31, and 31–35 will affect surveillance or management (i.e., will prompt colposcopy or excision procedures)
- Any female patient with genital warts (or the female partner of a male with genital warts) should undergo a Pap smear after diagnosis and annually thereafter
- Warts can be differentiated from corns by the disruption of skin lines and presence of "black dot" thrombosed blood vessels and dilated capillaries

TREATMENT & MANAGEMENT

- Most warts are self-limited and will disappear within 2 years
- If removal is desired, surgical excision is the treatment of choice
- Cryotherapy with liquid nitrogen may be used to lyse the HPV-infected keratinocytes
  - Cryotherapy and other office-based modalities should be repeated every 3–4 weeks
- Salicylic acid-containing products are usually disappointing as monotherapy but are useful adjuncts to maintain localized inflammation, destruction, and exfoliation of HPV-infected skin cells
- Other topically applied therapies that can be applied at office visits include Cantharone (0.7% cantharidin), podophyllin, and 100% trichloroacetic acid
- Recalcitrant warts require therapies such as squaric acid immunotherapy, intralesional bleomycin, pulsed-dye laser therapy, electrodessication-curettage, or oral cimetidine
- Imiquimod, a topical immunomodulator, has been approved by the FDA for treatment of genital warts and is a very effective agent; should be applied 3 days/week overnight for 8–12 weeks
- Gardasil vaccine is now FDA approved as a series of 3 shots used to prevent infection with HPV serotypes 6, 11, 16, and 18 in females aged 9–26
  - Thus, this vaccine may prevent the two HPV subtypes that cause most cases of cervical cancer and the two subtypes that cause most cases of genital warts

PROGNOSIS & COMPLICATIONS

- Many warts in immunocompetent patients will resolve in 1 to 2 years without treatment and weeks to months with treatment
- Cryotherapy, more so than other modalities, may result in hypopigmentation at the site due to melanocyte destruction
- Inadequate cryotherapy without a 2-mm rim of frost around the wart may result in a subsequently larger "ring wart" that may be more difficult to treat in the future
- Other topical treatments usually cause a transient, postinflammatory hyperpigmentation that will fade with time
- Periungal warts require special attention to avoid ablating the nail matrix (behind the lunula), which may result in either nail dystrophy or permanent loss of the nail plate

Cellulitis

INTRODUCTION

- Cellulitis is a common skin infection that extends to the dermis and subcutaneous tissue
- In 1996, cellulitis was estimated as the 28th most common discharge diagnosis in the U.S.; it has been reported as responsible for 2.2% of outpatient office visits
- Severe cases may result in systemic illness with hypotension or tachycardia
- The emergence of community-acquired methicillin-resistant *Staphylococcus aureus* (caMRSA) has changed the management of cellulitis and has resulted in more hospital admissions due to inappropriate outpatient antibiotic selection

ETIOLOGY, EPIDEMIOLOGY, & RISK FACTORS

- Cellulitis is defined as an infection of the dermis with some extension into the subcutaneous tissues
  - Usually develops on the extremities but has been documented on every area of the body
  - Occurs after the protective barrier of the skin (epidermis) has been compromised (e.g., due to trauma, ulcers, eczema), allowing bacterial access beneath the epidermis
  - Often, the portal of bacterial entry is unknown; however, the predilection of cellulitis to occur on areas exposed to the environment (e.g., hands, feet) supports the theory that disruption of the epidermis is essential in the development of cellulitis
- The majority of cases are caused by beta-hemolytic streptococci; however, *Staphylococcus aureus* and community-acquired MRSA have become more prevalent
- Factors that predispose to cellulitis include tinea pedis, diabetes mellitus, peripheral vascular disease, peripheral edema, trauma, bites, skin popping, immunodeficiency, and a prior history of cellulitis
- An important cellulitis-like syndrome is necrotizing fasciitis; it is a rapidly progressing soft tissue infection with rapid tissue destruction and bacterial spread along tissue planes and can result in thrombosis of blood vessels, systemic toxicity, and high morbidity and mortality

PATIENT PRESENTATION

- The hallmarks of cellulitis are erythema, pain, warmth, swelling, and tender regional adenopathy
- Develops over several days
- Cellulitis does not have well-defined borders (except erysipelas)
- Associated abscess formation is common in cases of *S. aureus* cellulitis
- Systemic symptoms (e.g., fever, chills, hypotension, tachycardia) are unusual unless bacteremia is present
- Signs and symptoms that suggest necrotizing fasciitis include pain out of proportion to physical examination, crepitus (i.e., subcutaneous air) on examination, bullae (especially hemorrhagic), rapid progression of erythema (minutes to hours), and fulminant course (rapid progression to shock)

DIFFERENTIAL DX

- Venous stasis disease
- Superficial thrombophlebitis
- Contact dermatitis
- Necrotizing fasciitis
- Chemical burn
- Deep venous thrombosis
- Allergic reaction
- Cutaneous abscess
- Angioedema
- Acute gout
- Drug reaction (erythema multiforme, Stevens-Johnson)
- Impetigo
- Insect bite
- Pyoderma gangrenosum
- Lyme disease
- Kawasaki's disease
- Cutaneous anthrax
- Osteomyelitis

DIAGNOSTIC EVALUATION

- Thorough history and physical examination
- Laboratory workup is indicated if the patient appears toxic, has history of recurrent infections, does not respond to therapy, or has significant animal or water exposure or if hospital admission is planned
  - Routine blood work (e.g., complete blood count, chemistries) are often more helpful to assess comorbid disease states (e.g., anemia, renal insufficiency) than cellulitis
  - Blood culture results are rarely positive (just 5% of outpatient cases); however, they should be sent prior to antibiotic administration in hospitalized patients to guide antimicrobial therapy in cases of antibiotic failure
- A wound culture is indicated if the cellulitis is associated with an abscess that can be drained or aspirated
- Plain films are warranted only if there is suspicion for a foreign body (e.g., needle fragment) or the presence of gas
- CT scan is used infrequently for cellulitis unless an underlying process is considered (e.g., necrotizing fasciitis, abscess)
- Arterial blood gas (ABG) and lactic acid level are indicated if there is suspicion for necrotizing fasciitis

TREATMENT & MANAGEMENT

- Initial antibiotic choice has changed recently due to the emergence of caMRSA
  - If caMRSA is not likely, treat with dicloxacillin or cephalexin
  - If caMRSA is a consideration, administer trimethoprim-sulfamethoxazole, clindamycin, doxycycline, or a third- or fourth-generation fluoroquinolone
  - If the patient is ill (e.g., hypotension, tachycardia), hospitalization and empiric treatment with vancomycin are warranted
- Antibiotic therapy should last at least 7–10 days
- Special antibiotic considerations
  - For penicillin-allergic patients, treat with clindamycin or levofloxacin
- For facial cellulitis (including preseptal), postsurgical cellulitis, and patients with diabetes or a bite wound, treat with amoxicillin-clavulanate
- Recurrent cellulitis (more than 2 episodes per year) can be treated with chronic, suppressive therapy with either penicillin V or clindamycin
- Adjunctive care may include elevation and immobilization of the affected limb, heat application, and sterile saline dressings
  - Administer tetanus prophylaxis for all bites and penetrating wounds
  - Ensure meticulous foot care in diabetics
  - May require hospitalization for IV antibiotics (e.g., cefazolin, ampicillin-sulbactam, vancomycin)

PROGNOSIS & COMPLICATIONS

- May progress to serious illness by contiguous spread or via the lymph or circulatory system; thus, compliance with a full course of antibiotics is necessary
- Cellulitis is generally a straightforward diagnosis without significant morbidity; however, it is imperative to ensure that a more sinister skin or soft tissue infection is not present when making this diagnosis
- Necrotizing fasciitis is uncommon (500–1500 cases annually in the U.S.) but carries a mortality rate of 30–40%, even if diagnosed in a timely fashion
- Complications include local abscess formation, osteomyelitis, joint infection, gas gangrene, bacteremia and metastatic infection, superinfection with gram-negative rods, thrombophlebitis, acute glomerulonephritis, and lymphedema

Scabies and Lice

INTRODUCTION

- Scabies and lice (pediculosis) are contagious infestations of the epidermis
- Although they can cause intense pruritus, they are usually benign conditions
- Approximately 300 million cases of scabies occur each year; in some areas of the world, scabies is a significant health problem, with an incidence as high as 100% in areas of South America; in the United States, scabies spreads quickly through nursing homes, hospitals, daycare facilities, and institutions
- Lice are endemic worldwide; cases of suspected lice infestations in school children affect 10% of young children and cause an estimated 12–24 million missed days of classes each year in the United States

ETIOLOGY, EPIDEMIOLOGY, & RISK FACTORS

- Scabies is caused by an 8-legged mite, *Sarcoptes scabiei*, which lives its entire life cycle in the human epidermis; it can survive for about 3 days when separated from the host
  - Transmitted via close contact or sharing of bedding or clothing
  - The pregnant females burrow into skin and deposit feces and eggs
  - After 3–4 days, the larvae burrow to the surface and mature
  - The classic infestation involves as few as 5–10 adult mites; crusted scabies can involve millions of mites (there are about 4700 mites in 1 gram of shedded skin)
  - Pruritus occurs due to a delayed hypersensitivity reaction that evolves after days-weeks
  - Increased risk in immunocompromised patients (2–4% of AIDS patients have scabies)
- Lice: *Pediculus humanus* var. *capitis* is the head louse; *Pediculus humanus* var. *corporis* is the body louse; *Pthirus pubis* is the crab louse that lives in pubic hair
  - Lice feed on blood from their host and inject saliva while feeding, which causes pruritus
  - Lice are transmitted through close contact or by fomites
  - On fomites, lice die within 1–2 days if they are not transmitted to a human contact
  - Body lice are associated with poor hygiene and infrequent clothing changes
  - Pubic lice are sexually transmitted
- Most common in young children ages 3–10, with higher incidence in girls and Caucasians

PATIENT PRESENTATION

- Scabies presents with generalized itching, especially at night
  - The web spaces of the hands, wrists, elbows, waist, and axillae are frequently involved
  - In men, scabies can involve the penis
  - In women, it can involve the breasts
  - Above the neck involvement is rare in adults
  - Crusted (Norwegian) scabies occurs in the immunocompromised and presents with thick, crusted lesions that can involve the face and scalp
- Head lice results in pruritus of the scalp; secondary infection can occur due to scratching
  - Inspection of hair can reveal live lice or nits
- Body lice presents with pruritus and excoriations; with chronic infestation, patients can develop postinflammatory pigmentation
- Pubic lice causes pruritus in pubic hair, axillae, eyelashes, and hair on the head

DIFFERENTIAL DX

- Infants: Infantile acropustulosis, atopic dermatitis
- Elderly: Bullous pemphigoid
- Immunocompromised: Seborrheic dermatitis, psoriasis, drug eruption, hyperkeratotic eczema
- Adults: Psoriasis, contact dermatitis, ichthyosis, Darier's disease
- Dried hair products, dandruff, other arthropods, and nonviable nits are frequently mistaken for active head lice infestations
- Systemic etiologies of pruritus (e.g., uremia, cholestasis)

DIAGNOSTIC EVALUATION

- History and physical exam focusing on interdigital spaces, wrists, periumbilical area, ankles, feet, and genitalia
- Scabies can be diagnosed by microscopic identification of the mite, egg, or scybala (mite pellets)
  - Skin scrapings (especially under the fingernails) using a drop of mineral oil on a sterile scalpel blade can be examined by a low-power microscope; adult mites may not be seen but the diagnosis can be made by the presence of eggs or fecal pellets alone; punch biopsies can reveal the mite
  - Empiric therapy without workup is reasonable in patients with symptoms consistent with scabies
- The CDC recommends basing the diagnosis of head lice on finding eggs within 6.5 mm of the scalp; other experts recommend treating only if a live louse is found
  - To find live lice, the hair should be combed with a fine-tooth "nit" comb; the comb should be placed at the crown and drawn down the scalp; after each pass with the comb, it should be examined for lice
  - Nits may persist for months after treatment and are not indicative of infestation

TREATMENT & MANAGEMENT

- In adults, the standard treatment for scabies is permethrin cream; the cream is applied to the body, avoiding the head and mucus membranes, and is washed off within 8–14 hours
  - Other options are 1% lindane (high toxicity) and 10% crotamiton cream
  - Newborns and pregnant women can safely use 5–10% precipitated sulfur in petrolatum
  - Ivermectin is not FDA approved for scabies but is becoming the preferred treatment and appears safe in children and pregnancy
- Crusted scabies can be treated with keratolytics to reduce the crusting, topical permethrin, and ivermectin; antibiotics are frequently used for suspected bacterial superinfection
- Linens should be washed in hot water, dry cleaned, or placed in plastic bags for 2 weeks; furniture and carpets should be vacuumed
- Lice can be treated with a variety of topical preparations
  - Topical options include malathion, permethrin, and pyrethrins
  - If infestation recurs, use a different insecticide; insecticide shampoos are less effective
  - Lindane 1% shampoo (contraindicated in lactating women or children younger than 2)
- Lice can be physically removed by wet-combing with nit combs, but this carries a higher failure rate
- Household members should be screened and treated; extensive cleaning of the home is not required, but combs and brushes should be washed in hot water for 20 minutes in dishwasher
- Itching can be treated with corticosteroid creams or an antihistamine (e.g., hydroxyzine)

PROGNOSIS & COMPLICATIONS

- Prognosis is good; occasionally, reinfestations occur, and scabies can be resistant to lindane, but permethrin is effective in these instances
- Itching may continue for weeks after eradication of mites and eggs of scabies because of delayed hypersensitivity response to antigens
- Secondary bacterial infection from excoriation may occur

Skin Cancer

INTRODUCTION

- Skin cancer is the most common cancer in the United States and worldwide; more than half of all new cancers in the U.S. yearly (>1 million) are skin cancers
- Basal cell carcinoma is the most common skin cancer, followed by squamous cell
- Most nonmelanoma skin cancers and early, thin (<1 mm in thickness) melanomas can be treated and cured with excisional surgery alone
- Malignant melanoma is the leading cause of skin cancer deaths
- Monthly patient-directed and yearly physician skin examinations are essential, particularly in patients with a history of skin cancer, a family history of skin cancer, or those with significant past sun exposure

ETIOLOGY, EPIDEMIOLOGY, & RISK FACTORS

- **Basal cell carcinoma** probably arises from pluripotent cells of the basal layer of epidermis
  - Characterized by slow, steady growth and rare metastasis, but local ulceration and tissue destruction may occur
  - Associated with sun exposure, fair complexion, radiation exposure, arsenic exposure, immunosuppression, xeroderma pigmentosum, or prior history of nonmelanoma skin cancer
  - Often seen on the face and neck
- **Squamous cell carcinoma** arises from keratinocytes in the skin and mucosa of the mouth and anus; it is generally a rapidly growing tumor but rarely metastasizes
  - Associated with sun exposure, irritants, burns (Marjolin ulcer), scars, chronic ulcers, HPV infection, hydrocarbons, and radiation
  - Appears on the ears, cheeks, lower lips, and back of hands
- **Malignant melanoma** arises from pigment-producing melanocytes
  - Risk factors include sun exposure, multiple or dysplastic nevi, early-life severe sunburn (especially in fair-skinned individuals), advancing age, large numbers of moles, family history, xeroderma pigmentosum, and familial atypical mole melanoma syndrome
  - Metastasizes to the liver, lung, brain, bone, adrenal, heart, and bowel
  - Usually arises on the head, neck, or extremities in men and trunk or thighs in women

PATIENT PRESENTATION

- Basal cell: Papule or nodular lesion with central erosion; may have stippled ulceration, waxy pearly edges, and telangiectasias
- Squamous cell: Small, hard, reddened, conical nodule with or without ulceration
- Melanoma: Solitary, flat or raised, macular or nodular lesion; satellite pigmentation (due to local metastases), erythema, ulceration, or bleeding may occur
  - Melanomas tend to display features of the mnemonic *ABCD*: Asymmetry in one axis, Border irregularity, Color changes (or more than one color, such as red, pink, brown, blue, or black), and Diameter greater than a pencil eraser
- Basal cell and squamous cell carcinomas tend to occur on sun-exposed areas such as the head, neck, or dorsal hands; melanomas may arise in any site, including sun-protected areas (e.g., palms, soles, nails, mouth, retina, vulva, perineum, CNS)

DIFFERENTIAL DX

- Benign nevi (moles)
- Metastatic skin cancer
- Seborrheic keratosis
- Dermatofibroma
- Cherry hemangioma
- Wart
- Seborrheic keratosis
- Actinic keratosis (precancerous)
- Skin tag
- Angioma
- Traumatized skin
- Cutaneous metastasis
- Fibrous papule
- Sebaceous hyperplasia

DIAGNOSTIC EVALUATION

- Skin biopsy must be performed immediately to establish the diagnosis
  - Removal in toto with a punch, shave, or excisional biopsy aids in establishing the depth of the tumor and its character (e.g., superficial vs. infiltrating)
  - Large pigmented lesions suspicious for melanoma that cannot be feasibly biopsied in toto should have either the darkest portion or the nodular/ulcerated portion biopsied
- Suspected or biopsy-proven squamous cell carcinomas and melanomas require a complete lymph node examination at the time of diagnosis or re-excision
- Squamous cell carcinomas with perineural invasion may require further imaging modalities (CT scan or MRI) to determine local extension; this should also be investigated if the patient complains of a history of local dysthesia or paresthesia
- Melanomas greater than 1 mm in Breslow's thickness or those less than 1 mm with lymphatic or vascular invasion or evidence of ulceration require a sentinel lymph node biopsy at the time of re-excision to rule out regional nodal disease; additionally, they require serum LDH assay for staging and chest X-ray or CT scan

TREATMENT & MANAGEMENT

- Biopsy-proven superficial basal and squamous cell carcinomas may be treated with 3 consecutive passes of electrodessication and curettage destruction
- Nodular or invasive basal and squamous cell carcinomas require complete excision using 4-mm margins beyond the clinically evident lesion
- Recurrent nonmelanoma skin cancers or those occurring in irradiated skin or in a cosmetically sensitive area (e.g., canthus, eyelid, nose, lip, or ear) may require Mohs' micrographic surgery
  - Mohs' surgery is a tissue-sparing excisional technique performed by a specialized dermatologist; it offers the highest cure rate for nonmelanoma skin cancers
- Melanoma in situ (limited to the epidermis) or lentigo maligna (melanoma in situ on sun-exposed skin) should be re-excised with 5-mm margins
- Melanomas less than 1 mm in Breslow's depth without lymphatic or vascular invasion may be excised completely with 1-cm margins
- Melanomas larger than 1 mm in Breslow's depth or those with lymphatic or vascular invasion require sentinel lymph node biopsies, usually performed at the time of complete re-excision, using 2-cm or greater margins
- Chemotherapy, interferon-beta, and interleukin-2 are commonly indicated for metastases

PROGNOSIS & COMPLICATIONS

- Both basal and squamous cell have better than 95% cure rate if detected and treated early
- More than 85% of patients with a biopsy-proven nonmelanoma skin cancer will eventually develop a second skin cancer, most commonly within 5 years of the initial diagnosis; monthly self skin exams and annual physician skin examinations are indicated
- Recurrent nonmelanoma cancers may require Mohs' surgery
- Most thin melanomas (<1 mm in Breslow's thickness) are cured with surgical excision using adequate margins and require no further workup; clinical lymph node and total-body skin examinations should follow every 6 months for 2 years, and then annually
- Intermediate (1–4 mm) melanomas and thick melanomas (thicker than 4 mm) and those with a positive sentinel lymph node biopsy require consultation with an oncologist

Opthalmology

Red Eye

INTRODUCTION

- Red eye is a common presenting complaint that may be caused by a multitude of conditions, most of which are benign; however, misdiagnosis of emergent conditions can result in loss of vision
- Red eye refers to hyperemia or infection of the superficial vessels of the conjunctiva, episclera, and sclera, and may be caused by disorders of these structures in addition to disorders of the cornea, iris, ciliary body, or ocular adnexa
- A careful history, visual acuity testing, and penlight examination may suggest the diagnosis or reveal "red flag" findings that warrant ophthalmologic referral

ETIOLOGY, EPIDEMIOLOGY, & RISK FACTORS

- Common etiologies include infections, inflammation, trauma, and glaucoma
  - Conjunctivitis: May be caused by allergies, viruses (e.g., adenovirus, herpes simplex, varicella), or bacteria (e.g., staphylococci, streptococci, pseudomonas)
  - Keratitis: Inflammation of the cornea due to herpes simplex, herpes zoster, bacteria, ultraviolet (UV) light, contact lenses, or dry eye syndrome
  - Anterior uveitis: Inflammation of iris and ciliary body; most often idiopathic but may be due to trauma, infection (e.g., TB, syphilis, herpes, Lyme), sarcoidosis, or connective tissue diseases (e.g., rheumatoid arthritis, SLE, RA, Sjögren's syndrome)
  - Scleritis: Inflammation of the sclera; may be the initial symptom of connective tissue disease or infection
  - Episcleritis: A benign, idiopathic inflammation near the sclera
  - Keratoconjunctivitis sicca (KS): A benign cause of dry, red eyes; may be due to drugs (e.g., antihistamines, anticholinergics), Sjögren's syndrome, or sarcoidosis
  - Subconjunctival hemorrhage: Benign rupture of small vessels due to underlying coagulopathy, trauma, coughing, or excessive eye rubbing

PATIENT PRESENTATION

- Pain, pruritus, discharge, sensation of foreign body, and photophobia are often present
- Keratitis: Pain, redness, tearing, decreased vision
- Uveitis: Pain, perilimbal injection
- Scleritis: Unilateral severe pain, decreased vision, and injection; no discharge
- Episcleritis: Mild pain, localized redness
- Subconjunctival hemorrhage: Painless localized hemorrhage
- Infectious conjunctivitis: Watery, purulent discharge with injection
- Allergic conjunctivitis: Severe itching, watery discharge with injection

DIFFERENTIAL DX

- Infection (conjunctivitis, blepharitis, dacrocystitis, endophthalmitis, orbital cellulitis)
- Allergic conjunctivitis
- Keratoconjunctivitis sicca
- Keratitis
- Anterior uveitis (iritis)
- Scleritis/episcleritis
- Subconjunctival hemorrhage
- Acute closed-angle glaucoma
- Entropion or ectropion
- Trauma (foreign body, corneal abrasion, globe injury)
- Corneal perforation
- Pterygium
- Chronic blepharitis
- Dry eye syndrome

DIAGNOSTIC EVALUATION

- Thorough history and ocular examination
  - Note onset, visual changes, pain, presence of photophobia or fever, history of head or eye trauma, prior eye surgeries, and use of contact lenses
  - Note characteristics of discharge clarity, color, and consistency
  - Note history of comorbid conditions (e.g., autoimmune disorders, hypertension, diabetes) that may have associated ocular symptoms
  - Physical examination should include testing for visual acuity, extraocular muscles, pupil reactivity and size, photophobia, disc assessment, and eyelid inspection
- Red flags that suggest the need for immediate ophthalmologic referral include corneal opacification, deep pain, acute vision changes, photophobia, nausea or vomiting, and blurred disc margins
  - Severe pain often indicates more serious conditions, such as elevated intraocular pressure, scleritis, infectious keratitis, and endophthalmitis
- Slit lamp examination with or without fluorescein dye
  - May help locate foreign bodies or corneal pathology
  - May show anterior chamber reaction/inflammation due to uveitis, keratitis, scleritis, corneal ulcer, or gonococcal or bacterial infection
- Laboratory studies may include culture and sensitivities for suspected infective causes, complete blood count and ESR for suspected inflammatory causes, rheumatoid factor and ANA for autoimmune causes

TREATMENT & MANAGEMENT

- Provide appropriate oral analgesics as needed
- Consider ophthalmologic referral, particularly for herpes simplex or herpes zoster keratitis or conjunctivitis, acute angle-closure glaucoma, scleritis, episcleritis, corneal ulcer, iritis, penetrating foreign bodies, and chemical injuries
- Avoid treating patients with steroid eye drops without consultation of an ophthalmologist
- Treat the underlying etiology as necessary
  - Allergic conjunctivitis: Avoid offending agents, cold compresses to eyes, NSAIDs, ocular decongestants, antihistamines
  - Viral conjunctivitis: Symptomatic relief (cool compress, artificial tears, topical antihistamine), and avoid spread with meticulous hand washing and hygiene
  - Bacterial conjunctivitis: Antibiotic eye drops; avoid neomycin
  - Subconjunctival hemorrhage: Cool compress; clears spontaneously in 1–2 weeks
  - Dry eye syndrome: Lubricating artificial tears
  - Foreign body of cornea or conjunctiva: Anesthetize with proparacaine, and remove with vigorous irrigation or cotton-tipped applicator using a slit lamp microscope; then treat with topical antibiotic drop
  - Corneal abrasion: Topical antibiotic drop or ointment and pressure patch if not contact lens wearer; refer to ophthalmologist if severe or any suspicion of infectious etiology

PROGNOSIS & COMPLICATIONS

- Many common causes of red eye are self-limiting and rarely cause permanent visual loss or complications
- Delay in diagnosis and referral of red flag conditions (e.g., infectious keratitis, acute angle-closure glaucoma, endophthalmitis) may lead to rapid, irreversible visual loss
- *Never* prescribe or distribute topical proparacaine or other anesthetic drops to treat eye pain because this will prevent corneal healing and eliminate the protective blink reflex and may cause severe allergic reactions
- Topical steroids have no role in the treatment of conjunctivitis without the supervision of an ophthalmologist; they can cause sight-threatening disease such as corneal melting, perforation, cataract, and glaucoma

Dry Eye

INTRODUCTION

- Dry eye is a common disorder caused either by decreased tear production or excessive tear evaporation
  - Affects 10–15% of adults
- The healthy tear film provides a smooth optical surface, allows for removal of debris, protects and prevents drying of the ocular surface, supplies oxygen and growth factors for the corneal epithelium, contains antimicrobial agents, and lubricates the cornea-eyelid interface
- The tear film is mechanically spread over the ocular surface by a neuronally controlled blink mechanism and is cleared through the nasolacrimal drainage system
- Disruption of these processes leads to the signs and symptoms of dry eye syndrome

ETIOLOGY, EPIDEMIOLOGY, & RISK FACTORS

- The tear film consists of three layers: A lipid layer produced by the meibomian (tarsal) glands, an aqueous layer produced by the main lacrimal glands and accessory lacrimal glands, and a mucin layer made by conjunctival goblet cells
  - The lipid layer prevents evaporation, contributes to the optical air-tear film interface, provides a hydrophobic barrier that prevents overflow tearing, thickens the aqueous layer, and prevents damage to the lid margin skin by tears
  - The aqueous layer supplies oxygen to the avascular corneal epithelium; contains antibacterial IgA, lysozyme, and lactoferrin; abolishes small irregularities of the corneal surface; and washes away debris and allows for passage of leukocytes after injury or infection
  - The mucin layer allows wetting of the hydrophobic corneal epithelium and provides lubrication
- Exposure to environmental extremes, temperate climates, low levels of humidity, or indoor heating during the winter can exacerbate symptoms
- Sjögren's syndrome is an aqueous deficiency state associated with xerostomia (dry mouth) and/or collagen vascular disease (e.g., rheumatoid arthritis, SLE, systemic sclerosis); it is thought to involve autoimmune infiltration of the lacrimal and salivary glands

PATIENT PRESENTATION

- Burning
- Dry sensation
- Photophobia
- Blurred vision
- Red eye (conjunctival injection)
- Decreased tear lake
- Increased tear breakup time
- Irregular corneal surface
- Epithelial corneal or conjunctival staining
- Mucus plaques

DIFFERENTIAL DX

- Tear-deficient dry eye: Sjögren's syndrome, lacrimal disease, impaired corneal sensation
- Evaporative dry eye: Blepharitis, meibomian gland disease, blinking disorders, disorders of the eyelid, globe congruity
- Drug-induced dry eye (e.g., oral contraceptives, antihistamines, phenothiazines)
- Conjunctival scarring: Ocular pemphigoid, Stevens-Johnson syndrome, trachoma, chemical burn)
- Lacrimal obstruction
- Blepharospasm
- Nocturnal lagophthalmos

DIAGNOSTIC EVALUATION

- Tear breakup time measures precorneal tear film stability
  - Instill fluorescein into the lower fornix, ask the patient to blink several times, and hold the eye open
  - Examine with broad-beam cobalt blue filter, and look for black spots or lines that represent a dry spot
  - Abnormal tear breakup time is defined as a time from last blink to first dry spot of less than 10 seconds
- Corneal or conjunctival staining with rose bengal, lissamine green, or fluorescein in a punctate pattern indicates a dry eye state and is usually seen in the area between the lids where evaporation is greatest; corneal filaments and mucus plaques will also be easier to see with these stains
- The Schirmer's test may be done with (basal tear production) or without (both basal and reflex tearing) proparacaine anesthetic
  - Fold a sterile filter paper strip at the wick end and place over the lower eyelid margin at the lateral two-thirds mark; the patient may gaze slightly upward or keep eyes gently closed
  - Remove strips after 5 minutes, and measure from the fold to the farthest extent of wetting: >10 mm is normal, 5–10 mm is borderline, and <5 mm indicates a dry eye state

TREATMENT & MANAGEMENT

- Avoid systemic medications that are known to decrease aqueous tear production, including diuretics, antihistamines, anticholinergics, and psychotropics
- Mild cases can be treated with artificial tears up 4 times daily, lubricating ointment at bedtime, hot compresses, and eyelid massage
- Moderate cases are treated with preservative-free artificial tears hourly, lubricating ointment at bedtime, and lower punctal plugs that provide reversible occlusion of tear drainage
- Severe cases may be treated as above, plus upper and lower punctal occlusion, sustained-release tear inserts, moist environment (e.g., humidifier, moisture shields), and tarsorraphy (to fuse the eyelids together)
- 0.05% cyclosporine A drops (Restasis) offer the first therapeutic treatment for patients with moderate to severe dry eye disease due to aqueous deficiency
  - Rule out ocular infection prior to use
- Mucolytic drops (acetylcysteine 5%) may be used for corneal filaments and mucous plaques

PROGNOSIS & COMPLICATIONS

- Severe dry eye predisposes to bacterial keratitis and sterile ulceration, which may lead to corneal perforation
- Filaments are comma-shaped strands of epithelial cells attached to the surface of the cornea over a core of mucus; filamentary keratopathy can be seen in severe dry eye states and can be quite painful due to firm attachment to the sensitive corneal epithelium
- Patients with Sjögren's syndrome have an increased incidence of lymphoma
- Contact lenses are discouraged in patients with dry eye due to the increased risk of corneal breakdown and infection

Visual Loss

INTRODUCTION

- Visual loss is a common presenting complaint that may occur as a result of numerous diseases of the eye and visual pathway
- Identifying the visual loss as acute or chronic, transient or persistent, sudden or gradual, monocular or binocular, painful or painless, and/or related to trauma can help to classify the disorder
- A careful history and directed ocular examination can often distinguish nonurgent conditions from sight-threatening disease necessitating urgent referral

ETIOLOGY, EPIDEMIOLOGY, & RISK FACTORS

- Differentiate rapid, acute vision loss from slow, chronic degeneration (e.g., commonly due to cataracts or diabetic retinopathy)
- Retinal detachment: Vision loss due to trauma or proliferative retinopathy
- Vitreous hemorrhage: Loss of vision due to bleeding within the globe secondary to coagulopathy, proliferative retinopathy, or trauma
- Central retinal artery occlusion (CRAO): Sudden, painless loss of vision caused by embolism, atherosclerosis, or temporal arteritis
- Central retinal vein occlusion (CRVO): Subacute, painless venous thrombosis or occlusion; associated with diabetes or hypertension (HTN)
- Temporal arteritis: Vasculitis of medium-sized arteries (especially the carotids) that affects patients older than 50
- Optic neuritis: Rapid, painful loss of vision due to optic nerve injury secondary to multiple sclerosis, connective tissue disease, sarcoidosis, viruses, or tuberculosis
  - Most common nontraumatic cause of vision loss in patients younger than 50

PATIENT PRESENTATION

- Brow ache, nausea, vomiting, and halos are often the presenting symptoms of glaucoma
- Flashing lights and new floaters suggest retinal pathology (e.g., retinal tear, vitreous hemorrhage, posterior vitreous detachment, retinal detachment)
- Sudden, severe, painless and persistent loss of vision may suggest a central retinal artery occlusion, vitreous hemorrhage, retinal detachment, retinal vein occlusion, ischemic optic neuropathy, or occipital stroke
- Temporal arteritis: Severe headache and tenderness over the temporal area, fever, malaise
- Optic neuritis: Painful; usually unilateral; afferent pupillary defect; normal funduscopy
- A painful red eye with purulent discharge may suggest infectious keratitis, especially in contact lens wearers

DIFFERENTIAL DX

- Transient vision loss: Papilledema, amaurosis fugax, migraine, vertebrobasilar artery insufficiency, orthostatic hypotension
- Acute, persistent visual loss:
  - Infectious keratitis, acute angle-closure glaucoma, vitreous or retinal hemorrhage, retinal detachment, retinal vascular occlusion, acute maculopathy, optic neuritis, ischemic optic neuropathy, occipital cortex infarction, endophthalmitis
- Chronic, progressive loss:
  - Refractive error, diabetic retinopathy, corneal opacity or scarring, cataract, vitreal opacity, macular degeneration

DIAGNOSTIC EVALUATION

- History should include age, onset, tempo of vision loss, history of trauma, associated headache, medications, past history (e.g., carotid or cardiac disease, HTN, diabetes, vertigo, migraine, syphilis, ocular, orbital, cranial radiation, keratoconus), family history of vision loss, alcohol and tobacco use
- Eye examination should include visual acuity, color vision, blood pressure, refractive error, cranial examination, cranial nerve innervation, intraocular pressure, ocular media opacity (for corneal edema, dystrophy, anterior chamber or vitreous cells, cataracts), and fundus and optic disc exam
- Confrontation visual field testing: Look for peripheral vision loss by testing each quadrant with finger counting, and matching your left eye with the patient's right eye and vice versa
- Swinging flashlight test for afferent pupillary defect
  - Marcus-Gunn pupil: The pupil inappropriately dilates to direct light but has an appropriate consensual response (i.e., constricts when the light is shined in the other eye)
  - Present in optic nerve injury (e.g., optic neuritis) and temporal arteritis
- Using a penlight, examine the conjunctiva and iris, assess for opacity (whitening) of the cornea, and stain with fluorescein to evaluate for a corneal abrasion
- Ophthalmoscopy: Using the direct ophthalmoscope, assess the red reflex (loss indicates media opacity), optic disc, retinal vessels, and macula
- Consider a contrast CT/MRI of the orbits and head, carotid Doppler, echocardiogram, ERG, and VEP (retinal dystrophies, optic neuropathies, nonphysiologic)

TREATMENT & MANAGEMENT

- Infectious keratitis: Often warrants corneal cultures and aggressive broad-spectrum topical antibiotics to protect vision; refer these patients to ophthalmology emergently
- Acute angle-closure glaucoma can cause rapid optic nerve damage; refer these patients emergently for intraocular pressure-lowering medications
- Endophthalmitis, whether from blood-borne, postsurgical, or surface pathogens, requires emergent referral for intravitreal and/or parenteral antibiotics
- Retinal detachment, often presenting with visual loss, flashes, floaters, and visual field loss, should be referred emergently for evaluation and surgical repair
- Central retinal artery occlusion: Ocular massage in hopes of dislodging the embolus
- Giant cell arteritis: High-dose steroids to prevent loss of vision in the unaffected eye
- Other vascular occlusions, vitreous or retinal hemorrhage, acute maculopathy, optic neuritis, and occipital cortex infarction may be referred on an urgent basis
- Many chronic causes of visual loss (e.g., refractive error, cataracts, glaucoma) may be referred on a nonurgent basis
- Transient, bilateral visual loss that lasts seconds and is positional may be a sign of increased intracranial pressure; if present, neuroimaging is indicated to assess for mass lesions
- Migraine may be managed by avoiding triggers (e.g., oral contraceptives, alcohol, caffeine), correction of refractive error, and abortive and prophylactic medications

PROGNOSIS & COMPLICATIONS

- Early, accurate diagnosis and timely treatment are critical in cases of acute vision loss; emergent ophthalmology consultation is necessary
- Detection of ocular diseases such as glaucoma, cataracts, diabetic retinopathy, and macular degeneration may provide the primary care physician the opportunity to refer the patient nonurgently for vision-saving treatment
- True emergencies requiring immediate management and referral include acute central retinal artery occlusion, ischemic optic neuropathy due to giant cell arteritis, infectious keratitis, acute angle-closure glaucoma, endophthalmitis, and retinal detachment

Eye Pain

INTRODUCTION

- Ocular and periorbital pain may result from stimulation of trigeminal nerve fibers anywhere within the eye, surrounding tissues, deep orbit, or the base of the anterior and middle cranial fossae
- A directed eye examination and history of the pain will likely reveal the cause (if the pain originates from the eye itself)

ETIOLOGY, EPIDEMIOLOGY, & RISK FACTORS

- Pain fibers of the eye, orbit, and face project to the spinal nucleus of cranial nerve V and originate from 3 major divisions of the trigeminal nerve (ophthalmic, maxillary, and mandibular)
- Epidemiologic clues can suggest the etiology:
  - The most common etiology in patients older than 50 is giant cell arteritis
  - The most common etiology in young women (18–45) is optic neuritis, which is often associated with multiple sclerosis or infections (e.g., measles, mumps, chickenpox, zoster, mononucleosis, tuberculosis, syphilis, encephalitis)
  - Previous trauma to eye (e.g., fingernail, tree branch) suggests corneal abrasion, recurrent erosion, or corneal ulcer
  - Participation in high-risk activities without protective eyewear (e.g., metal grinding, landscaping) suggests foreign body in the cornea, conjunctiva, or intraocular
  - Previous eye surgery suggests endophthalmitis
  - History of connective tissue disease (e.g., rheumatoid arthritis, SLE, Wegener's granulomatosis, polyarteritis nodosa, ankylosing spondylitis), reactive arthritis, psoriasis, gout, Behçet's syndrome, inflammatory bowel disease, or infections suggests uveitis, episcleritis, or scleritis

PATIENT PRESENTATION

- Associated symptoms may include red eye, discharge, pain with reading or visual tasks (asthenopia), a foreign body sensation (feels like grain of sand or something poking the eye), diplopia (double vision), ptosis (drooping eyelid), or proptosis (bulging eye)
- Jaw claudication (pain with chewing), scalp tenderness (i.e., tenderness upon combing hair), headache, fever, malaise, and proximal muscle and joint aches suggest giant cell arteritis
- Cloudy cornea, halos, nausea and vomiting, headache, and mid-dilated fixed pupil suggest acute angle-closure glaucoma
- Pain with eye movements, loss of visual acuity and color vision, altered perception of movement, and worsening of symptoms with exercise or increased body temperature suggest optic neuritis

DIFFERENTIAL DX

- Corneal abrasion
- Recurrent erosion syndrome
- Corneal ulcer or infiltrate
- Dry eye syndrome
- Conjunctivitis
- Blepharitis
- Foreign body
- Episcleritis, scleritis, uveitis
- Endophthalmitis
- Acute angle-closure glaucoma
- Optic neuritis
- Giant cell arteritis
- Orbital or cavernous sinus syndrome
- Preseptal or orbital cellulitis
- Orbital pseudotumor
- Cranial nerve palsy
- Sinusitis
- Refractive error

DIAGNOSTIC EVALUATION

- History and physical examination will often reveal the etiology
  - Important historical clues include distinguishing constant versus episodic pain, time of day (morning vs. late day), association with reading or computer use, and presence of redness, foreign body sensation, jaw claudication, scalp tenderness, headache, visual loss, diplopia, proptosis or ptosis, or prior trauma or surgery
- Each patient requires a complete ophthalmic examination
  - Loss of visual acuity suggests an ocular or neural cause (refer to *Vision Loss* entry)
  - Defect of confrontation visual fields suggests visual pathway disease
  - Penlight examination may reveal conjunctival hyperemia or injection (seen in corneal disease, dry eye, conjunctivitis, foreign body, uveitis, episcleritis, scleritis, endophthalmitis, acute angle-closure glaucoma), ptosis (cranial nerve III palsy), or proptosis (seen in Graves' disease and orbital or cavernous sinus disease)
  - Eyelid swelling suggests orbital infection or an inflammatory process
  - A relative afferent pupillary defect may be present in optic neuritis
  - Reduced eye movements may occur with Graves' disease, orbital inflammation or tumor, or cranial nerve III, IV, or VI palsy
- If corneal disease is suspected, examine the eye after staining with fluorescein
- Ophthalmoscopy may reveal reduced red reflex in keratitis and endophthalmitis or swelling of the optic nerve in optic neuritis

TREATMENT & MANAGEMENT

- Giant cell arteritis: Immediately begin high-dose systemic corticosteroids to prevent visual loss and refer to an ophthalmologist or oculoplastic surgeon for definitive diagnosis via temporal artery biopsy
- Corneal abrasion: Rule out infection (seen as opacity of the cornea, which prevents view of the underlying iris), use fluorescein to measure the size and location of the abrasion, and use topical antibiotic drops or ointment until healed and no fluorescein staining occurs
- Recurrent corneal erosion: Same therapy as corneal abrasion; may require sodium chloride drops or ointment to speed healing; if not responsive to treatment, may need bandage contact lens, anterior stromal puncture, or PTK excimer laser treatment
- Foreign body: Fluorescein often aids in finding foreign bodies; use a topical anesthetic followed by irrigation, a cotton tipped applicator, and/or needle with slit lamp biomicroscope to remove corneal or conjunctival foreign bodies; if metallic, may need an ophthalmic burr to remove residual rust ring; treat residual corneal abrasions as above
- Dry eye: Artificial tears, lubricants, punctal occlusion (refer to *Dry Eye* entry)
- Episcleritis: Artificial tears may be sufficient; severe cases should be referred to an ophthalmologist for topical steroids
- Suspected cases of uveitis, scleritis, endophthalmitis, corneal ulcer or infiltrate, acute angle-closure glaucoma, cranial nerve palsy, orbital or cavernous sinus disease, or optic neuritis should be referred to an ophthalmologist immediately

PROGNOSIS & COMPLICATIONS

- The presence of "red flag" findings (e.g., visual loss, diplopia, ptosis, proptosis) requires emergent referral to an ophthalmologist

Glaucoma

INTRODUCTION

- Glaucoma is the second leading cause of blindness in the United States and the third most common cause worldwide
- Up to 3% of elderly individuals have glaucoma
- Approximately 100,000 persons in the U.S. are legally blind due to glaucoma
- Glaucoma is the most common form of optic neuropathy, presenting with characteristic cupping of the optic disc and visual field defects; elevated intraocular pressure is common, but not necessary for diagnosis
- Early detection and treatment with medications and surgery can prevent permanent peripheral vision loss and blindness

ETIOLOGY, EPIDEMIOLOGY, & RISK FACTORS

- Glaucoma occurs due to elevated intraocular pressure (either acute or chronic) that results in corneal edema, optic nerve damage, and blindness if not corrected
- Intraocular pressure depends on the production and drainage of aqueous humor (normal is 10–21 mmHg); aqueous humor is normally produced by the ciliary body in the posterior chamber, circulates to the anterior chamber, and is reabsorbed by the trabecular meshwork
- The drain, or angle, spans 360° around the eye located between the cornea and the iris
- Open-angle glaucoma is a chronic disease of inadequate trabecular reabsorption of aqueous humor; it may be asymptomatic until significant optic nerve damage has occurred
  - Risk factors include advanced age, African-American race, family history, diabetes mellitus, severe myopia, and steroid use
- Closed-angle glaucoma is caused by a narrowed anterior chamber that prevents aqueous humor from reaching the trabecular meshwork (i.e., the drain is closed); it is a medical emergency that results in a rapid increase in intraocular pressure and severe symptoms
  - Risk factors include Asian descent, family history, hyperopia, and prior uveitis
  - Some medical illnesses and medications increase the risk (secondary glaucoma), including diabetes, endocrine disease, trauma or surgery, brain tumor, or drugs (e.g., steroids, atropine, antidepressants, anxiolytics, sympathomimetics, antihistamines, mydriatics)

PATIENT PRESENTATION

- Most patients with open-angle glaucoma are asymptomatic except for gradual vision loss
  - Peripheral vision loss begins early but often goes unrealized; central vision is preserved until late; most patients lack pain and ocular symptoms
- Acute angle-closure glaucoma may present with severe eye pain, eye redness, headache, blurry vision, halos around lights, nausea and vomiting, and abdominal pain
  - On ocular exam, the globe is firm to palpation, the cornea is cloudy, and the pupil is minimally reactive
- Chronic angle-closure glaucoma may present only with vague eye pain
- Characteristic visual field losses may include arcuate scotoma, nasal step, altitudinal defects, or advanced constriction with central island of vision
- Elevated intraocular pressure may or may not be present

DIFFERENTIAL DX

- Red eye (e.g., infection, uveitis, allergy, abrasion, trauma)
- Headache (e.g., migraine, cluster, tension, temporal arteritis)
- GI causes of nausea/vomiting
- Vision loss (e.g., vascular occlusion, retinal injury)
- Secondary glaucoma
- Normal tension glaucoma (optic nerve damage and visual field loss despite normal intraocular pressure)
- Congenital glaucoma
- Physiologic cupping of the optic nerve without visual loss
- Ischemic optic neuropathy
- Retinal degenerative disease

DIAGNOSTIC EVALUATION

- Screening should be routinely performed in high-risk patients (e.g., older adults, African-Americans, those with positive family history)
  - Screening entails measurement of intraocular pressure by tonometry, ophthalmoscopy to examine the appearance of the optic nerve head, and formal visual field testing by perimetry
  - Asymptomatic, chronically elevated intraocular pressure does not necessary indicate glaucoma (i.e., glaucoma cannot be diagnosed unless optic nerve damage is present)
  - The cup-to-disc ratio (horizontal and vertical diameter of the cup compared to the overall diameter of the optic disc) is directly correlated with glaucomatous damage (ratio greater than 0.5 is worrisome); asymmetry in optic nerve cupping between the two eyes is also suggestive
- The flashlight test is positive in angle-closure glaucoma
  - Hold the light at the temporal limbus, and shine medially
  - If the nasal half of the iris is shadowed, the angle is narrowed, and glaucoma is likely
- Ophthalmologists can use a technique called gonioscopy to examine the drain of the eye, in which a special contact lens is placed on the topically anesthetized cornea
- Steroids (ophthalmic, systemic, or nasal) can cause steroid-induced glaucoma, which is more common in patients with a family history, diabetics, African-Americans, and patients with primary open-angle glaucoma

TREATMENT & MANAGEMENT

- Treatment is aimed at decreasing intraocular pressure by minimizing aqueous humor production and increasing outflow
  - Topical beta-blockers (e.g., timolol, betaxolol) and carbonic anhydrase inhibitors tend to reduce the production of aqueous humor
  - Miotics (e.g., pilocarpine) and prostaglandin analogs (e.g., latanoprost) facilitate outflow drainage
  - Adrenergic agonists (e.g., apraclonidine, brimonidine) may decrease production and facilitate drainage
- Marijuana has been shown to decrease intraocular pressure; however, side effects and legal issues limit its use
- If medical therapy is not effective, laser or surgical options may be necessary
- Any patient with one or more of the following findings should be referred to an ophthalmologist: Intraocular pressure greater than 21 mmHg, difference in intraocular pressure of 5 mmHg or more between the two eyes, optic cup diameter greater than one-half the disc diameter, significant asymmetry of cupping between the two eyes, family history of glaucoma or other significant risk factors, or symptoms of acute angle-closure glaucoma

PROGNOSIS & COMPLICATIONS

- All patients with acute angle-closure glaucoma require emergent ophthalmology consultation and admission
- Glaucomatous visual loss is usually irreversible
- If intraocular pressure is lowered substantially, progressive visual field loss may be prevented; routine screening and early diagnosis and management can prevent blindness
- Topical medications may have systemic side effects: beta-antagonists may cause bradycardia, bronchial constriction, depression, and impotence; alpha-agonists used alongside MAO inhibitors can cause hypertensive crisis, dry mouth, dry eye, and hypotension; carbonic anhydrase inhibitors may cause hypokalemia, GI symptoms, and bitter taste and are contraindicated in patients with sulfa allergy; miotics may cause headache and brow ache

Cataract

INTRODUCTION

- A cataract is an opacification or discoloration of the natural crystalline lens of the eye that focuses light onto the retina
- Cataracts are the leading cause of preventable blindness worldwide and the most common cause of decreased vision uncorrectable by eyeglasses in the United States; furthermore, cataract removal and implantation of an intraocular lens is the most common surgical procedure performed in the United States
- Symptoms depend on the density and location of the lens opacity
- It is important to rule out other contributing causes of visual loss, such as glaucoma, macular degeneration, and diabetic retinopathy

ETIOLOGY, EPIDEMIOLOGY, & RISK FACTORS

- The crystalline lens has 3 functions: to maintain its own clarity, to focus light onto the retina, and to provide accommodation as part of the near reflex
- The lens has no blood supply and no innervation after fetal development; thus, it depends on the aqueous and vitreous humor to meet its metabolic needs
- The lens continues to grow throughout life; no cells are lost, but new fibers are laid down while older layers become more compact and centralized; thus, the lens becomes denser and more opacified with age, ultimately obstructing incoming light rays
- Virtually all persons of advanced age have some degree of cataract, including 50% of individuals 65–74 and 70% of individuals over 75
- 1.5 million cataract extractions are performed annually in the United States; it is perhaps the most effective surgical procedure performed in medicine
- Cataract formation may be related to congenital, genetic, disease-related (e.g., uveitis, diabetes, trauma, radiation), drug-induced (e.g., steroids, miotics), nutritional, and age-related factors

PATIENT PRESENTATION

- Decreased vision
  - Severity depends on the location and type of cataract
  - Nuclear cataracts often cause more difficulty at distance, with some patients having a "myopic shift" of their lens prescription, which may improve the ability to see near objects (e.g., reading)
- Glare is characteristically seen in posterior subcapsular and cortical cataracts
  - May be debilitating despite seemingly adequate visual acuity
- Loss of contrast sensitivity
- Monocular diplopia (a "ghost image" is seen)
  - As opposed to binocular diplopia, the image remains even when the opposite eye is covered
- Color changes: Objects tend to appear yellow or browner than normal

DIFFERENTIAL DX

- Glaucoma
- Macular degeneration
- Diabetic retinopathy
- Chronic progressive visual loss: Refractive error, ocular media disturbance, retinal detachment, macular degeneration, optic neuropathy
- Leukocoria (white pupil) in a child: Retinoblastoma, persistent fetal vasculature, trauma (child abuse), retinopathy of prematurity, toxocariasis, Coats' disease, coloboma (absence of eye wall or eye structure), vitreous hemorrhage

DIAGNOSTIC EVALUATION

- Work-up of visual loss includes the basic ocular examination with special attention to visual acuity at distance and near, pupil examination, and ophthalmoscopy
  - Be sure to assess for other causes of visual loss, such as macular degeneration and diabetic retinopathy, that would limit visual rehabilitation
  - No amount of cataract can explain a relative afferent pupillary defect; if present, be sure to rule out other significant causes of vision loss, such as optic neuropathy or diffuse retinal vascular pathology
- An ophthalmologist can use specialized equipment to assess visual loss with careful refraction, slit lamp examination, indirect and direct ophthalmoscopy, brightness acuity, and potential acuity estimation
- Direct ophthalmoscopy allows the examiner to estimate the density of the cataract
  - The examiner's view into the eye is similar to the patient's view out of it
  - Focal lens opacification appears as black against the red reflex
  - A very dense cataract results in the appearance of a white pupil (leukocoria) and absence of the red reflex
  - Cataract is only one cause of leukocoria, which is a significant finding in infants that should prompt evaluation for retinoblastoma

TREATMENT & MANAGEMENT

- Nonsurgical management to improve visual function includes eyeglasses for distance and near vision, increased ambient lighting, and pupillary dilation
- No medication has been found to effectively delay or reverse cataract formation in humans
- Often, the only effective management option for cataracts is surgical removal and implantation of an intraocular lens
  - Cataract extraction is typically an elective procedure and is indicated when the patient desires improved visual function and if correction of visual limitations outweighs the known risks and complications of surgery
  - Surgical removal consists of a small corneal incision at the junction of the cornea and sclera, careful removal of the lens material with an ultrasonic handpiece (phacoemulsification), and placement of an intraocular lens implant
- Laser surgery may be needed after cataract surgery to remove residual posterior capsular material that may opacify (often called "second cataract")

PROGNOSIS & COMPLICATIONS

- Mature cataracts may cause inflammation and glaucoma if not removed
- Cataract surgery has an excellent success rate: >90% of otherwise healthy eyes achieve 20/40 or better vision following surgery
  - In patients with comorbid conditions (e.g., diabetic retinopathy, glaucoma, age-related macular degeneration), the rate is still excellent: 85–90% achieve 20/40 or better vision
  - Patients show significant improvement in many quality-of-life parameters, including community and home activities, mental health, driving, and life satisfaction
- Complications rates are low: Clinically significant opacification of the posterior lens capsule is common (20%) but not serious; less than 1.5% of patients develop dislocation of the implant, elevated intraocular pressure, cystoid macular edema, or retinal detachment

Macular Degeneration

INTRODUCTION

- Age-related macular degeneration (AMD) is the leading cause of legal blindness in people older than 65 in the United States
- It is generally a slowly progressive, binocular condition that preferentially affects central vision (the macula)
- Primarily affects patients over the age of 50

ETIOLOGY, EPIDEMIOLOGY, & RISK FACTORS

- The pathogenesis of AMD is not completely understood, but genetics and choroidal blood flow are felt to play a role in the development and progression of disease
- Drusen represent localized yellow deposits between the retinal pigment epithelium and the underlying Bruch's membrane, which provides a barrier between the retina and the choroids
  - Drusen occur in nonexudative ("dry") AMD
- When Bruch's membrane is disrupted, new vessels may grow under the retina from the underlying choroidal vessels (called choroidal neovascularization); the new vessels leak and cause subretinal fluid, blood, and exudate to accumulate, ultimately leading to fibrovascular scarring
  - Choroidal neovascularization occurs in exudative ("wet") AMD
- A small percentage of patients (about 10%) develop exudative ("wet") AMD, which accounts for the majority of cases of visual loss and may be amenable to laser or photodynamic therapy if diagnosed early
- More than 2% of individuals over 65 are blind in one eye due to macular degeneration
- Risk factors for AMD include advancing age, family history, tobacco use, and cardiovascular factors including hypertension

PATIENT PRESENTATION

- The majority of cases of nonexudative AMD are asymptomatic
  - Patients may have mild distortion or visual loss with drusen
  - Difficulty with reading or recognizing details may occur if extensive retinal pigment epithelial atrophy occurs
  - Blind spots (paracentral or central scotomata) may occur
- Abrupt visual loss or visual distortion (metamorphopsia, or seeing a straight line as wavy) suggests exudative AMD
- Poor depth perception may occur in cases of unilateral disease
- Micropsia (objects appear smaller in the affected eye)
- Formed hallucinations in the blind field of vision may occur (Charles Bonnet syndrome)

DIFFERENTIAL DX

- Nonexudative ("dry") AMD (including drusen and retinal pigment epithelial alterations or atrophy)
- Exudative ("wet") AMD (including choroidal neovascularization, pigment epithelial detachment or tear, subretinal hemorrhage, and fibrovascular scar formation)
- Choroidal neovascularization due to trauma
- Myopic degeneration
- Inherited central retinal dystrophies
- Toxic retinopathies
- Ocular histoplasmosis syndrome
- Inflammatory maculopathies

DIAGNOSTIC EVALUATION

- Visual acuity testing
- Amsler grid testing is used to screen for changes related to metamorphopsia (visual distortion)
  - The patient examines a grid of black lines on a white background at reading distance
  - Distortion is described as bent, distorted, or missing lines
  - This test may be given to the patient to monitor at home; if changes are noted, they should be re-examined by an ophthalmologist
- Ophthalmoscopy to identify drusen, retinal pigment epithelial alterations, or complications of exudative AMD
- Fluorescein angiography may be indicated to identify, locate, and classify choroidal neo-vascularization (appears as bright spots of leakage)

TREATMENT & MANAGEMENT

- Smoking cessation is strongly recommended
- Modification of cardiovascular risk factors (e.g., aggressive control of blood pressure)
- There is no known treatment for nonexudative AMD
- The use of antioxidants such as zinc, beta-carotene, vitamin C, and vitamin E may help patients at high risk of progression of AMD
- Laser photocoagulation has been shown to be effective in reducing the risk of severe visual loss in patients with well-demarcated choroidal neovascularization outside the fovea (the center of the macula)
- Photodynamic therapy uses a light-activated dye (verteporfin) to close the new vessels without damaging adjoining retinal tissue
  - May be used for patients with well-demarcated choroidal neovascularization of the fovea because traditional laser use in this area would cause a permanent blind spot in the center of vision; however, results are temporary, and several treatments are necessary
- Patients with significant visual loss will benefit from low-vision evaluation and assisting devices, such as magnifiers, illumination, closed-circuit television, and telescopes
- In cases of more severe involvement of the dominant eye, occlusion of the eye may allow for better reading

PROGNOSIS & COMPLICATIONS

- The majority of individuals with nonexudative AMD have a good prognosis
- Patients may be reassured that, even though AMD may cause them to lose reading vision, they will not lose peripheral vision
- The risk of choroidal neovascularization is 10–15% over 5 years in patients with bilateral drusen; unfortunately, not all cases of choroidal neovascularization are amenable to laser and/or photodynamic therapy
- Fibrovascular scarring is a late complication of untreated choroidal neovascularization and is permanent; thus, early referral and prompt treatment for abrupt visual changes is warranted
- New treatment modalities under investigation include macular translocation, submacular surgery, and antiangiogenic drug therapy

Infectious Conjunctivitis

INTRODUCTION

- The conjunctiva is a thin, vascular epithelial tissue that is tightly adherent to the inner aspect of the eyelids (the palpebral conjunctiva) and loosely adherent to the sclera (the bulbar conjunctiva); conjunctivitis is a nonspecific inflammation of the conjunctiva resulting in infection of the blood vessels and often discharge and discomfort
- Conjunctivitis is the most common cause of ocular inflammation and "red eye"
- Trachoma is a chronic conjunctivitis caused by *Chlamydia*; it is the most common cause of blindness worldwide
- Infectious conjunctivitis may carry significant morbidity if therapy is delayed; fortunately, most cases of conjunctivitis are self-limiting, requiring only symptomatic care

ETIOLOGY, EPIDEMIOLOGY, & RISK FACTORS

- Typically spread from person-to-person by contact (e.g., a handshake followed by self-inoculation by rubbing eyes or nose) or via fomites (e.g., clothing, towels, utensils)
  - Trachoma in developing countries may be spread by flies or genital-to-eye contact
- Bacterial etiologies are common, including *Staphylococcus aureus*, *Streptococcus pneumoniae*, *Haemophilus influenzae*, *Neisseria gonorrhoeae*, *Chlamydia trachomatis*, and *Neisseria meningitidis*
- Viral etiologies include adenovirus, enterovirus, coxsackievirus, vaccinia virus, molluscum contagiosum, herpes simplex virus types 1 and 2, varicella-zoster virus, Epstein-Barr virus, human papillomavirus, congenital rubella, influenza viruses, and measles
- Toxic conjunctivitis may occur due to neomycin, aminoglycosides, atropine, and other topical medications, as well as cosmetics and preservatives
- Seasonal allergic conjunctivitis (hayfever) is common and usually due to exposure to airborne allergens; allergic conjunctivitis may also occur due to rubbing the eyes with allergen (e.g., cat dander)
- Immunogenic conjunctivitis is associated with systemic immune disorders (e.g., Graves' disease, rheumatoid arthritis, Sjögren's syndrome, SLE, Wegener's granulomatosis, relapsing polychondritis, polyarteritis nodosa)

PATIENT PRESENTATION

- If visual acuity is acutely and significantly reduced, conjunctivitis is extremely *unlikely*
- *Hyperemia of the conjunctiva*
- Nonspecific symptoms (e.g., tearing, irritation, stinging, burning, photophobia)
- Pain, particularly the sensation of a foreign body, suggests corneal involvement
- Discharge may occur as purulent (severe bacterial conjunctivitis), watery (allergic and viral conjunctivitis), mucoid (dry eye), mucopurulent (mild bacterial and chlamydial conjunctivitis)
- Sticky eyelids when the secretions dry up
- Loss of the normal transparency of the conjunctiva

DIFFERENTIAL DX

- Other causes of red eye (refer to *Red Eye* entry)
- Uveitis
- Endophthalmitis
- Acute angle-closure glaucoma
- Trauma
- Sicca syndrome
- Meibomian gland carcinoma
- Scleritis
- Keratitis
- Blepharitis
- Stevens-Johnson syndrome
- Ocular cicatricial pemphigoid
- Graft-versus-host disease
- Parinaud's oculoglandular syndrome
- Molluscum contagiosum
- Pediculosis (lice, crabs)

DIAGNOSTIC EVALUATION

- Generally a clinical diagnosis
  - Examination is similar to the workup for red eye
  - Visual acuity is generally normal in uncomplicated conjunctivitis
  - Pupil examination to compare the relative size of pupils and reactivity to light; rule out a mid-dilated, fixed pupil as occurs in acute angle-closure glaucoma
  - Penlight examination
  - Categorize discharge as purulent, watery, mucoid, or mucopurulent
  - Detect corneal opacity and irregularity, and stain with fluorescein to look for disruption of the corneal epithelium
  - Assess for "red flags," such as anterior chamber blood (hyphema) or pus (hypopyon), proptosis, and limitation of eye movement
- Mild conjunctivitis is not routinely investigated and is often treated empirically and symptomatically
- In severe conjunctivitis, cultures should be taken from the inferior and superior tarsal conjunctiva; however, this should not delay initiation of therapy

TREATMENT & MANAGEMENT

- Mild bacterial and viral conjunctivitis are self-limited
- Topical therapy for 7–10 days may be used for bacterial conjunctivitis
  - Gram-negative bacterial conjunctivitis: Topical aminoglycosides (gentamicin or tobramycin)
  - Gram-positive bacterial conjunctivitis: Topical erythromycin, bacitracin, or multiple antibiotics (polymyxin, bacitracin, trimethoprim, and/or neomycin)
  - If broad-spectrum antibiotics are needed, use a topical fluoroquinolone
- Gonococcal conjunctivitis requires urgent parenteral therapy with a broad-spectrum cephalosporin and frequent ocular lavage
- Chlamydia conjunctivitis (inclusion conjunctivitis) is treated with doxycycline or erythromycin for 7 days
- Allergic conjunctivitis is treated with cool compresses, artificial tears, topical and systemic antihistamines, olopatadine (for itching), and avoidance of allergens
- Viral conjunctivitis is self-limited but extremely contagious
  - Avoid spread by frequent hand washing, not sharing towels, not rubbing at eyes, and not participating in school, work, or daycare as long as discharge is present (10–12 days)
  - Cool compresses and artificial tears may give symptomatic relief

PROGNOSIS & COMPLICATIONS

- Nearly all cases resolve without complications
- Serious conjunctivitis with common or virulent pathogens can result in severe complications, including chronic or recurrent conjunctivitis, corneal ulceration and perforation, keratitis/endophthalmitis, and ocular destruction with blindness of the affected eye
- Ophthalmologic referral for patients with "red flags" (e.g., vision loss, proptosis, limitation of eye movement, corneal involvement, hypopyon), *Neisseria* and neonatal conjunctivitis, contact lens-related keratitis, recent eye surgery, history of foreign body injury, or conjunctivitis that does not respond to treatment within several days

Hordeolum and Chalazion

INTRODUCTION

- A hordeolum ("stye") is painful, localized infection of an eyelash follicle
  - It is most often infectious, usually caused by *Staphylococcus aureus*
- *Arises from the meibomian (posterior) or Zeis (anterior) sebaceous glands*
- A chalazion is a slowly enlarging nodule on the eyelid that is not caused by infection
  - It is the result of a granulomatous inflammatory reaction and may persist for weeks or even months

ETIOLOGY, EPIDEMIOLOGY, & RISK FACTORS

- Hordeola may be internal or external and are usually caused by *S. aureus*
  - An external hordeolum arises from blockage and infection of the Zeis or Moll sebaceous glands
  - An internal hordeolum is a secondary infection of the meibomian glands in the tarsal plate
  - *S. aureus* causes 75–95% of cases; rarely, other causative organisms include strepto-cocci, gram-negative enteric organisms, or mixed bacterial flora
- Chalazion results from obstruction of a sebaceous gland (either meibomian or Zeis) that is associated with surrounding chronic inflammation due to extravasated lipids
  - A chalazion may also occur following the acute inflammation of a hordeolum, in which case the lesion becomes less painful and eventually painless
- Hordeola are found more frequently in patients with diabetes or other debilitating illnesses, chronic blepharitis, and seborrhea
- Chalazia often occur in patients with blepharitis, seborrheic dermatitis, or acne rosacea
  - There may also be a correlation with elevated serum lipid levels
  - More commonly affects males, possibly due to androgenic hormones

PATIENT PRESENTATION

- Hordeolum usually presents with abrupt onset of pain, swelling, and erythema of the eyelid
  - An external hordeolum points toward the skin surface of the eyelid and may spontaneously drain
  - An internal hordeolum may point toward the conjunctival side of the eyelid and may cause conjunctival inflammation
- Chalazia are usually rubbery, cystic, and non-tender on palpation
  - When the upper lid is involved, vision is often temporarily blurred
  - It is usually a painless, rounded, slowly enlarging, subcutaneous lid mass that may wax and wane in size
  - May rupture posteriorly (resulting in a poly-poid conjunctival mass of granulation tissue on the conjunctiva) or anteriorly (resulting in a subcutaneous mass)

DIFFERENTIAL DX

- Conjunctivitis
- Corneal abrasion
- Recurrent chalazia may be caused by an underlying seba-ceous gland carcinoma

DIAGNOSTIC EVALUATION

- History and physical examination are sufficient for diagnosis; no lab studies are necessary
  - Completely examine the eye and conjunctival surface: Examine the eyelids for crusting, irregularity, lash loss, misdirected eye lashes, or lesions; invert the eyelid to visualize the palpebral conjunctiva; examine the preauricular nodes to assess for infection (nodes should not be swollen)
  - In both conditions, infection of the conjunctiva is a common secondary finding, but no intraocular pathology should be found
  - Presence of fever or distant nodes is not consistent with a stye or chalazion
  - Hordeolum: Examination reveals a localized tender area of swelling with a pointing eruption either on the internal or on the external side of eyelid (occasionally, the hordeolum points on both sides); the hordeolum appears at the lid's edge, while the chalazion does not
  - A chalazion is a palpable, usually nontender nodule on the eyelid; it is nonerythematous and nonfluctuant
- Eye cultures are of little clinical value (although hordeola are likely caused by *S. aureus*, eyelid cultures are more likely to reveal *Staphylococcus epidermidis*)

TREATMENT & MANAGEMENT

- Hordeola are usually self-limited and will eventually drain by themselves
  - Warm compresses are the mainstays of treatment
  - Antibiotics are indicated only when inflammation has spread beyond the immediate area of the hordeolum; topical antibiotics may be used for recurrent lesions and for those that are actively draining; systemic antibiotics are indicated if signs of bacteremia are present or if the patient has tender preauricular lymph nodes (in which case, the problem is no longer a simple stye)
  - If the patient does not begin to respond to conservative therapy (as above) within 2–3 days, or if the problem is not completely resolved within 1–2 weeks, an ophthalmologist should be consulted
  - Large hordeola may require drainage by an ophthalmologist
- Chalazia may resolve spontaneously or may require ophthalmologic therapy
  - Treated with hot compresses to encourage localization and drainage
  - Since chalazia are sterile inflammations, topical antibiotics are not usually helpful; however, many physicians recommend their use in patients with a minor infection
  - Chronic chalazia may be treated by an ophthalmologist using an intralesional corticosteroid injection or surgical drainage
  - Chalazia persisting for more than 3 months may require incision and curettage

PROGNOSIS & COMPLICATIONS

- Hordeolum: Untreated, the disease may spontaneously resolve, or it may progress to chronic granulation and formation of a chalazion
  - Most morbidity is secondary to improper drainage, such as disruption of lash growth, lid deformity, or lid fistula; in extreme cases, the infection can spread to involve the entire lid and even the periorbital tissues and must be managed as periorbital cellulitis
- Chalazion: May progress to a painless granuloma that may be disfiguring cosmetically
  - Can become quite large and cause visual disturbances by deforming the cornea (more typical of upper lid chalazia than of lower lid chalazia)
  - Most morbidity occurs due to secondary infection caused by improper drainage
- Both conditions usually resolve with conservative management, but recurrences may occur

Optic Neuritis

INTRODUCTION

- Optic neuritis is an autoimmune demyelination of the optic nerve that causes varying degrees of central vision loss, usually of one eye
- Often presents as a manifestation of multiple sclerosis
  - Up to 60% of affected individuals develop clinical multiple sclerosis within 15 years of the initial attack
- May be associated with viral, demyelinating, vasculitic, or granulomatous processes
- Visual prognosis is generally excellent

ETIOLOGY, EPIDEMIOLOGY, & RISK FACTORS

- Most commonly associated with multiple sclerosis
  - Up to 60% of patients with optic or retrobulbar neuritis will develop multiple sclerosis; thus, neuroimaging is performed to detect those patients at risk for multiple sclerosis and treatment with IV and oral steroids is initiated if there is associated CNS demyelinating disease on MRI
- May infrequently occur as a manifestation of connective tissue disease, autoimmune diseases, granulomatous diseases (e.g., sarcoidosis, tuberculosis, syphilis, cryptococcosis), or postviral infection (e.g., measles, mumps, chickenpox, mononucleosis, herpes zoster, encephalitis)
- May also occur secondary to contiguous inflammation of meninges, orbit, globe, or sinuses
- Optic neuritis is the most common optic neuropathy of early adulthood
- Typically affects individuals of ages 18–45
- Most common in young females
- Devic's disease is a rare condition in which bilateral optic neuritis is followed by transverse myelitis (demyelination of the spinal cord)

PATIENT PRESENTATION

- Loss of vision over hours to days
  - Usually unilateral vision loss, but may be bilateral
  - Central visual field is lost
  - May be subtle or profound
- Pain in or around the eye that may or may not be exacerbated by eye movement
- Loss of color vision
- Reduced perception of light intensity
- Other focal neurologic signs may occur, including weakness, numbness, and tingling; these may suggest a second demyelinating lesion or multiple sclerosis
- Altered perception of moving objects or seeing two-dimensional objects in three dimensions (Pulfrich phenomenon)
- Worsening symptoms with exercise or increase in body temperature (Uhtoff's sign)
- Preceding flu-like viral illness is common

DIFFERENTIAL DX

- Ischemic, toxic, or metabolic optic neuropathy
- Transient obscuration due to papilledema
- Severe hypertension
- Compressive optic neuropathy (e.g., orbital tumor, glioma, meningioma)
- Brain tumor
- Leber's optic neuropathy
- Neuroretinitis
- Acute demyelinating encephalomyelitis
- Devic's disease
- Paraneoplastic or neoplastic disease
- Central retinal artery occlusion

DIAGNOSTIC EVALUATION

- Detailed history and review of systems to identify previous neurologic events or symptoms of systemic disease
- Each patient should have a complete neurologic and ophthalmic examination including visual acuity, color vision exam, papillary exam, and visual field exam
- Ophthalmoscopy: 35% of patients have a swollen optic disc with or without flame-shaped hemorrhages
  - The presence of an exudate in macular star formation indicates neuroretinitis, which is usually associated with cat-scratch disease (*Bartonella henselae*), virus, syphilis, or Lyme disease, rather than demyelination
- Consider MRI of the brain and orbits
  - For patients with classic demyelinating lesions on MRI, minimal additional workup is needed
- Screening for connective tissue disease may include ESR, ANA, SS-A antibodies, anticardiolipin antibodies, angiotensin-converting enzyme, C-ANCA antibodies, and paraneoplastic antibodies

TREATMENT & MANAGEMENT

- Isolated optic neuritis is treated with observation alone
- Steroids are controversial but are often administered (high doses for moderate to severe disease, varying doses for milder disease)
  - It is unclear whether steroids prevent subsequent development of multiple sclerosis
  - Do not use oral steroids alone as a primary treatment due to an increased risk of recurrence
- Consider IVIG, plasmapheresis, or immunosuppressives for severe disease
- Consider immunomodulators for cases associated with multiple sclerosis

PROGNOSIS & COMPLICATIONS

- Nearly 90% of patients have full or near-complete recovery of vision; however, patients often note other residual visual deficits, such as defects of color vision, contrast sensitivity, depth perception, light brightness, and peripheral vision
- Optic neuritis recurs in about 25% of cases
- If cerebral MRI suggests multiple sclerosis at the onset of optic neuritis, 50–90% will develop multiple sclerosis within 5–10 years; if cerebral MRI is negative at onset of optic neuritis, 10% will develop multiple sclerosis within 5 years and 20% within 10 years
- Patients with CNS demyelination on MRI or abnormal neurologic examination should be referred to a neurologist
- Patients on steroids should be followed closely due to an increased risk of glaucoma

Uveitis and Iritis

INTRODUCTION

- Uveitis is inflammation of the uveal tract, which consists of the iris (iritis), ciliary body (cyclitis), and the choroid; it is often isolated but may be associated with infectious, traumatic, neoplastic, or autoimmune diseases
- Anterior uveitis (iritis, iridocyclitis) presents with the triad of pain, redness, and photophobia
- Diagnosis depends on slit lamp examination; thus, referral to an ophthalmologist is necessary if clinical features are suggestive
- Treatment consists of steroids, cycloplegics, and, in severe cases, systemic immunosuppressive medications

ETIOLOGY, EPIDEMIOLOGY, & RISK FACTORS

- Acute cases (lasting weeks to months) may be idiopathic or associated with trauma, ankylosing spondylitis, inflammatory bowel disease, reactive arthritis (including Reiter's syndrome), psoriatic arthritis, Behçet's disease, Lyme disease, medications (e.g., sulfa drugs, cidofovir, rifabutin), leptospirosis, Kawasaki disease, or rickettsial disease
  - Up to 12% of patients with ulcerative colitis and 3% of patients with Crohn's disease develop anterior uveitis
  - 50–60% of patients with acute iritis may be HLA-B27 positive, and HLA-B27 is positive in 90% of ankylosing spondylitis and reactive arthritis patients
- Chronic cases (lasting 3 months to years) that are nongranulomatous are associated with juvenile rheumatoid arthritis
  - Onset of uveitis in patients with juvenile rheumatoid arthritis may occur up to 25 years after developing joint disease
- Chronic, granulomatous cases may be associated with sarcoidosis, herpes simplex, varicella zoster, syphilis, and tuberculosis

PATIENT PRESENTATION

- Ocular pain
- Photophobia
- Tearing
- Miosis
- Blurred vision
- Red eye
- Ciliary flush (injection of vessels primarily at the limbus where the sclera meets the cornea)

DIFFERENTIAL DX

- Other causes of red eye (refer to the *Red Eye* entry)
- Retinal detachment
- Intraocular tumor (retinoblastoma in children, malignant melanoma in adults)
- Intraocular foreign body
- Juvenile xanthogranuloma
- Intraocular foreign body
- Sclerouveitis
- Endophthalmitis

DIAGNOSTIC EVALUATION

- A careful history and review of systems is an important step in determining the etiology
- Slit lamp examination is necessary to evaluate for irregular pupil due to scarring to the lens (synechiae), cellular deposits on the back of the cornea (large collection of cells indicate granulomatous disease, individual cells indicates nongranulomatous disease), cells and protein debris in aqueous humor, iris nodules (indicate granulomatous iritis), high or low intraocular pressure, hypopyon (layering of cells in the anterior chamber), cystoid macular edema of the fovea, or cataracts
- There is no standard battery of tests; the diagnostic approach is tailored for each patient
  - The first occurrence of unilateral, nongranulomatous disease does not require further workup
  - If bilateral, granulomatous, or recurrent, then testing for specific diagnoses is performed based on history; testing may include complete blood count, ESR, HLA-B27 assay, angiotensin-converting enzyme, ANA, RPR, FTA-ABS, PPD with anergy panel, chest X-ray, and Lyme disease titer

TREATMENT & MANAGEMENT

- Urgent referral to an ophthalmologist if iritis is suspected
- Ophthalmologic treatment may include steroids (topical, systemic, or injections) to reduce inflammation; cycloplegics/mydriatics to prevent the pupil from scarring and to relieve photophobia; systemic immunosuppressives (e.g., methotrexate, azathioprine, cyclosporine, tacrolimus) for severe, refractory inflammation; topical glaucoma agents if intraocular pressure is markedly elevated; or oral antibiotics to treat associated infections
- Referral to a rheumatologist, internist, or dermatologist may be indicated to help manage systemic disease, if present
- Daily follow-up is indicated during the acute phase

PROGNOSIS & COMPLICATIONS

- Adequate control of inflammation is the key to prevent damage to the uveal vasculature, which may result in chronic, refractory disease
- Chronic or recurrent iritis may cause band keratopathy, cataract, glaucoma, macular edema, membrane formation, or end-stage shrinkage of the eye (phthisis bulbi)

Index

Chronic inflammatory demyelinating polyneuropathy, 127
Chronic kidney disease, 168–169
Chronic obstructive pulmonary disease, 76–77
Chronic pelvic pain syndrome, 162–163
Chylothorax, 88
Ciclopirox, 257
Cinarizine, 123
Ciprofloxacin
 gonorrhea treated with, 149, 165
 prostatitis treated with, 162
 urinary tract infections treated with, 171
Cirrhosis, 28–29
Clarithromycin, 35
Claudication, 44
Clindamycin
 cellulitis treated with, 267
 vaginal cream, 211
Clomiphene, 185, 219
Clonidine, 251
Clopidogrel, 44
Closed-angle glaucoma, 282
Cluster headache, 121
Colon cancer, 116–117
Colonic peristalsis, 12
Community-acquired pneumonia, 80–81
Congestive heart failure, 50–51
Conjunctivitis, 274–275, 288–289
Constipation, 12–13
Contact dermatitis, 246
Continuous positive airway pressure, 91
Corneal abrasion, 275, 281
Corneal erosion, 281
Coronary artery bypass grafting, 61
Coronary artery disease, 40, 60–61
Corticosteroids
 acne vulgaris treated with, 255
 acute gouty arthritis treated with, 237
 asthma treated with, 79
 chronic obstructive pulmonary disease treated with, 77
 Cushing's syndrome treated with, 199
 fever reduction using, 223
 inflammatory bowel disease treated with, 25
 intranasal, 105
 multiple sclerosis treated with, 137
 myasthenia gravis treated with, 139

optic neuritis treated with, 293
osteoarthritis managed using, 225
polymyalgia rheumatica treated with, 231
pruritus treated with, 247
psoriasis treated with, 261
rhinitis treated with, 105
Sjögren's syndrome managed using, 241
systemic lupus erythematosus treated with, 235
temporal arteritis treated with, 29
urticaria treated with, 249
Cortisol, 198
Cortisol-releasing hormone stimulation test, 199
Cough, 68–69
Crohn's disease, 24–25
Cromolyn, 105
Cryotherapy, 265
Cushing's syndrome, 198–199
Cyclophosphamide, 29, 233, 235
Cycloplegics, 295
Cyclosporine
 psoriasis treated with, 261
 systemic lupus erythematosus treated with, 235
 uveitis treated with, 295
Cyclosporine A, 233, 277
Cyproheptadine
 atopic dermatitis treated with, 259
 urticaria treated with, 249
Cystitis, 155, 170–171

D2 receptor antagonists, 11
Danazol, 185
Deep venous thrombosis, 56–57, 82–83
Defecography, 13
Dementia, 128–129
Depression, 6–7
Dermatomyositis, 242–243
Desloratadine, 249
Desmopressin, 109, 177
Detrusor hyperreflexia, 156
Devic's disease, 292
Dexamethasone, 183
Dexamethasone suppression test, 199
Diabetes insipidus, 176
Diabetes mellitus, type 2, 188–189
Diabetic ketoacidosis, 186–187
Diabetic nephropathy, 168, 188–189